AF822041

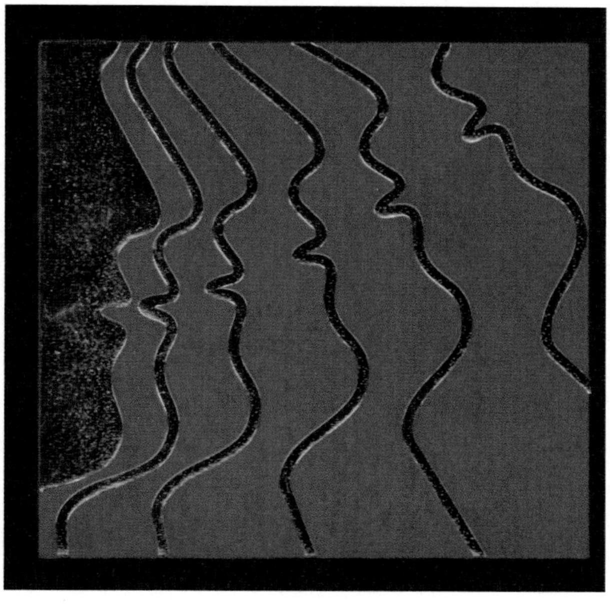

Chemical Peeling Wounding Spectrum*

Superficial wounding (to the stratum granulosum–papillary dermis)

- *Very light*—stratum corneum exfoliation or stratum granulosum depth
  - TCA, 10%-20% (TCA, superficial), resorcin, Jessner's solution, salicylic acid, solid CO_2, α-hydroxy acids, tretinoin
- *Light*—stratum basale or upper papillary dermal depth
  - TCA, 35%, unoccluded, single or multiple frost

Medium-depth wounding (through the papillary dermis to the upper reticular dermis)

- Combination Peels, single or multiple frost
  - CO_2 + TCA, 35%
  - Jessner's + TCA, 35%
  - Glycolic acid + TCA, 35%
- TCA, 50%, unoccluded (TCA, deep), single frost
- Full-strength phenol, 88%, unoccluded
- Pyruvic acid

Deep-depth wounding (to the midreticular dermis)

- Baker's phenol, unoccluded
- Baker's phenol, occluded

*Depth is dependent on prepeel skin defatting preparation, wounding agent strength or amount applied, and skin thickness or location. Clinical reepithelialization may depend on skin location and the character of the dermal pathology, which determine the degree of inflammatory response evoked.

CHEMICAL PEELING

and RESURFACING

CHEMICAL PEELING *and* RESURFACING

HAROLD J. BRODY, M.D.

Clinical Professor

Department of Dermatology

Emory University School of Medicine

Atlanta, Georgia

Second Edition

Mosby

An Affiliate of Elsevier Science

Chemical Peeling and Resurfacing

3rd Edition

Preface
to the Third Edition

The third edition of Chemical Peeling and Resurfacing is a unique departure from the printed edition of previous years. The availability of textbooks through the internet means that the material in the second edition will be available to all that wish to see it for the foreseeable future. All of the techniques in the second edition are still valid and true. There are three new developments that have occurred in the last decade that are mentioned in this preface that are worth the attention of the reader. Other than that, the refinements in the field have been minor. The marketing of lasers that allegedly rise to the standards and results of chemical peeling allegedly without complications has been the chief reason for the decline in awareness of peeling to the general public and cosmetic physicians alike. In truth, lasers that accomplish the results of superficial peeling are expensive and unnecessary. Devices that accomplish the reduction of mild wrinkling without significant pigmentary change are impressive though more expensive than peeling. And finally, devices that produce elimination of deep wrinkling and significant photodamage in one treatment without any downtime or complications have not yet been developed. Chemical resurfacing still produces stunning results with little cost and a healthy risk/benefit ratio. The change is in the perception of the media and communications of the twenty-first century that bends medicine towards the proprietary, be it in devices or in topicals related to resurfacing, in the case of the latter, most of which are not necessary. A case may be made that devices are simpler than the techniques in this textbook and that the public deserves mass production of these devices in the name of youth. Equitability has never been a human right.

The following advances in chemical peeling are significant in the last decade:

Hetter's landmark publication in 2000 describes a series of phenol/croton oil formulas designed to be applied to moderately photoaged skin. The formulas are thoroughly investigated histologically based on photoaging and application to different cosmetic units. They eliminate the heavier application and taping that could be used to regulate penetration of the Baker/Gordon formula. The work is based on the premise that croton oil is the active ingredient in the formula and phenol is the carrier. Higher concentrations of croton oil make it possible to use a weaker strength of phenol in the formula, reducing systemic effects of phenol toxicity. Addition of 0.2% croton oil increases phenol peel depth by 20%. The phenol concentration is not the important variable. Hetter's 1.2% croton oil concentration formula is a strength for moderately photodamaged perioral skin as opposed to the 2.1% croton oil concentration of the traditional Baker/Gordon formula, originally used for severe photodamage.

Hetter's Perioral Peel for Moderate Wrinkled Skin	
Phenol, USP, 88%	3cc(55%)
Tap Water	2cc
Septisol soap	8 drops
Croton oil	3 drops (2.1%)

All techniques have merit, and unoccluded Baker/Gordon formula produces an excellent peel as long as the wound depth is deep enough to efface defects. It is easier to selectively tape very severe, thick, actinically damaged skin and rest assured that the deepest peel possible is produced over these areas. The Hetter formula is ideal for less photodamaged perioral skin. The phenol formulas for the other facial cosmetic units are less necessary with TCA peeling being safe and available. [1]

The treatment of pigmented disorders in Asian skin has been complicated by the difficulty in toleration of hydroquinone compounds by the patients. Yoshimura has suggested alternating the application of a hydroquinone *bleaching* formula containing tretinoin applied for four weeks and then a *healing* formula without tretinoin applied for four weeks, modified by patient tolerance. This allows more time for the skin to recover from sometimes increasing erythema that becomes uncomfortable or produces paradoxical hyperpigmentation. Elimination of the tretinoin from the Bleach-Eze formula for the *healing* formula is a modification of this technique. Though the hydrocortisone could be eliminated in both formulas, since it is the weakest of all cortisone creams, we choose to leave it in the formula. The concept has been helpful in heavily pigmented skin types.

The author suggests carefully applying tretinoin gel separately and then hydroquinone and lactic acid combination as the *bleaching* formula and eliminating the tretinoin and using hydroquinone and ascorbic acid combination as the *healing* formula. This may be more effective, but this concept has been an assistance in bleaching with peeling for melasma.[2]

Lee's pioneering technique of applying 100% TCA with a sharp wooden toothpick-type applicator to icepick scars has been a revolutionary treatment for all skin types prior to resurfacing. In a series of Korean patients, this focal treatment application, called Chemical Reconstruction of Skin Scars(CROSS Technique,) has produced 82-94% improvement when repeated one to six times every one to three months. It is important to exercise care in applying the TCA exactly inside the pits and not on the surrounding skin and in selecting icepick scars and not pseudo-icepick scars because widening of the scar may occur with either miscalculation. We have utilized this technique on all Fitzpatrick skin types I-VI without complication. This histologically proven procedure has eliminated dermabrasion and punch grafting in many patients.[3] [4]

The epidemic of non-physicians performing epidermal and dermal chemical peels in spas, salons and walk-in clinics has produced a considerable increase in complications from chemical peeling. Scarring and pigmentary problems have produced lawsuits and dissatisfaction with the scope of practice of medicine laws in many states. The American Society for Dermatologic Surgery Public Safety Campaign has surveys that demonstrate the complications of the non-physician practice of medicine. The invasion of living skin by chemical surgery continues to be the cosmetic practice of medicine. This data is available through the website of the organization, www.asds.net.

It is my hope that this third edition of readily available educational material in this textbook will be preserved for future generations so that they may understand the science that produced the cost-effective techniques to improve wrinkles, actinic keratoses, pigmentary problems and scars.

Harold J. Brody, M. D.
Atlanta, Georgia
www.atlantadermatology.com
2008

---

[1] Hetter GP: An Examination of the Phenol-Croton Oil Peel: Parts I-IV. Plast Reconstr Surg 2000;105:227, 240, 752, 1061.

[2] Yoshimura K, Sato K, Aiba-Kojima E, Matsumoto D, Machino C, Nagase T, Gonda K, and Koshima I: Repeated Treatment Protocols for Melasma and Acquired Dermal Melanocytosis. Dermatol Surg 2006;32:365-371.

[3] Lee J, Chung W, Kwahck H and Lee K: Focal Treatment of Acne Scars with TCA: Chemical Reconstruction of Skin Scars Method(CROSS). Dermatol Surg 2002; 28:1017-1021.

[4] Yug A, Lane J, Howard M, Kent D: Histologic Study of Depressed Acne Scars Treated with Serial High-Concentration Trichloroacetic Acid. Dermatol Surg 2006;32:985-990.

Dedication

Man is a vain animal. From the time of the ancient Egyptians to the present, through all cultures and through the span of centuries, mankind has been preoccupied with youth and physical appearance. At some point in the lifetime of every man or woman, concern with the quality of his or her skin becomes a priority regardless of concomitant inappropriate clothing, tussled hairstyle, or apparent tooth decay. Undesirable pigmentation and scarring may affect the economic opportunities and mental stability of the contemporary individual as much as they did the ancient Egyptian, whose vitiligo marked him a "leper." Thus, the heritage of chemical peeling in the 1990s is predicated upon the legacy left to us from those peacocks of the past, those artistic scientists and scientific artists who helped develop our present methodology.

This book is indebted to them.

Harold J. Brody, M.D.

The elder I wax, the better I shall appear.

Shakespeare: *Henry V,* Act V, Scene 2

Mislike me not for my complexion,
The shadow'd livery of the burnish'd sun.

Shakespeare: *The Merchant of Venice,* Act II, Scene 1

Preface *to the Second Edition*

Since the publication of the first edition of this text, the more broad and marketable title, chemical resurfacing, is being increasingly used by more writers. Instructional courses at the American Academy of Dermatology beginning in 1997 have expanded in terminology to encompass courses in chemical and physical resurfacing. While concentrating on chemical peeling or resurfacing, comparisons in the text with the CO_2 resurfacing lasers and dermabrasion are increasingly referenced in this second edition. There is no question of the firm foothold of chemical resurfacing as a clinically effective and cost-effective method for the treatment of skin defects in the face of heavy marketing of excellent new laser techniques.

The 1991 practice marketing survey of the American Society for Dermatologic Surgery[1] (ASDS) revealed that **chemical peeling** was among the top 10 dermatologic surgical procedures performed. A more marketable term, **chemical resurfacing,** has been used by some writers. Among dermatologists who had been in practice more than 10 years, the percentage performing chemical peeling rose 20% from 29% in 1986 to 49% in 1991. A survey of 80 ASDS members at the annual meeting in 1995 revealed that 30% of them make greater than 20 recommendations for topical α-hydroxy acids per week. **Combination skin resurfacing** using several different techniques with chemical resurfacing or physical agents such as laser or dermabrasion resurfacing on different facial cosmetic units is becoming more common.

In fact, national projections based on a survey of 1100 members of the American Academy of Cosmetic Surgery, a multidisciplinary cosmetic surgery group, showed that chemical peel was second only to sclerotherapy in the top 10 cosmetic surgery procedures of 1994, an increase of 291% from 1990 through 1994.[1] Concurrent with this increase has been considerable variation in peeling techniques, ensuring better safety, fewer complications, and more predictable results.

The increase in marketing of unproven chemical peel techniques and the projectile advertising of glycolic acid have led to the need for a textbook devoted to both the scientific aspects of peeling and also to an attempt to dispel the hype that accompanies any new procedure or process that is introduced to the public through the communications media. This book concentrates on scientific peels, ethics, and the medical literature. Some unethical proprietary peel programs and aesthetician-cosmetologic superficial wash peels marketed and named without scientific substantiation are not included unless directly applicable to the practice of medicine.

Since publication of the first edition of *Chemical Peeling,* there has been a plethora of new book chapters, scientific articles, booklets, and treatment variations on chemical peeling. I have been fortunate enough to edit many of these and unfortunate enough to examine many litigious cases of peel complications. As director of the first Chemical Peeling Symposia at the American Academy of Dermatology, as chairman of the task force on clinical usage of α-hydroxy acids for the American Society for Dermatologic Surgery, and as task force chairman for the Guidelines of Care for Chemical Peeling for the American Academy of Dermatology,[2] I have tried to incorporate into this book the many lessons learned from investigations on these assignments. This second edition also incorporates the additional discipline, which has led to the addition of more than 165 new references, 60 new illustrations, and more than 20 new subsections within the chapters.

In addition to imparting a more user-friendly format to the book through illustrative referenced examples throughout, progress and new knowledge are the impetuses to the production of this second edition.

Harold J. Brody, M.D.

1. ASDS 1991 Practice Profile Summary, Committee on Practice Marketing, 930 North Meacham Road, Schaumburg, IL 60173.
2. Bates B: Peel and dermabrade away managed care blues, *Skin Allergy News*, 26(11):20, 1995.
3. Guidelines/Outcomes Committee, American Academy of Dermatology: Guidelines of care for chemical peeling, *J Am Acad Dermatol* 33:497-503, 1995.

Preface *to the First Edition*

Chemical peeling, also called chemexfoliation, chemosurgery, or dermapeeling, is the application of one or more exfoliating agents to the skin, resulting in destruction of portions of the epidermis and/or dermis with subsequent regeneration of new epidermal and dermal tissues. These application techniques produce a controlled wound with instant vascular coagulation resulting in skin rejuvenation with reduction or disappearance of actinic keratoses and changes, pigmentary dyschromias, rhytides, and selected superficial depressed scars.

The level of expertise in chemical peeling has improved greatly in the last 5 years due to the demand of today's population for correction of photodamage and the expectation of "excellent" versus "adequate results. The response of dermatologic surgery to this need has resulted in peeling methodology that combines the old with the new and places us on a path of objectivity which supplements clinical observations with adjunctive histologic depth evaluation.

In a 1984 study, the American Academy of Dermatology (AAD)[1] was surveyed with a 52% response rate, and this study revealed that 24% of dermatologists were performing trichloroacetic acid (TCA) peels, 7% were performing phenol peels, and 8% were performing other resorcinol-based peels, for an average of 13%. When the American Society for Dermatologic Surgery (ASDS)[2] was surveyed 5 years later in 1988 with a return rate of 98%, 46% of the ASDS members were performing chemical peels. The frequency of peeling has increased. Concurrent with this increase has been considerable variation in peeling techniques, ensuring better safety, fewer complications, and more predictable results. A comparison of the two studies can be made on the basis of the excellent return rate of the ASDS study and on the basis that roughly one third of the AAD membership is made up of the ASDS membership, presumably roughly the respondents in the initial study. A more detailed survey is in progress.

It is my hope that this book will satisfy the need for a reference source on the wealth of knowledge that exists in chemexfoliation at this time. This book will also serve as an impetus for future research in the field and as a guide to dermatology residents who are beginning their training as well as more expert dermatologic surgeons who are advancing their knowledge in chemical peeling techniques.

Harold J. Brody, M.D.

1. Tromovitch TA, Stegman SJ, Glogau RG: A survey of dermatologic surgery procedures, *J Dermatol Surg Oncol* 13:763-766, 1987.
2. Hanke CW, Bailin PL: Current trends in the practice of dermatologic surgery, *J Dermatol Surg Oncol* 16:130-131, 1990.

Acknowledgments *to the Second Edition*

The birth of the second edition of this text was sparked by new knowledge culled from attendance at meetings with evaluation of scientific sessions and presentations accompanied by discussion sessions with dermatologists and surgeons in cosmetic surgery specialties worldwide. Physicians share their knowledge and expertise through the medical literature and in devoting their time to academic teaching. The second edition's critical reevaluation is indebted to reviewers. Thanks to Richard Glogau and Seth Matarasso, Chapters 4, 5, and 7; Larry Moy, Chapter 4; Diane Baker, Chapters 4 and 5; William Coleman, Chapter 6; Elizabeth McBurney and John Yarborough, Chapters 9 and 10; William H. Beeson in facial plastic surgery, Chapter 7; and pathologists Marian Finan, Al Solomon, and Tom Wade, Chapter 2.

Thanks to Darren L. Casey, my new associate in clinical practice of dermatology and dermatologic surgery, who read and critiqued the entire manuscript. Special kudos to Jon Adams, who also read the entire manuscript with his expertise in publications and communications.

My colleagues on the board of directors of the American Society for Dermatologic Surgery serve as an inspiration to me for their tireless devotion to the promotion of ethical cosmetic medicine and surgery and academic excellence. I am indebted to all of those who have served on the board in recent years, especially June Robinson, Bill Hanke, Bill Coleman, Pat Lillis, Rhoda Narins, Darrell Rigel, Randy Roenigk, John Skouge, Rick Glogau, John Yarborough, Neil Swanson, Elizabeth McBurney, Duane Whitaker, Lynn Drake, Mitch Goldman, Steve Mandy, and Bob Weiss.

Incredible technological advances in the Macintosh Performa computer and the Crawford W. Long hospital library at Emory University in Atlanta made the second edition information much easier to consolidate.

Again my deepest thanks to my immediate and extended family, who shared my time commitment in writing this book. They understand dedication, and they taught the principle to me.

Harold J. Brody, M.D.

Acknowledgments *to the First Edition*

This book was written with the assistance of my two associates in dermatology, Chenault W. Hailey and Robert A. Clark, whose input and sharing of patients make the learning of new knowledge a challenge.

I shall always be indebted to my teachers who encouraged me to write in the beginning. Fred F. Castrow and Robert M. Fine were instrumental in my first publishing efforts in dermatology. I performed my initial chemical peel as a resident in 1976 with Hiram M. Sturm, who eased the usual trepidation of the novice peeler. Additional Emory faculty members, Henry Earl Jones and Sidney Olansky, were inspirational in their instruction of dermatology.

Deep and sincere thanks go to my colleagues in dermatologic surgery who encouraged and supported me in writing this book, especially Richard Glogau, Pamela Baj, and Seth Matarasso. C. William Hanke, June Robinson, John Yarborough, Bill Coleman, and Elizabeth McBurney inspired confidence at every opportunity.

The invaluable assistance of the following dermatologists and dermatologic surgeons as reviewers, revisionists, and proofreaders were Seth Matarasso, Chapters 1, 6, 9 and 10; Richard Glogau, Chapters 2, 4, 7, and 10; Diane Baker and Thomas D. Griffin, Chapter 5; Roger Ceilley, Chapters 8 and 10. Special thanks to Mary Spraker and Robert A. Clark, who read the entire manuscript and provided special support.

Thanks also to dermopathologists Marian Finan, Tom Wade, and Al Soloman, who provided assistance, revision, and suggestions on the important chapter on histopathology. Blake Goslen and Howard Maibach reviewed and examined Chapter 3 on wound healing. Gloria Graham's input into the cryosurgical aspects of peeling was much appreciated.

Special thanks go to William H. Beeson, our friend and colleague in facial plastic surgery, for his revisional suggestions in Chapter 7 on deep peeling.

I am especially indebted to Marilynne McKay, who was accessible at any time of day or night to get me out of a computer hassle with the Macintosh SE, on which this book was ably written.

Grateful admiration to Lyn Ross at Personal Aesthetics in Atlanta for her openess and sharing about her profession as an aesthetician and the positive relationship with dermatology.

Thanks to my office staff, nurses, and assistants, especially Sharyn Whitmire, Debbie Lamb, Teresa Tippitt Stuart, and Jean Moss, who heard unceasingly about "the book" and assisted me with illustrations and projects.

The staff at the medical library of Crawford W. Long Hospital of Emory University in Atlanta were always ready to help me obtain obscure articles and literature searches to prepare the manuscript. Thanks especially to Vijay, George, Gladys, Carolyn, and Arlene.

Finally, my deepest thanks to the two most important and inspirational teachers that I have met in my career, and who are also the two individuals who taught me the most about patients, chemical peeling, and dermatology: my associate Chenault Hailey and the late Samuel J. Stegman. Dr. Stegman's influence on my approach to academia in general as well as chemical peeling cannot be overstated.

Last, but by no means least, my family—both immediate and extended—receives the lion's share of the gratitude: Betty, Amy, Jon, Russell, and Jerry rearranged their time for me. Very special thanks are due to my mother and late father to whom I owe my inherent talents. Without the attentions and compromises of my family, I would not be who I am, and this book would not have been written.

Harold J. Brody, M.D.

Table of Contents

1 History of Chemical Peels

The ancient Egyptians used animal oils, salt, and alabaster to aesthetically improve the skin.[1,2] When the ancient Egyptian woman bathed in sour milk to produce smooth skin, she unknowingly utilized lactic acid, an α-hydroxy acid. Poultices containing mustard, sulfur, and limestone were used later. The Turks used fire to singe the skin in an attempt to induce light exfoliation. Indian women mixed urine with pumice for skin application. In Europe, Hungarian gypsies passed their particular formulas down from generation to generation.

Dermatologists pioneered skin peeling for therapeutic benefit (Table 1-1). In 1882, P.G. Unna, a German dermatologist, described the properties of salicylic acid, resorcinol, phenol, and trichloroacetic acid (TCA). George Miller MacKee, a dermatologist who eventually became chairman of the dermatology department at New York University (NYU), began using phenol peels for acne scarring in 1903 and published his results in 1952 with Florentine Karp. They managed a phenol clinic in the 1940s at NYU.[4] During the first half of the twentieth century, sporadic reports on peeling appeared in textbooks and the early American medical literature. A colleague of Mackee's, George Henry Fox, wrote of the treatment of facial freckles with phenol in his textbook in 1905.[5]

During World War I, phenol solutions were an acceptable treatment for gunpowder burns of the face. Dr. la Gassé noted that an injured area that was treated with phenol and covered with adhesive tape healed with cosmetic improvement. His techniques of 1918 wartime France were brought to the United States by his daughter Antoinette, who practiced lay peeling near Los Angeles in the 1930s and 1940s to improve scarring and wrinkles.[6] Francis and Miriam Maschek, lay peelers in south Florida, probably learned portions of the technique from her and from her protégé Cora Galenti of Los Angeles. The House of Renaissance was one of several salons operating at the time in Florida. In addition, the salons sometimes served as fronts for physicians performing massive silicone injections.

Dr. H.O. Bames, a Los Angeles physician who became one of the first plastic surgeons, wrote about both superficial face peeling with resorcinol and deep face peeling with phenol for wrinkles covered with adhesive plaster in 1927.[7,8] He described phenol complications, the use of thymol iodide powder, and the importance of dividing the facial peel into halves separated by a week's time.

In 1941, Eller and Wolff[9] summarized the peeling formulas available for exfoliation at that time (Table 1-2). Sulfur and resorcinol pastes were described, probably originally derived from the Egyptian, Babylonian, and Indian use of pumice on the skin to cause stratum corneum exfoliation. Phenol, salicylic acid combinations, and carbon dioxide snow peels were detailed, and the dangers of renal phenol toxicity as well as the importance of degreasing the skin before

TABLE 1-1.
Skin Peeling Investigators in Medical History

INVESTIGATOR AND DATE	ADVANCE
Unna, 1882	Salicylic acid, resorcin, phenol, and TCA* descriptions (Ref. 3)
Fox, 1905	Phenol for facial freckles
Bames, 1927	Resorcinol and occluded phenol face peels for cosmesis
Mackee, 1903-1952	Phenol for scarring
Eller and Wolff, 1941	Sulfur, resorcinol, salicylic acid, phenol lotions, CO_2 slush
Monash, 1945	TCA peeling
Urkov, 1946	Resorcinol, lactic acid, salicylic acid, phenol, cantharidin
Combes, 1960	Buffered phenol
Brown, 1960	Phenol histology and buffered formulas
Ayres, 1960	TCA for actinic damage
Baker and Gordon, 1961	Phenol formula, saponified
Litton, 1962	Phenol formula, nonsaponified
Sperber, 1965	Buffered phenol formulas
Resnik, Lewis, and Cohen, 1976	TCA peeling
Stegman, 1980-1982	Histologic comparison of wounding agents
Van Scott and Yu, 1984	α-Hydroxy acids
Brody and Hailey, 1986	Medium-depth peeling
Monheit, 1989	Medium-depth peeling variation
Coleman and Futrell, 1994	Medium-depth peeling variation

**TCA,* Trichloroacetic acid.

peeling agent application were noted. β-Naphthol peeling pastes for acne treatment had been utilized since the early part of the century.

In 1946, Urkov[15] described dermatologic exfoliation by methods including occluded phenol. He also described superficial exfoliation by applying a mixture of resorcinol with lactic and salicylic acids under occlusion. Cantharidin was employed under an occlusive dressing for deeper exfoliation. Winter[16] in 1950 used phenol in ether to remove freckles. The work of Ayres[14,17] in the 1960s combined the TCA experiments of Monash in 1945[18] with his own conclusions based on clinical experience and histology of both TCA and phenol. He felt that TCA was the more caustic agent. Sultzberger and others[19] at NYU began to treat acne scars. Dr. Max Jessner utilized his salicylic acid, lactic acid, and resorcinol combination at NYU.

In the late 1950s and early 1960s, the detailed studies on phenol formulas and toxicities by Brown and co-workers[11] and the nonsaponified phenol formula of Litton[13] were products of the renaissance in peeling that occurred in the early 1960s. Adolph Brown, a maxillofacial surgeon, and his wife, Marthe Brown, a dermatologist, performed histologic studies, sparked by lay peelers and their formulas in Los Angeles. Dr. Clyde Litton, in West Virginia, met Miami lay peelers and worked to modify their formulas. Sir Harold Gillies, an otolaryngologist, used phenol and tape in the midfifties.[20] Combes and co-workers[21] and Sperber[12] attempted to produce a buffered phenol formula that would prove less caustic than full-strength phenol.

Simultaneously in the early 1960s, Dr. Thomas Baker, a plastic surgeon in Miami, became aware of a lay peeler who was using a mystery formula to perform peels that seemed to produce incredible results for the treatment of wrinkles. Lay operators of this time would not reveal their exact formulas but gave skeletal information. Complications in the form of scarring and sloughs were

TABLE 1-2.

Significant But Outdated Formulas in the Anthropology and Evolution of Chemical Peeling

FORMULA	INGREDIENT	AMOUNT	DATE
Unna's peeling paste	Resorcinol	40 g	
	Ichthammol	10 g	
	Petrolatum	10 g	
	Zinc oxide paste	40 g	Early 1900s (Ref. 9)
Lassar's peeling paste	β-Naphthol	10 g	
	Sulfur	50 g	
	Soft soap	20 g	
	Petrolatum	20 g	Early 1990s (Refs. 9,10)
Original peeling paste	Resorcinol	40 g	
	Zinc oxide	5 g	
	Kaolin	5 g	
	Petrolatum liquid	4 g	
	Anhydrous lanolin	12 g	
	Petrolatum	q.s. ad* 80 g	
Original resorcinol lotion	Resorcinol	60 cc	
	Salicylic acid	30 cc	
	Lactic acid	30 cc	
	Oil of rose	0.195 cc	
	Ethyl hydrate	240 cc	1930s
Phenol peel lotion	Phenol	30 g	
	Salicylic acid	6 g	
	Alcohol, 95%	64 g	1930s and 40s (Ref. 9)
Brown's phenol formula	Phenol	60%-95%	
	Saponated cresol solution	0.3% (buffer)	
	Olive oil or sesame oil	0.25%	
	Distilled water	q.s. ad 100%	1960 (Ref. 11)
Sperber's "buffered" phenol†	Phenol	15 ml	
	Sodium salicylate	0.05 ml	
	Camphor	0.025 ml	
	Anhydrous glycerine	1.25 ml	
	Ethanol, 100%	0.50 ml	1963 (Ref. 12)
Litton's phenol mix (requires heat for dissolving)	First		
	Phenol crystals	1 lb	
	Distilled water	8 cc	
	Glycerine	8 cc	
	Heat and liquify		
	Then		
	Liquified phenol	4 oz	
	Croton oil	1 cc	
	Distilled water	4 oz	1962 (Ref. 13)
Dennie's freckle formulas (determined by Ayres to be comparable to liquid phenol 88%) alone	Phenol	33⅓%	
	TCA*	33⅓%	
	Alcohol	33⅓% (q.s. ad 100 cc)	1960 (Ref. 14)

q.s. ad, Quantity sufficient to add up to; *TCA,* trichloroacetic acid.

†See the section on croton oil addition in Chapter 2 for "buffers" clarification.

frequent sequelae, and physicians were doubtful that a peel could accomplish significant results until Baker and Gordon presented a patient at a national plastic surgery conference in 1972 who had had good results from a peel documented by before-and-after photographs. From their experience with lay peelers, the work of Doctors Brown and Brown, and their own research in 1961,[22,23] they developed a saponated formula that is still in use today.

The 1970s provided an environment for dermatologists, plastic surgeons, and otolaryngologists to perform full-face peels with either TCA or phenol. Resnik and co-workers[24] published their experiences with TCA during this period. Horvath[25] used a superficial resorcinol, salicylic acid, and lactic acid peel earlier used by Dr. F.C. Combes and Dr. Max Jessner at NYU. Dupont and co-workers[26] followed phenol peels with dermabrasion, and Stagnone[27] followed TCA peels with dermabrasion and coined the term *chemabrasion*. These variations were attempts to further refine methodology in order to improve skin texture. Neither of them is used extensively today.

Stegman's work in the 1980s[28,29] on both the animal and the human model compared the histologic depth of both chemical wounding agents and dermabrasion, paving the way for chemical peeling in a controlled and scientific fashion. These excellent histologic concepts for the evaluation of peeling influenced Brody and Hailey, who combined two superficial agents, solid carbon dioxide followed by TCA, to produce a medium-depth peel in 1986.[30] Monheit[31] in 1989 employed another medium-depth technique utilizing resorcinol, salicylic acid, and lactic acid (Jessner's solution) followed by TCA.

Van Scott and Yu[32] began investigating the α-hydroxy acids (AHAs) in the late 1970s. Their experimentation with these chemicals as superficial peeling agents came to fruition in the 1980s. As the 1990s have unfolded, the AHAs have become an addition to the peel spectrum with widespread attention from the communications media, an event unprecedented in the history of chemical peeling. They have been combined with TCA for medium-depth peeling by Coleman and Futrell.[33] With Glogau's sensible photoaging classification[34] and the depth knowledge of wounding techniques, peeling can be accomplished with more technical accuracy than at any point in history. The introduction of the resurfacing lasers used in combination with or in addition to peeling agents heralds a new era. The scientific, histologic, and clinical evaluation and comparison of the newer agents and techniques with existing agents will be the work of the future.

Double, double, toil and trouble;
Fire burn and cauldron bubble.

SHAKESPEARE: *MACBETH*, ACT 4, SCENE 1

REFERENCES

1. Bryan CP: *Ancient egyptian medicine; the Papyrus Ebers* (translation), Chicago, 1974, Ares, pp. 158-161.
2. Ebbell B: *Papyrus Ebers* (translation), Copenhagen, 1937, Ejnar Munksgaard.
3. Letessier SM: Chemical peel with resorcin. In Roenigk RK, Roenigk HH, edtiors: *Dermatologic surgery*. New York, 1989, Marcel Dekker, p. 1017.
4. Mackee GM, Karp FL: The treatment of post acne scars with phenol, *Br J Dermatol* 64:456-459, 1952.
5. Fox GH: *Photographic atlas of the diseases of the skin*, vol 2, Philadelphia, 1905, Lippincott. pp. 119-120.
6. Gross BG, Maschek F: Phenol chemosurgery for removal of deep facial wrinkles, *Int J Dermatol* 19:159-164, 1980.

7. Bames HO: Truth and fallacies of face peeling and face lifting, *Med J Record* 126:86-87, 1927.
8. Marmelzat WL: A historical review of chemical rejuvenation of the face. In Kotler R, editor: *Chemical rejuvenation of the face,* St Louis, 1992, Mosby, pp. 16-17.
9. Eller JJ, Wolff S: Skin peeling and scarification, *JAMA* 116:934-938, 1941.
10. Hemels H: Percutaneous absorption and distribution of 2-naphthol in man, *Br J Dermatol* 87:614, 1972.
11. Brown AM, Kaplan LM, Brown ME: Phenol induced histological skin changes: hazards, techniques, and uses, *Br J Plast Surg* 13:158, 1960.
12. Sperber PA: Chemexfoliation in treatment of acne scarring, *Tex State J Med* 59:496, 1963.
13. Litton C: Chemical face lifting, *Plast Reconstr Surg* 29:371, 1962.
14. Ayres S: Dermal changes following application of chemical cauterants to aging skin, *Arch Dermatol* 82:578, 1960.
15. Urkov JC: Surface defects of skin: treatment by controlled exfoliation, *Ill Med J* 89:75, 1946.
16. Winter L: Method of permanent removal of freckles, *Br J Dermatol Syphil* 62:83, 1950.
17. Ayres S: Superficial chemosurgery in treating aging skin, *Arch Dermatol* 82:125, 1962.
18. Monash S: The uses of diluted trichloroacetic acid in dermatology, *Urol Cutan Rev* 49:119, 1945.
19. Sultzberger MB, Wolf J, Vitten VH, et al: *Dermatology diagnosis and treatment,* St Louis, 1961, Mosby.
20. Gillies HD, Millard DR: *The principles and art of plastic surgery,* Boston, 1957, Little, Brown, p. 403.
21. Combes FC, Sperber PA, Reisch M: Dermal defects: treatment by a chemical agent, *N Y Physician Am Med* 56:36, 1960.
22. Baker TJ: Chemical face peeling and rhytidectomy, *Plast Reconstr Surg* 29:199, 1962.
23. Baker TJ, Gordon HL: The ablation of rhytides by chemical means: a preliminary report, *J Fla Med Assoc* 48:541,1961.
24. Resnik SS, Lewis LA, Cohen BH: Trichloroacetic acid peeling, *Cutis* 17:127-129, 1976.
25. Horvath PN: The light peel, *Bull Assoc Milit Dermatol* 18:2, 1970.
26. Dupont C, Ciaburro H, Prevost Y, et al: Phenol skin tightening for better dermabrasion, *Plast Reconstr Surg* 50:588, 1972.
27. Stagnone JJ: Chemabrasion, *J Dermatol Surg Oncol* 3:217, 1977.
28. Stegman SJ: A study of dermabrasion and chemical peels in an animal model, *J Dermatol Surg Oncol* 6:490, 1980.
29. Stegman SJ: A comparative histologic study of the effects of three peeling agents and dermabrasion on normal and sundamaged skin, *Aesthetic Plast Surg* 6:123, 1982.
30. Brody HJ, Hailey CW: Medium depth chemical peeling of the skin: a variation of superficial chemosurgery, *J Dermatol Surg Oncol* 12:1268, 1986.
31. Monheit G: The Jessner's + TCA peel: a medium depth chemical peel, *J Dermatol Surg Oncol* 15:945, 1989.
32. Van Scott EJ, Yu RJ: Hyperkeratinization, corneocyte cohesion and alpha hydroxy acids, *J Am Acad Dermatol* 11:867-879, 1984.
33. Coleman WP, Futrell JM: The glycolic acid + trichloroacetic acid peel, *J Dermatol Surg Oncol* 20:76-80, 1994.
34. Glogau RG: Chemical peeling and aging skin, *J Geriatr Dermatol* 2(1):30-35, 1994.

2 Histology and Classification

Histology has been the mainstay of assessing the efficacy of wounding agents from a scientific standpoint. From a clinical standpoint, the expected improvement of a wrinkle, a scar, or an actinic keratosis after different depths of peeling may not be in question, but the selection of exactly which agent or technique to use depends on an understanding of the depth of the wound so as to choose an agent that is not needlessly deeper than the defect itself. For example, peeling a very mildly sun-damaged patient for freckles alone (epidermal lesions) with a deep wounding agent such as Baker's phenol compromises that skin unnecessarily when a medium-depth agent would have yielded the same results with no deeper reticular dermal damage or melanin reduction from phenol. Peeling rhytides of varying severity necessitates adequate penetration through an adequate amount of dermal elastic fiber damage. In addition, proper defatting preparation of the skin can increase wound depth. This does not diminish the value of our knowledge because in many cases it is duplicated by multiple studies by investigators over many decades (Fig. 2-1). The dermis may be between 20 and 30 times as thick as the epidermis, and it is in this layer that most important changes occur to demonstrate peel results.

Anatomically the skin of the **face** differs from nonfacial skin by the relative number of pilosebaceous units per cosmetic unit. The nose and forehead have more sebaceous glands than do the cheeks or temples. The **eyelid** skin has a relatively flat dermal-epidermal junction with a thinner but denser dermis that is composed of a delicate network of spongy fibrous connective tissue. The little fat that is present is closer to the surface, as is the underlying muscle.

In chemical peels, the difference in appearance between sun-damaged nonfacial skin vs. facial skin is a function of anatomic area as well as metabolic factors of the wounding agent. (See the section on trichloroacetic acid metabolism in Chapter 5.) The dermis of extensor surfaces is usually thicker than that of flexor surfaces. The dorsum of an actinically damaged **hand** may reflect the atrophic process of age more than the face does. Atrophy in this area may be more clinically and histologically obvious because of a paucity of subcutaneous fat and pilosebaceous units (Fig. 2-2, *A* and *B*). This may affect selection of wounding agents for use in this location because with aging the dermis may be significantly attenuated and wounding agents may be more destructive because they are metabolizd less rapidly. Fewer adnexal structures exist to promote reepithelialization. However, the actual role of "thin skin" in choosing wounding agents may not be of practical value because scarring may occur in "thick-skinned" areas of the face and spare the areas that display a thinner dermis.

The dermis of the **back** is very thick and has dense dermal collagen. Although relatively more resilient than other body areas, it is capable of

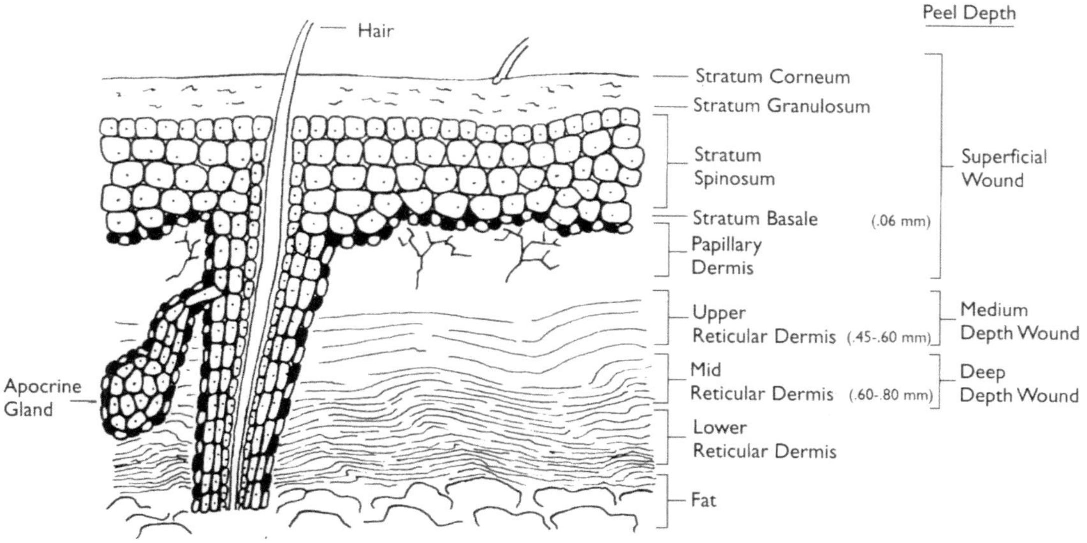

FIG. 2-1. Diagram of the skin showing the wounding depth of superficial, medium-depth, and deep-depth peels.

A 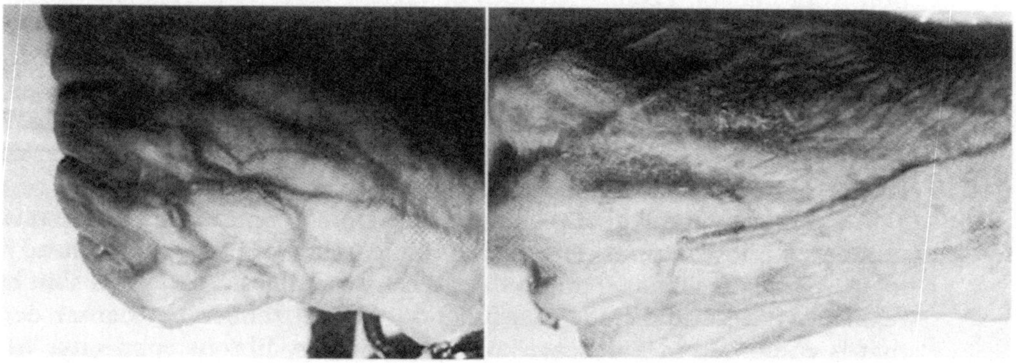 B

FIG. 2-2. A, Senile atrophy of the hand of an 83-year-old with little photodamage. The thin dermis and epidermis reveal the vasculature. **B,** Senile atrophy of the hand of an 81-year-old with severe photodamage. Additional lentigos, pigmented keratoses, xerosis, and ecchymosis are present.

scarring with high-strength TCA and phenol in the absence of preexisting acne scarring. Our clinical impression, although not proven, is that the presence of acne scarring in the dermal matrix on the back either retards wounding agent penetrability or impedes the inflammatory response of higher-strength TCA so that there is a relative skin resistance in peeling scars in this area.

In glycomethacrylate sections, the **epidermis of sun-damaged skin** is characterized by a compact, laminated, or gelatinous stratum corneum, sometimes containing vesicles full of proteinaceous material from the enlarged stratum lucidum.[1] There may be no clear transition between the two strata. In the malpighian layer, cell heterogeneity, vacuolization, dysplasia, and individual cell necrosis are common. Intercellular and intracellular vacuoles are present, especially in the melanocytes and keratinocytes of the stratum basale, with a loss of cell polarity. The number of Langerhans' cells is reduced. Flat-

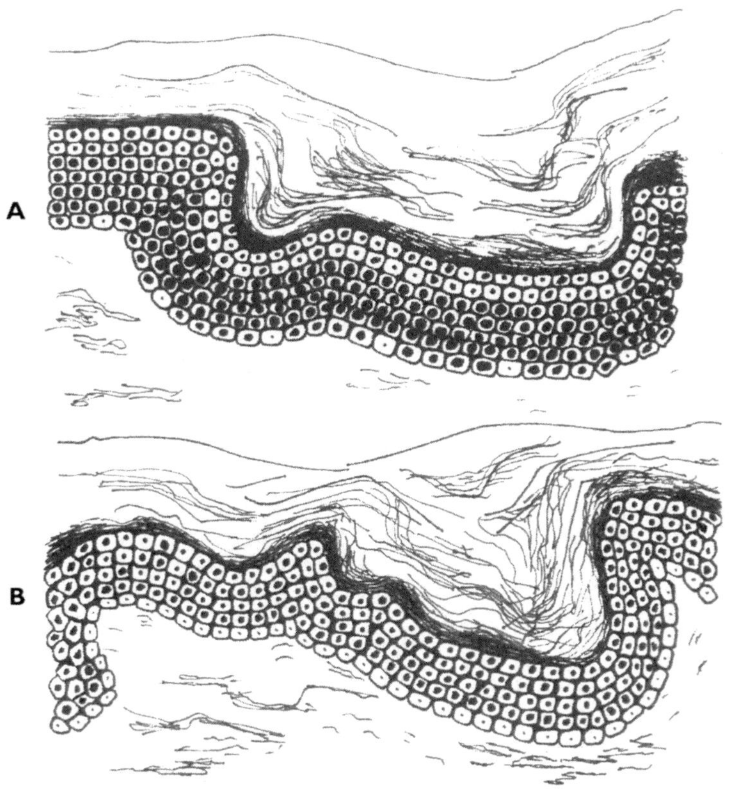

FIG. 2-3. Histology of freckle (ephelides) **(A)** showing an increase in the melanin content of the basal cell layer cells but no increase in the numbers of melanocytes and solar lentigo **(B)** showing the basal cell layer almost completely replaced by melanocytes. Both require full epidermal peeling for total elimination (see text).

tening of the dermal-epidermal junction and effacement of the rete ridge pattern occur in intrinsically aging skin regardless of photodamage.

Melanin granules contribute to the pathology of **freckles,** or **ephelides,** and are erratically distributed throughout the epidermis with the greatest accumulation being in the basal and suprabasal keratinocytes, similar to non–sun-damaged skin. Melanocytes in the basal layer may focally increase and form clinical **solar lentigos** (Fig. 2-3). Increased melanin is present in both the melanocytes and basal keratinocytes with slight rete ridge elongation and occasional upper papillary dermal melanophages. Peeling through the entire epidermis is required to remove these epidermal lesions.

The **dermis** shows disparate degrees of elastic tissue changes, with both elastic fiber breakdown in the form of fibrorhexis and fibrolysis and the formation of amorphous elastotic masses. Macrophages among these elastotic masses contain coarse granules. Reticulin fibers increase in areas of fiber breakdown and predominate around the masses, which are supported by a delicate collagenous fiber scaffolding. As elastotic material accumulates, it crowds out all the collagenous fibers, which are resorbed. As the elastotic material itself is resorbed, collagen fiber whisps replace them. The total volume of dermis seems to gradually diminish so that with severe photodamage the epidermis rests directly on the middermis with neither a papillary dermis nor a Grenz zone. The epidermis is too ample for the shrinking dermis, and this results in small wrinkles[1] (Fig. 2-4, *A* and *B*).

Perspective on Sundamaged histology

An understanding of the histology of sun-damaged skin helps explain the subsequent combined degeneration of the epidermal and dermal systems into the clinical forms of actinic damage familiar to the clinician. As ***epidermal maturation becomes aberrant*** there is a loss of translucency and the appearance of dry, rough, and dull skin with the evolution of keratoses, ephelides, solar lentigos, and comedones. ***Dermal collagen and elastin degeneration*** results in the appearance of wrinkles, creases, folds, and furrows (see Fig. 4-2). As the ***melanin system becomes disordered,*** blotching, freckles (ephelides), lentigines, and pigmented actinic and seborrheic keratoses become evident, and melasma and postinflammatory hyperpigmentation are aggravated. All of these are amplified by ***irregularities in papillary dermal blood flow*** causing telangiectasias and microangiomas with resulting erythema and ecchymosis.[2]

Although no histologic correlate of wrinkles has been established, they are probably the result of a reduction in dermal collagen, both from decreased formation of collagen I and increased extracellular breakdown of collagen I by collagenase. This biosynthetic alteration in sun-damaged skin may produce wrinkles.

A

B

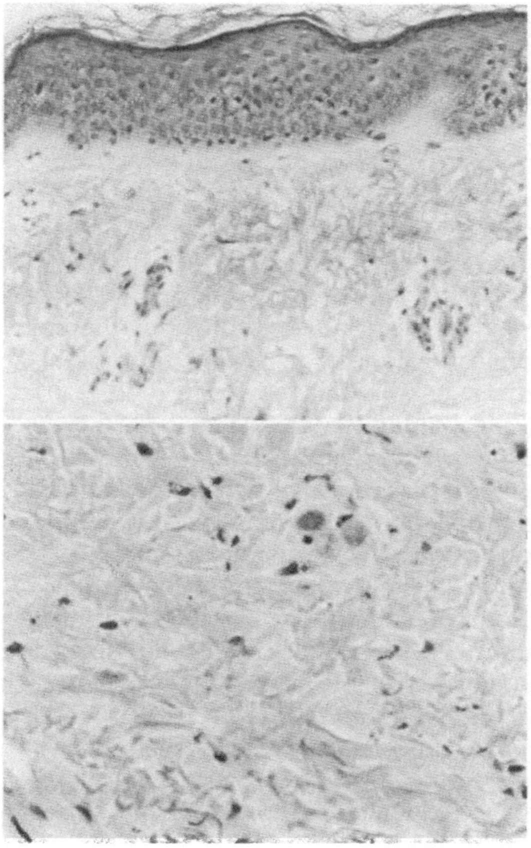

FIG. 2-4. Photomicrographs showing histologic changes of photodamaged skin (see text). **A,** Epidermis, 10×. **B,** Dermis, 10×. *(Courtesy of Dr. Marian Finan.)*

CHEMICAL PEELING

Epidermal Injury—Superficial Wounding

Epidermal injury without clinical vesiculation is evident from **Jessner's solution** (JS), also called a **Combes' peel**. This combination of resorcinol plus salicylic and lactic acids in alcohol solution shows only stratum corneum separation with upper epidermal intraepithelial and intercellular edema when the wounding agent is applied as three coats with two cotton-tipped applicators (Fig. 2-5).[3] No dermal changes are apparent.

In a similar fashion, α-**hydroxy acids,** specifically **glycolic acid,** create corneocyte detachment at the junction with the stratum granulosum resulting in desquamation at the lower, newly forming levels of the stratum corneum in concentrations of up to 20%. This more uniform dyscohesion of the stratum corneum may be unique to this class of compounds and is not produced by skin irritation or by keratolysis, the elimination of the stratum corneum from the outermost level downward. Keratolysis is the mechanism of salicylic acid, a β-hydroxy acid. In concentrations of 70% or higher, epidermolysis occurs below the level of the stratum corneum.[4]

Glycolic acid 70% applied to non–sun-damaged guinea pig skin for 15 minutes causes dermal necrosis equivalent to the depth of 35% to 45% TCA, demonstrating the time dependency of the agent.[5] Both 50% and 70% glycolic acid along with 12% lactic acid produce increases in papillary dermal collagen on skin biopsy at 21 days after peeling in the minipig. When compared with agents such as TCA and phenol, which cause collagen deposition in concert with more inflammation, these AHAs cause disproportionate papillary dermal collagen deposition if left on minipig skin for 15 minutes.[6] They may directly stimulate cell growth and protein synthesis without causing actual damage. This study is limited by its short duration (3 weeks) and the long duration of pigskin application time clinically unapplicable to humans. Glycolic acid causes an increase in collagen synthesis by human skin fibroblasts in tissue

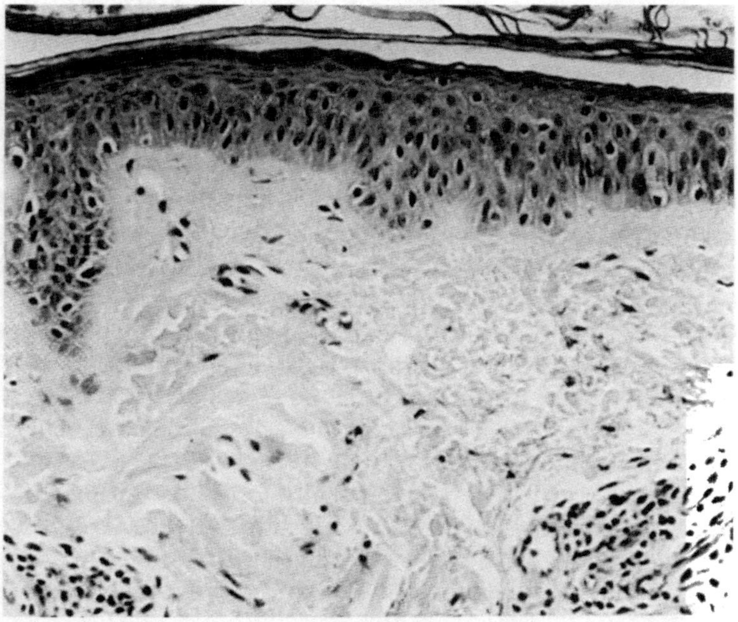

FIG. 2-5. Epidermal edema 2 days after peeling with Jessner's solution.

culture.[7] Histologic comparison of 50% vs. 70% glycolic acid peels using varying pH in two patients suggests that a more acidic pH below 2.0 and a higher concentration are two factors that induce more skin necrosis in peeling.[8] With AHA cream application of less acidic pH, increased dermal glycosaminoglycan deposition is histologically noted.[9] Application of the AHA cream study to repetitive peeling is uncertain, but it may suggest less dermal benefit to increased direct tissue damage. Comparative long-term maintenance of dermal collagen is not known with different wounding agents.

Application of AHA cream produces specific skin effects. Seventeen patients applied 25% glycolic acid lotion (five patients), 25% lactic acid lotion (five patients), and 25% citric acid lotion (seven patients) with a pH of 3.5 to photoaged facial and forearm skin for 6 months as compared with placebo. Light microscopic and ultrastructural changes include enhanced rete ridge pattern, more orderly pattern of differentiation and polarity of basal keratinocytes, 25% increase in epidermal and papillary dermal thickness, increase in dermal mucin ground substance, improved elastic fiber quality with increased length but less fragmentation, and a non–statistically significant increase in density of collagen fibers.[10] There was no increase in elastic fiber quantity, and the quality of elastic fibers is subject to different interpretation by dermatopathologists. No inflammation or edema was seen, and there were increases in mast cell degranulation and expression of factor XIIIa transglutaminase in dermal dendrocytes. The benefits of AHAs may be the result of the activation of dermal dendrocytes through cytokine release such as mast cell tumor necrosis factor alpha.[11]

Ultrastructrually, there are decreased desmosomal attachments and tonofilament aggregation on electron microscopy (EM) with some suggestion of increase in anchoring fibrils. Dermal dendrocytes were increased in size with dilation of rough endoplasmic reticulum, representing activation. (For histologic correlation of AHA cream applications, see the section on AHAs in Chapter 5.)

Tretinoin, when used consistently on the skin in a concentration of 0.1% for greater than 4 months,[12] produces a compaction of actinically damaged stratum corneum. A homogeneous layer that contains a glycosaminoglycan (GAG)-like material replaces the basket-weave pattern. Pretherapy dysplastic changes in keratinocytes are not seen in the epidermis following tretinoin therapy (Fig. 2-6, *A* and *B*). Melanocytic hyperplasia is in tretinoin-treated skin. Widened vascular lumina are found in the dermis, and whether this represents dilation of vessels or true induced angiogenesis cannot be determined. Electron microscopy reveals increased collagen formation with increased fibroblasts that are undetectable by the light microscope. Continued treatment beyond 1 year substantially widens the papillary dermal Grenz zone and pushes down the old elastotic tissue to create a sharp interface between old and new tissue. Tretinoin seems to have no effect on the elastotic tissue itself at 6 months as revealed by collagen and elastic stains.[13] After 48 weeks there is a small but significant reduction of elastic tissue corresponding to a relative increase in collagen tissue.[14]

Treatment with 0.1% tretinoin daily for 12 weeks on photodamaged and photoprotected human skin shows an 80% increase in type I collagen formation as compared with a 14% decrease with vehicle treatment.[15] Tretinoin directly induces collagen synthesis and decreases collagen breakdown by inducing tissue inhibitors of collagenase. Both of these factors may contribute to tretinoin's improvement of photoaged skin.

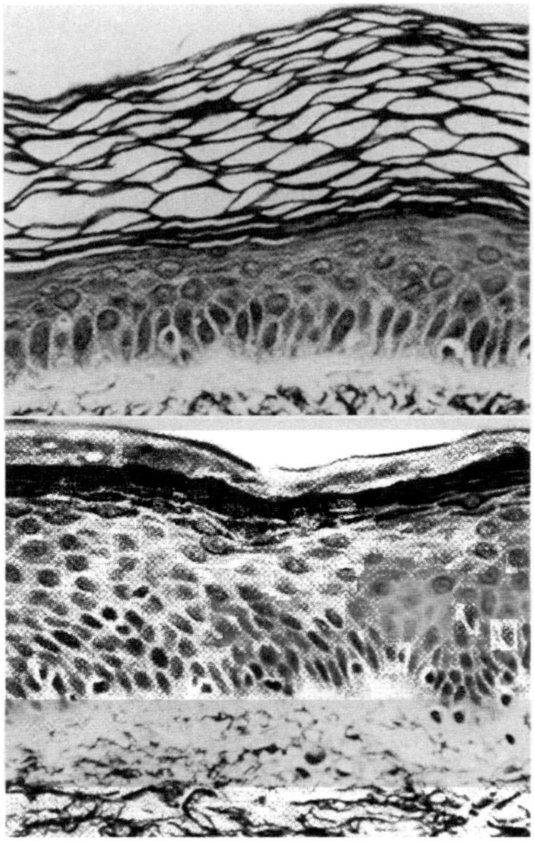
A

B

FIG. 2-6. Tretinoin-treated forearm skin before therapy **(A)** and after 4 months of therapy **(B)**. These changes after 6 months may largely revert to baseline after 1 year of topical therapy, suggesting that the early histologic changes may be due to retinoid effect for which accommodation occurs. Clinical improvement continues in spite of the reversion of epidermal histology. *(From Weiss JS, Ellis CN, Headington JT, et al: JAMA 259:527-532, 1988.)*

The epidermal hyperplasia, increase in granular layer thickness, and appearance of compact orthokeratosis seen at 24 weeks of tretinoin treatment return to baseline and reverse after 48 weeks of treatment, suggesting that continued clinical improvement is not histologically correlated. The initial epidermal alterations may reflect a retinoid effect for which accommodation occurs. Epidermal melanin content continues to decrease through 48 weeks of treatment, however, consistent with clinical pigmentary lightening.[14]

Double-blind, vehicle-controlled comparisons of 0.1% and 0.025% tretinoin creams on photodamaged facial skin for 48 weeks reveal no significant difference between the two concentrations in improvement of stratum corneum compaction, spongiosis, and epidermal cell thickness. Granular layer thickness is significantly increased with 0.1% tretinoin application.[16] (For effects on reepithelialization, see Chapter 3 and the section on tretinoin in Chapter 5.)

Solid carbon dioxide (CO_2) applied to the skin for 15 seconds produces complete epidermal necrosis with pronounced dermal edema. A mixed inflammatory infiltrate is seen, but there is no collagen destruction[3] (Fig. 2-7). After reepithelialization, elastic stains do not show changes in the elastic tissue, thus confirming epidermal injury alone. A comparison of solid CO_2

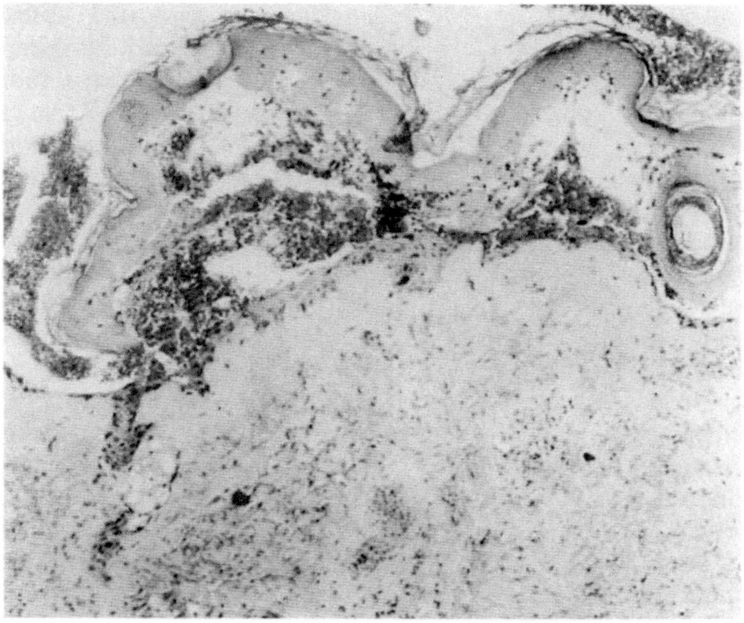

FIG. 2-7. Epidermal necrosis 2 days after peeling with CO_2 (hematoxylin-eosin [HE] stain).

with JS in the human model shows CO_2 with 20 seconds of hard pressure to be a vesiculating agent producing complete epidermal necrosis as opposed to JS, which does not vesiculate or cause epidermal necrosis. At day 7 after peeling, parakeratin remains in the stratum corneum of CO_2-treated skin, thus indicating incomplete healing as opposed to JS-applied skin. A single application of CO_2 is therefore a more superficially aggressive modality than JS.

Upper Dermal Injury—Medium-Depth Wounding

Dermal injury, both upper dermal (medium-depth wounding) and middermal (deep wounding), is sustained by a number of viable wounding agents and combination techniques. The range of injury from the lower papillary dermis into the upper reticular dermis is classically defined by the wounding agent TCA, 40% to 60%. Stegman[17] compared TCA with full-strength phenol, Baker's phenol, and dermabrasion in sun-damaged and non–sun-damaged skin on the human neck. Occlusion was also studied. Trichloroacetic acid, 40% to 60%, produced epidermal necrosis, papillary dermal edema and homogenization, and a sparse lymphocytic infiltrate in the midreticular dermis 3 days after peeling. Findings in sun-damaged skin were similar to non–sun-damaged skin in that the elastotic band that occurs in sun-damaged skin did not seem to offer a barrier to wounding. The progression or graduation of wound depth was similar when comparing TCA with full-strength phenol or Baker's phenol solution on sun-damaged and non–sun-damaged skin.

Ninety days after peeling, Stegman[17] observed a normal-appearing zone of expanded papillary dermis that he referred to as a **Grenz zone**. The thickness of this Grenz zone varied with the strength of the wounding agent used and with the depth of the wound produced. A band of thick amorphous brown fibers was present in the middle-to-upper dermis. This band when stained with both elastic stain and colloidal iron displayed large amounts of elastotic-

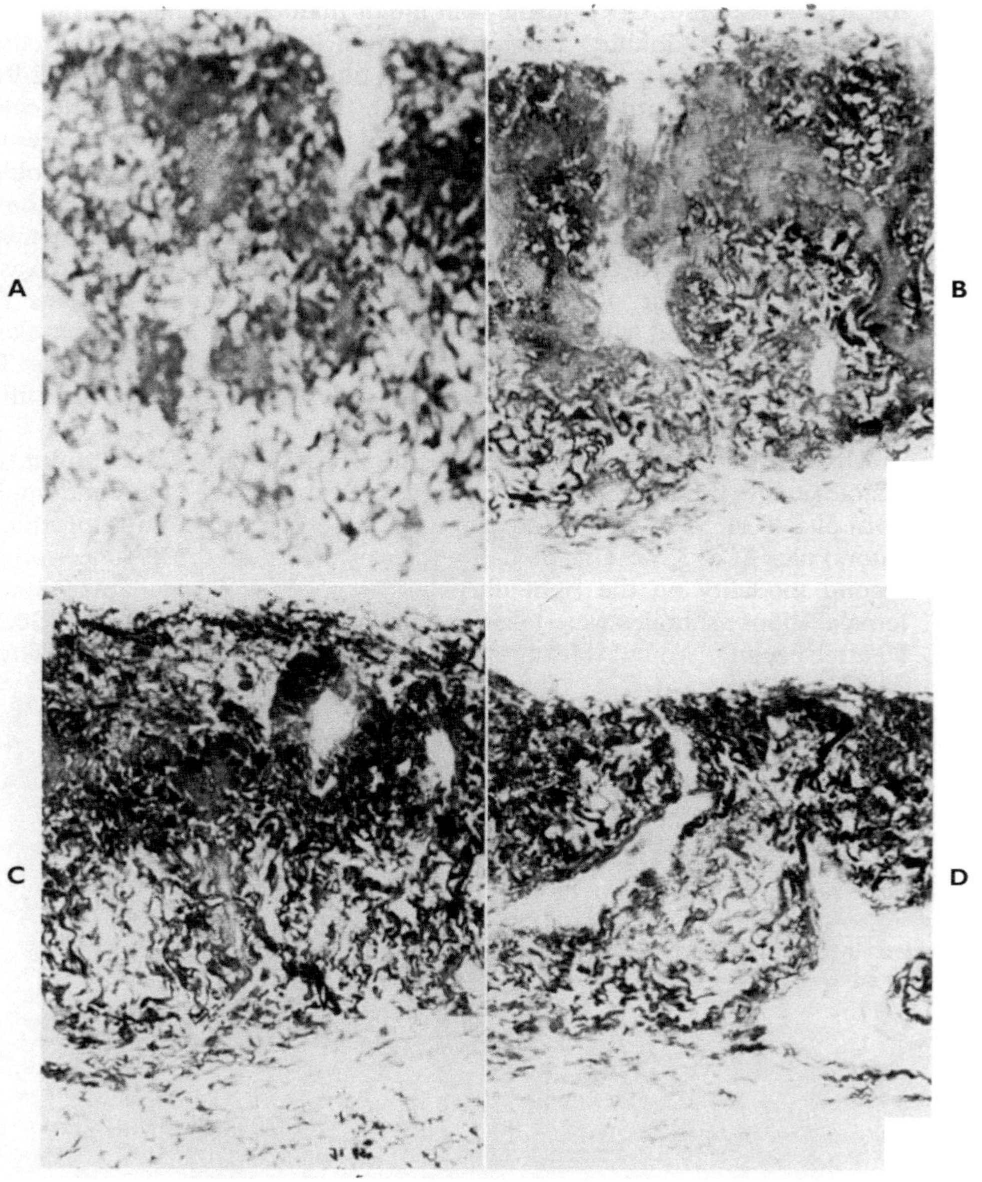

FIG. 2-8. Non–sun-damaged skin, elastic stain. **A,** normal control. **B,** Sixty days after treatment with 100% phenol, unocccluded. **C,** Sixty days after treatment with 100% phenol occluded for 24 hours. **D,** Sixty days after treatment with Baker's formula occluded for 24 hours. *(From Stegman SJ: Aesthetic Plast Surg 6:123-135, 1982).*

like fibers and GAGs. The thickness and depth of staining of this band increased with the strength of the wounding agents, specifically TCA, unoccluded full-strength phenol, Baker's phenol solution, Baker's phenol under occlusion, and dermabrasion. The band was only faintly present in the TCA peel sections. This description of dermal changes constitutes the essence of the histology of dermal chemical peeling as we understand it (Fig. 2-8). See also Fig. 3-3.

Glycosaminoglycans play a major role as the ground substance of the dermal matrix in providing hydration for the skin because of their water-binding capacity. Any modality, including chemical peeling, that stimulates the accumulation of GAGs in the skin might maintain normal hydration and counteract fine wrinkling. This accumulation is independent of the clinical appearance of sagging skin associated with altered elastic fibers (Fig. 2-9).

Studies on **medium-depth peeling** with the combination of solid carbon dioxide followed by TCA, 35%, demonstrated a peel depth slightly greater than that in Stegman's study of 60% TCA alone[18] (Fig. 2-10). Although problems exist in comparing two patients with one patient, the combination of the two agents on a human model seems to produce a wound of similar thickness to full-strength phenol. In Stegman's case, the TCA dermal elastotic band was the most weakly staining of all wounding agents. Unoccluded CO_2 plus TCA-treated skin stained with ease, however, and showed an obvious elastic-staining dermal band as well as heavy GAGs. This confirmed CO_2 plus TCA, 35%, to be a greater wounding agent than 60% TCA alone, although still not as potent as Baker's solution (Fig. 2-11).

This author compared two **medium-depth peeling agent combinations** histologically: solid carbon dioxide (hard pressure, 15- to 20-second application) plus TCA, 35%, vs. JS (four coats applied with two cotton-tipped applicators) plus TCA, 35%.[3] One modality was performed on the left cheek and the second modality on the right cheek of a moderately sun-damaged white female. Biopsy samples were taken prepeel (control) and at days 2, 7, 30, and 90 after peeling. Wound thickness was determined by measuring the distance

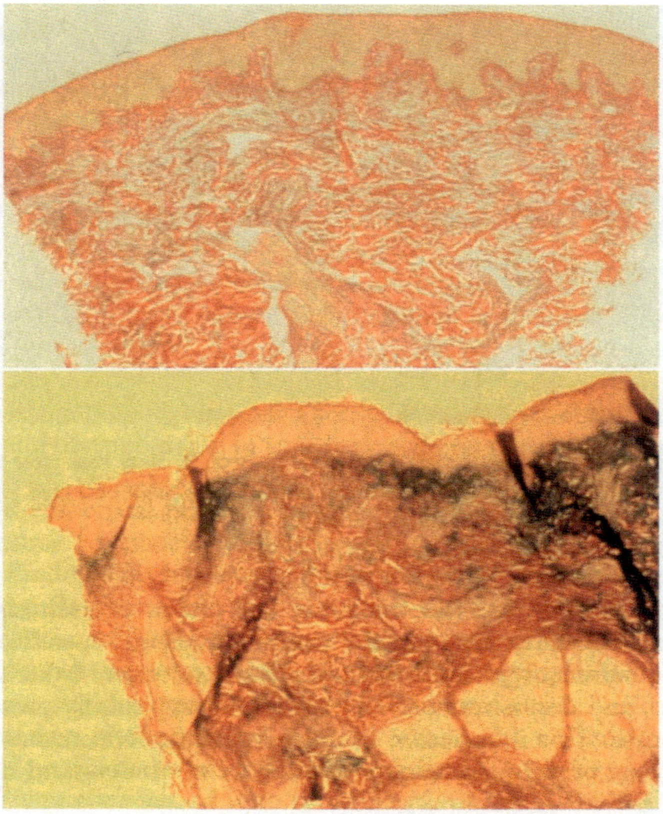

A

B

FIG. 2-9. A, Non–sun-damaged skin before a medium-depth CO_2 plus TCA peel. **B,** Ninety days after CO_2, hard, plus TCA, 35%. More GAG and mucin deposition is apparent (colloidal iron stains).

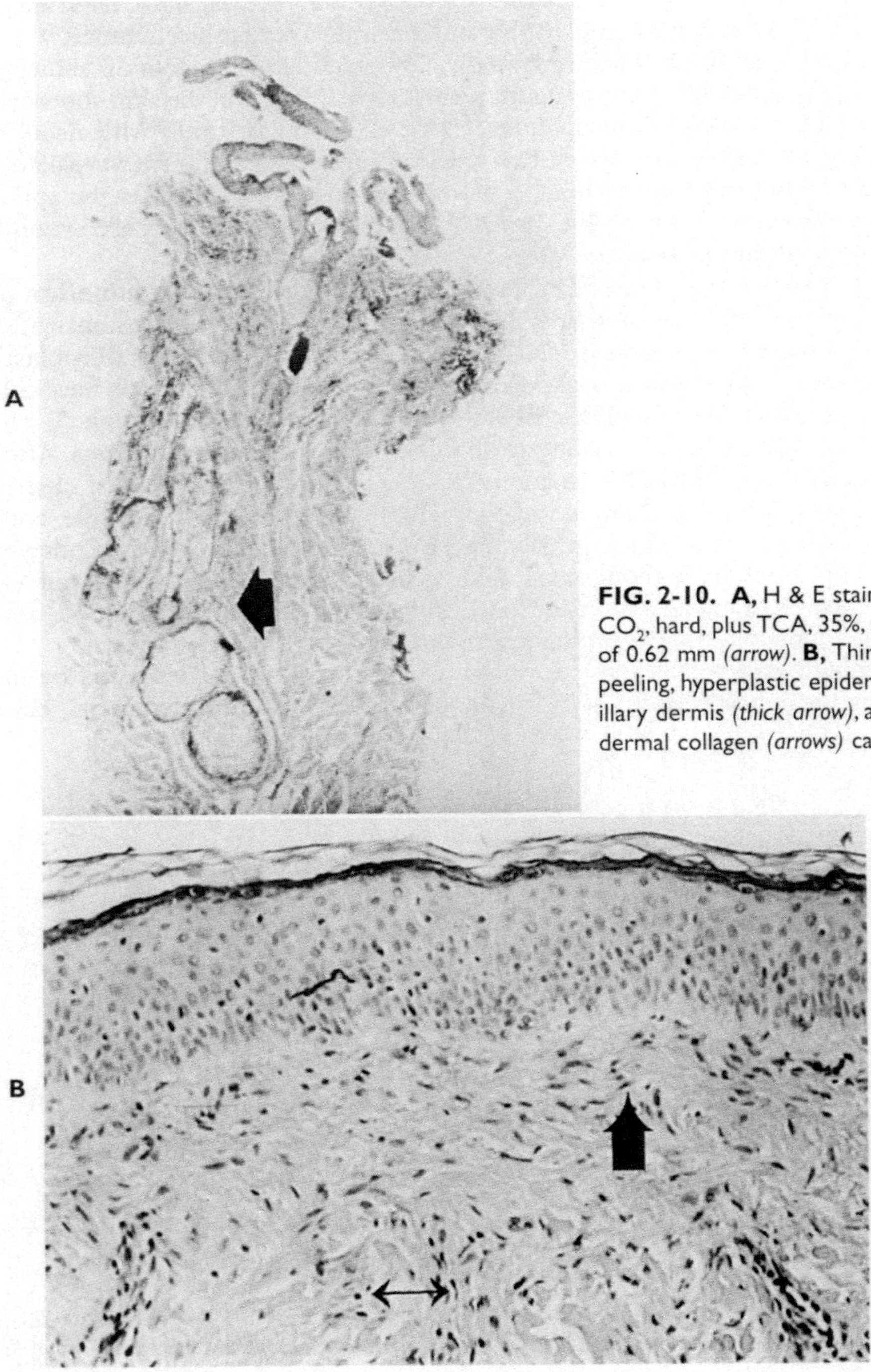

FIG. 2-10. A, H & E staining 5 days after CO_2, hard, plus TCA, 35%, shows a peel depth of 0.62 mm *(arrow)*. **B,** Thirty days after peeling, hyperplastic epidermis, thickened papillary dermis *(thick arrow)*, and new reticular dermal collagen *(arrows)* can be seen.

from the basement membrane to the depth of the wound in the dermis by using a calibrated ocular reticle (Fig. 2-12).

When measurements in wound depth, the time to return to normal epidermal thickness, depth of the Grenz zone, and thickness of the dermal elastotic band were compared, the wound depth was greater for CO_2 plus TCA, and there was prolonged epidermal healing time with wider and deeper staining of the reticular elastotic band for CO_2 plus TCA as opposed to JS plus TCA 90 days after peeling. The difference of 0.06 mm between dermal elastotic band measurement of the two peels is probably not a significant depth difference.

Stegman and Brody have separately performed skin biopsies 30 minutes after deep phenol and medium-depth peels, respectively, and the skin shows no recognizable histologic abnormalities. However, ultrastructurally with electron microscopy, tonofilament dissolution with varying degrees of intracytoplasmic organelle disintegration has been demonstrated at 10 minutes after the application of medium-depth peeling agents.[19] Whether these changes are synonymous with keratinocyte death is not clear.

Nelson and co-workers[20] have shown that **ultrastructural examination** of actinically damaged skin 3 months after a JS plus 35% TCA peel demonstrated a marked decrease in intracytoplasmic vacuoles. Mature activated fibroblasts with more cytoplasm and organelles were immersed in abundant new collagen deposition. Dermal elastic fibers were rare (Fig. 2-13, *A* through *D*).

Collagen fibers before peeling were disordered with poor striations. After peeling, collagen fibrils lay in more organized parallel arrays with clearly defined striations. The diameter of individual fibrils was more variable, consistent with recent production of collagen by activated fibroblasts. Collagen striation periodicity is reduced in collagen after peeling (Fig. 2-13, *E* and *F*).

The degree of epidermal insult that results in the most linear, cleanest, and deepest penetration of wounding agent without scarring is not known.

Brodland and co-workers[21] investigated depths of wounds created by increasing the concentrations of TCA from 20% to 80% in a minipig model. They

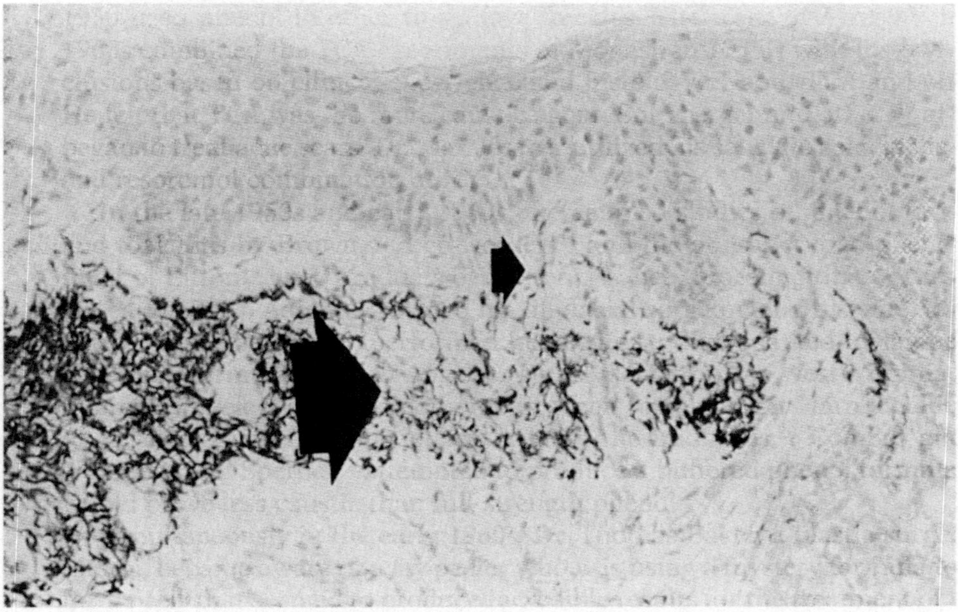

FIG. 2-11. Elastic staining 90 days after CO_2 plus TCA, 35%, peel shows a papillary dermal Grenz zone *(small arrow)* with a middermal elastic band *(large arrow)*.

A

B

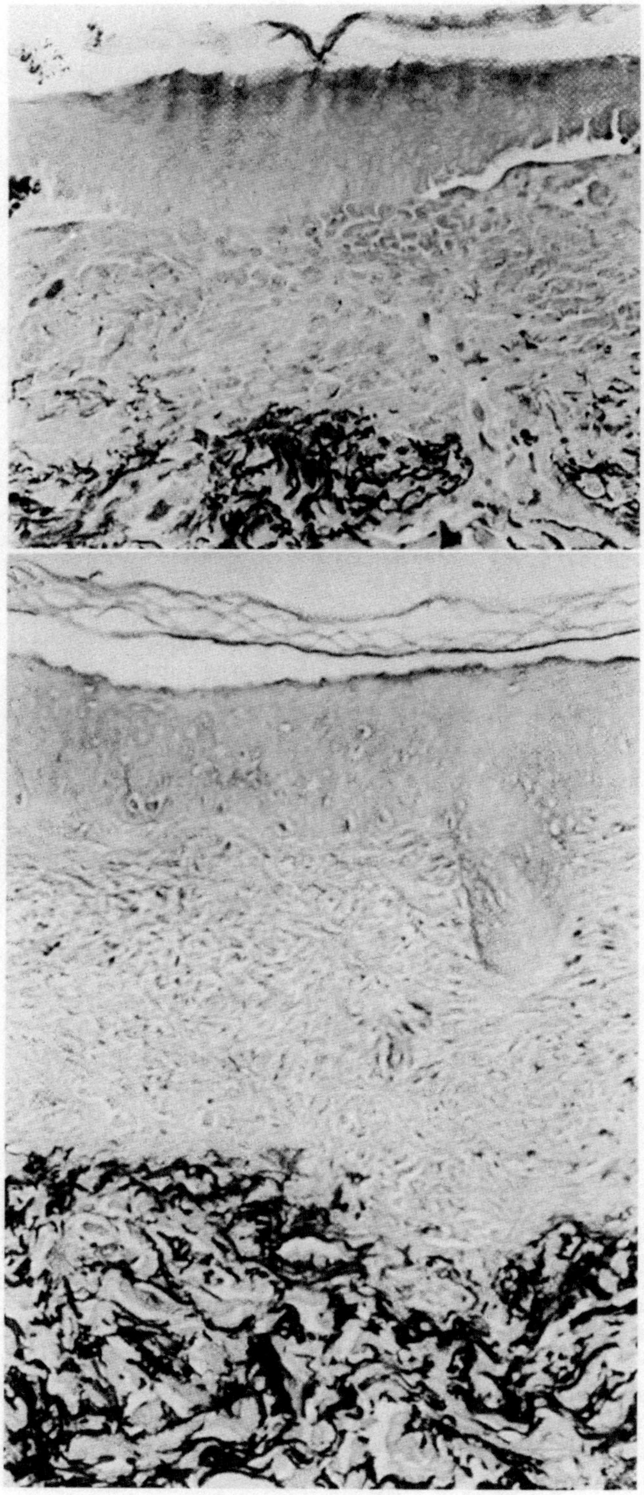

FIG. 2-12. Elastic stain. **A,** Three days after peeling with JS plus TCA (three consecutive TCA applications) there is a focal dermal absence of elastic fibers. **B,** Thirty days later.

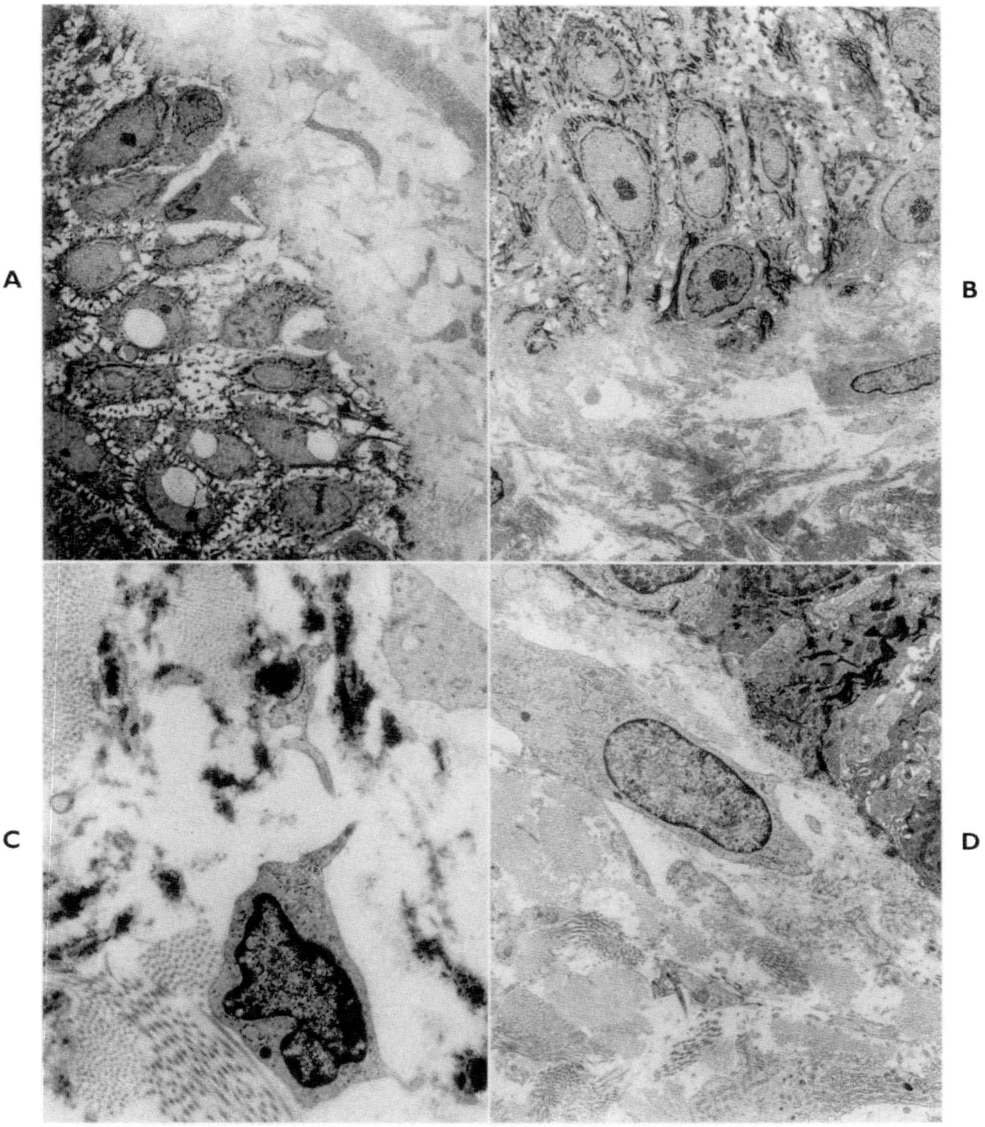

FIG. 2-13. **A,** Electron micrograph of skin before peel shows epidermal spongiosis, intracytoplasmic vacuoles, and intracellular epidermal and dermal edema. **B,** Specimen 3 months after peel shows marked decrease in intracytoplasmic vacuoles, compared with **A**. **C,** Skin before peel reveals inactive fibroblast with few organelles and scant cytoplasm. **D,** Examination 3 months after peel shows activated fibroblasts with more cytoplasm and organelles, compared with **C**.

(Continued)

E 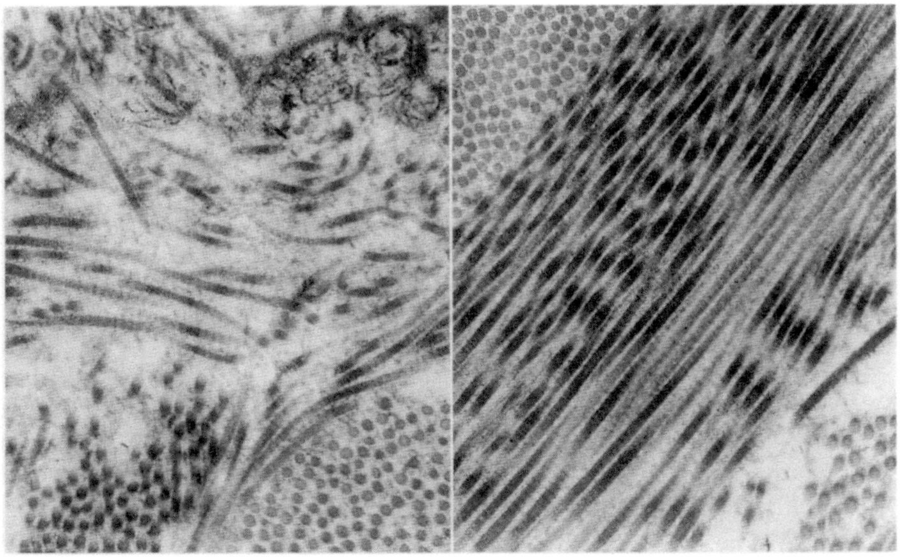 F

FIG. 2-13. cont'd., **E,** Ultrastructure before peel reveals disordered, edematous collagen with uniform fibril diameter but poorly defined cross-striations. **F,** Collagen structure 3 months after peel shows fibers in more organized parallel arrays with clearly defined cross-striations. *(From Nelson BR, Fader DJ, Gillard M, et al: J Am Acad Dermatol 472-478, 1995.)*

found that the depth of tissue necrosis increased with the concentration of TCA. A minimum concentration of 35% was necessary to cause complete epidermal necrosis with a single application. An inverse relationship of wound depth to epidermal thickness was found such that when the rete ridges on the minipig were thicker, the amount of dermal necrosis was less. This confirms that hypertrophic actinic keratoses may require a higher concentration of TCA for complete epidermal destruction. This may have relevance when we use prepeeling epidermal preparatory agents that thicken or freshen the epidermis, although the response on human skin may not correlate exactly with the minipig. They also found that serial peeling with 20% TCA every 2 weeks for three applications produced possible papillary dermal remodeling.

Coleman and Futrell[22] compared histologic depth of **70% glycolic acid** applied for 2 minutes on undefatted preauricular skin **followed by 35% TCA** and found penetration through the papillary dermis to the upper reticular dermis at 24 hours after peeling. In comparison at 90 days after peeling, the papillary dermal Grenz zone was not as thick as previous medium-depth combinations, suggesting that this peel does not wound as deeply as CO_2 + TCA.

Tse and co-workers[23] compared the effects of 70% glycolic acid (GA) applied for 2 minutes plus TCA, 35% to the right Glogau type III photoaged face vs. JS applied with two cotton swabs plus TCA, 35% to the left face in 13 patients of Fitzpatrick types I through III. The patients were pretreated for 2 weeks with tretinoin cream, and all wounding agents were applied with two cotton-tipped applicators after cleansing with isopropyl alcohol followed by acetone. Skin biopsies at 7, 30, and 60 days were evaluated by two independent investigators. The GA + TCA peel caused a slightly thicker Grenz zone (mean = 0.053 mm) 60 days after peel than the JS + TCA peel (mean = 0.048 mm), although this was not statistically significant. The GA + TCA peel caused more neoelastogenesis on elastic stain (15% of patients) than the JS + TCA peel (7%), and the JS + TCA peel resulted in more papillary dermal fibrosis (38%), neovascularization (46%) and inflammatory infiltrate (85%)

than the GA + TCA peel (23%, 23%, and 69%, respectively). Neovascularization suggests repair after injury and predates fibrosis. There was less erythema clinically after GA + TCA, perhaps related to less inflammation. Although the deepest medium peel, the CO_2 + TCA peel, requires 90 days for collagen reorganization, this study evaluates a 60-day comparison and demonstrates only slight differences between the peels. Although both peels are effective in this study in treating actinic damage, varying techniques for the prepeel defatting and application of the GA, JS, and TCA may affect histologic results.

Occlusion of Trichloroacetic Acid

Tape occlusion of TCA does not increase penetration in the minipig model of Brodland and co-workers[21] or the human model of Stegman.[17] This could be due to interstitial humidification by prevention of transepidermal water loss, which leads to increased interstitial water content in the epidermis and, consequently, more rapid neutralization of TCA by the serum. It is possible that the adhesive itself neutralizes the acid.

Peikert and co-workers[24] studied other occlusive modalities besides tape in a controlled study of 50% TCA application to alopecic scalp skin. Bacitracin ointment produced equal or greater necrosis if applied immediately or 4 hours after peeling. There was greater necrosis with Vigilon applied immediately and lesser necrosis with Vigilon applied 4 hours after peeling or Tegaderm secured immediately after peeling. Both Vigilon and Tegaderm are occlusive to water and permeable to oxygen. Therefore the type of occlusion and the time of application are factors in TCA wounding. Ointment will not compromise peel depth.

Pyruvic Acid

Griffin and co-workers[25] at the American Academy of Dermatology in 1989 and 1990 have described preliminary findings employing pyruvic acid, an α-keto acid, as a peeling agent. One hundred percent pyruvic acid produced epidermal and dermal necrosis in a human model in 30 to 60 seconds and is unsuitable as a peeling agent. When diluted to concentrations between 50% and 80% with ethyl alcohol, more even epidermal necrosis, papillary dermal homogenization, and penetration to the reticular dermis were noted progressively. The addition of croton oil produced a greater inflammatory response. Lower concentrations in the range of 60% wound the skin more evenly and predictably than in the range of 80%. Scarring and hypopigmentation are recognized, and the frequency is unknown. (See also the section on pyruvic acid in Chapter 6.)

Multiple Frosting Applications

The depth of wounding from three consecutive applications of TCA at 10-minute intervals is definitely greater than a single frost. This is confirmed histologically in the human model by deeper wound thickness, greater epidermal hyperplasia, and a more intensely staining dermal elastotic band[3] (Fig. 2-14). The average wound depth difference is 0.25 mm greater with multiple frosts. Stegman[26] in 1980 demonstrated that multiple Baker's phenol applications produced deeper wounding in the guinea pig.

Middermal Injury—Deep Wounding

Evaluation of phenol and phenol formula peeling has been described by numerous authors in the past 30 years on the minipig as well as on the human

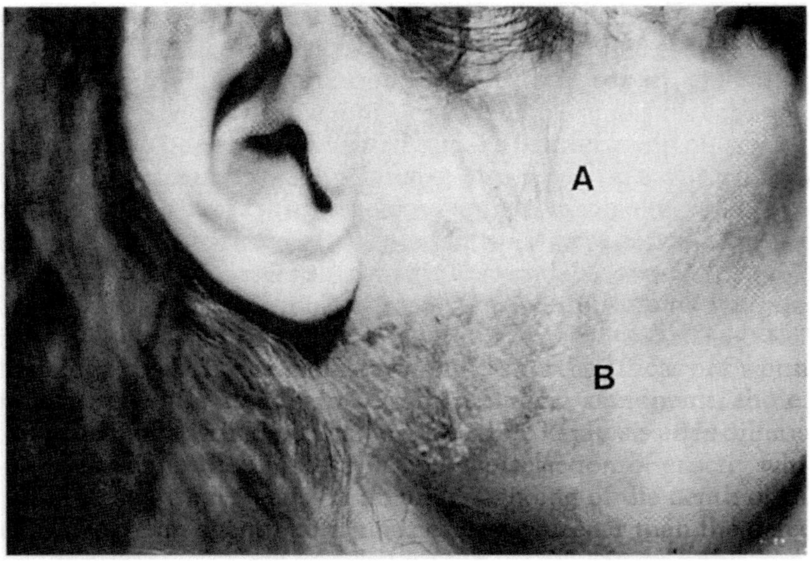

FIG. 2-14. A human cheek 7 days after a JS plus TCA peel. Three consecutive applications of TCA from the lower rim of the earlobe to the mandible exhibit a prolonged healing time.

model. MacKee and Karp[27] in 1952 performed a biopsy on a back 1 month after six monthly treatments of phenol. Collagen bundles in the upper dermis were compact and arranged parallel to the surface.

In 1960 Ayres[28] found similar findings when applying **phenol** to neck skin: a 0.3 to 0.4 mm subepidermal new collagen band arranged horizontally. This new collagen in the papillary dermis is probably responsible for the lessening of wrinkles. Brown and co-workers[29] in 1960 treated rabbit ears with phenol and described thickening of the dermis with fibers in compact layers parallel to the surface.

In 1962, Litton[30] described the results on a single subject at 48 hours, 3 weeks, and 3 months after a phenol peel. He described an increase in the number and thickness of collagen fibers.

Spira and co-workers[31] in 1970 applied phenol to the thighs of six paraplegics and evaluated different concentrations of phenol. They also noted dermal thickening with new collagen deposition. Concentrations of phenol higher than 50% did not appear to extend the depth of destruction. One hundred percent phenol produced only slightly more destruction than 25%.

Baker and co-workers[32] in 1974 performed biopsies on facial skin from 22 patients who had undergone peeling up to 13 years earlier. Increased dermal elastosis was found with diminution of the quantity of melanin granules in the basal layer of the epidermis, and the histologic changes persisted for years. After chemical peeling the elastic fibers were increased in quantity and were oriented in bizarre directions.[33]

In 1977 Behin and co-workers[34] applied Baker's solution to minipig skin and observed a zone of new collagen in 2 weeks that increased in thickness up to 16 weeks. Elastic fibers were less than in untreated skin. The new collagen was wider and thicker in peeled skin as compared with dermabraded skin, possibly suggesting that peeling might be more effective for actinically damaged aging skin.

Stegman's comparative histology[17] in 1982 of deep-peeling agents and medium-peeling agents is described in the section on upper dermal injury.

Kligman and co-workers[35] in 1985 performed biopsies on strips of skin of patients who had been peeled with Baker's solution 1.5 to 20 years earlier. In contrast to the abnormal elastotic appearance of unpeeled skin, a new parallel collagen band approximately 2 to 3 mm wide was present in the dermis. Many fine elastic fibers formed a dense network in the band of regenerated collagen, and there was a decrease in ground substance in the papillary dermis. The atrophic, cytologically atypical epidermis thickened and normalized.

Melanocytes were not eliminated and were spottily increased. Melanin synthesis was impaired, but melanin granules were found in the epidermal cells, and this accounts for hypopigmentation, not depigmentation. The changes persisted as long as 20 years after deep peeling. Brown and co-workers[36] in 1960 contrasted the histology of human eyelid skin before and 15 years after peeling. The epidermis was more acanthotic, and the dermis was much more dense, with laminated connective tissue arranged parallel to the surface.

Croton Oil Addition

Significantly, the evaluation of human skin for up to 3 months after peeling by Spira and associates[31] did not find any additional penetration grossly or histologically with the addition of croton oil to Baker's formula. Stegman[26] showed in 1980 on the minipig that croton oil may increase penetration of phenol, but this was based on two photomicrographs 2 days after wounding. Perhaps only an increase in inflammatory response may be illustrated. Ninety-day studies were not performed.

The use of additives such as cresol (methyl phenol) or olive oil to phenol to "buffer" the phenol solution and thus achieve greater or less penetration through surface tension alteration was initially described by Brown and co-workers[36] in the early days of investigation of the evolution of the present-day phenol formula. Spira and co-workers[31] felt that there is little evidence to substantiate these buffers, and they have fallen into disuse. (See Chapter 1 for Sperber's buffered phenol formula and the box on page 166 on hypopigmentation.)

Occlusion of Phenol

Occlusion of phenol with adhesive tape has been shown to histologically increase the penetration of wound depth in the dermis by Spira and co-workers[31] in 1970 on the legs of humans and by Stegman in 1980 on the guinea pig[26] and in 1982 on the human model.[17] A clinical model substantiating its increased depth properties has been noted by Stegman when a 2-inch portion of a taped mask became loose and necessitated repeeling of this single area because of the reappearance of rhytides after healing. Occlusion with petrolatum ointment does not produce the depth of occlusion as tape.

Studies performed by Zukowski, and co-workers[37] on non–sun-damaged minipig skin demonstrated no depth difference in occlusion with adhesive tape or bacitracin ointment. However, juvenile minipig skin cannot be equated with previous histologic and clinical studies on actinic human skin. A single human patient or single minipig are limitations of all these analyses.

Dermal Healing after Local Skin Flaps and Chemical Peeling

Hayes and co-workers[38] on the guinea pig and Davies and co-workers[39] on the rat model have done studies on dermal healing after local skin flaps and simultaneous chemical peeling with Baker's solution. Studies on the guinea pig confirm that there is an increased risk of contracture and scar with a chemical peel over a flap as compared with deep granulation tissue without scarring when a

Perspective on Histologic Correlation

Based on wound depth changes, a spectrum classification can be formulated. (See the box on p. 26.) The continuum of destruction of the epidermis and dermis may vary according to prepeel skin defatting, wounding agent strength or amount applied, and skin thickness or location. The healing process is similar only in that reformation of a less cytologically atypical epidermis is generated from the epidermal appendages. Reepithelialization may differ and depends on the skin location (e.g., the face vs. the back or neck) and the character of the dermal pathology (e.g., degree of actinic elastotic change or scarring) with ensuing evocation of inflammatory response. (See the section on Reepithelialization and the summary in Chapter 3 for additional discussion.)

The wounding depth alone of a wounding agent is not sufficient to always predict the frequency of complications. A classification based on histologic depth of injury is only a rough guideline to communicate about peeling agents. Any peeling agent can produce complications, although some of the untoward effects may be predictable in their frequency from depth. (See the section on scarring in Chapter 8 for additional discussion.)

Superficial wounding is defined as the wounding of portions of the epidermis alone or completely through the epidermis into the papillary dermis. Exfoliation may slough only the stratum corneum and stratum granulosum. ***Medium-depth wounding*** extends through the papillary dermis down to the upper portion of the reticular dermis, and ***deep-depth wounding*** extends to the midreticular dermis. (For the selection of proper wounding agent for peeling for varying indications, see the section on indications and wounding agent selection/application concepts and perspective: how to peel, in Chapter 4.)

flap is raised alone. They hypothesize that the upper reticular dermis responds to injury by realignment or replacement of its collagen without contracture, similar to the papillary dermis. The deep reticular dermis, however, responds to injury by scar tissue formation, presuming a compromise of nutrient supply. This may explain a greater risk of scarring with a deeper reticular dermal insult.

The study of Davies and co-workers[39] on rats showed a decrease in hair follicles and adnexa when more dermis was involved, as well as upper dermal lamination of new collagen, similar to the human model. Both lidocaine injection, with or without epinephrine, and flap elevation were risk factors that produced more penetration with peeling by Baker's formula.

Comparison of Dermal Peeling with the Carbon Dioxide Laser[40,41]

Histologic comparison of chemical peeling with the high energy short-pulse CO_2 resurfacing laser is variable based on the laser system, number of passes, pattern generator, increasing doses of laser energy, overlapping of pulses and the parameters used. A single or double pass with the superpulse Sharplan laser at 400 mJ, 10 W, 0.33-second interval in sun-protected and sun-exposed periauricular skin produces a depth of injury approximating that typically seen with medium-depth chemical peels. Wound healing at 90 days occurs in a similar fashion as with chemical peeling but perhaps with less inflammation. Precise depth of vaporization can be difficult to measure. Laser-tissue interaction with collagen results in clinical heat-induced collagen contraction, which alters visible dermal thickness as well.[42]

Chemical Peeling Wounding Spectrum*

Superficial wounding (to the stratum granulosum–papillary dermis)
Very light—stratum corneum exfoliation or stratum granulosum depth
TCA, 10%-20% (TCA, superficial), resorcin, Jessner's solution, salicylic acid, solid CO_2, α-hydroxy acids, tretinoin
Light—stratum basale or upper papillary dermal depth
TCA, 35%, unoccluded, single or multiple frost
Medium-depth wounding (through the papillary dermis to the upper reticular dermis)
Combination Peels, single or multiple frost
CO_2 + TCA, 35%
Jessner's + TCA, 35%
Glycolic acid + TCA, 35%
TCA, 50%, unoccluded (TCA, deep), single frost
Full-strength phenol, 88%, unoccluded
Pyruvic acid
Deep-depth wounding (to the midreticular dermis)
Baker's phenol, unoccluded
Baker's phenol, occluded

*Depth is dependent on prepeel skin defatting preparation, wounding agent strength or amount applied, and skin thickness or location. Clinical reepithelialization may depend on skin location and the character of the dermal pathology, which determine the degree of inflammatory response evoked.

There may be a limit that resides within the upper reticular dermis after which further significant tissue coagulative changes from each pass with the laser are small. The first pass may encompass 100 μm of coagulative necrosis; successive passes may achieve only 80, 40, and 30 μm, respectively. As in peeling, the technique specificity is operator dependent.

A study of the Ultrapulse 5000 Coherent Laser at increasing energy levels from 150 to 450 mJ per pulse and increasing up to three passes compared with 35% TCA, dermabrasion, and Baker-Gordon phenol formula was undertaken in a porcine model with biopsies of a single application of peeling agent and laser parameters at 7, 21, and 42 days.[42] There was no spot size overlapping, and saline skin wipes were used between passes. Up to 250 mJ with two passes approximated the depth of 35% TCA in the porcine model. Both reepithelialization in 7 days and healing comparable with dermabrasion were discovered with laser treatment of 250 to 450 mJ and two to three passes. Baker's phenol application was slower than the laser to reepithelialize and slower to heal, indicating deeper depth than the laser parameters studied. The healing time of the single Baker's phenol application in this study is considerably slower than previous similar studies.[17,26,34] None of the healing times in the pig are clinically equivalent to human skin healing in which both the laser and the phenol formula may take about 10 to 14 days to reepithelialize. The results extrapolated to humans are dependent on operator techniques of the laser with overlapping spot size, the peeling agents, and dermabrasion. (For additional discussion, see Chapters 7 and 10). See the Perspective on deep peeling in Chapter 7 and the section on combining chemical resurfacing with laser resurfacing in Chapter 10.

CLASSIFICATION OF WOUNDING AGENTS AND TECHNIQUES

Dermal wounding agent strength is based on evaluating the reaction at its peak by noting the depth of the wound as opposed to the depth of inflammation. Although the wound may reepithelialize in 7 to 14 days depending on the residual hair shafts and sebaceous glands, dermal thickening and collagen production does not begin until the inflammatory reaction subsides. This begins about 2 weeks after treatment and ends 60 to 90 days later. These time frames were demonstrated by Spira and co-workers,[31] Litton,[43] Brown and co-workers,[29,36] Baker and co-workers,[32,33] Behin and co-workers,[34] and Stegman[17,26] for deep peeling. Medium-depth human histologic studies by this author[3,18] and Stegman[17] show that dermal elastic-staining fibers have not completely reincorporated at 30 to 60 days. They organize closer to 90 days after peeling. Because wound depth alone does not evaluate the later healing phases, that is, the degree of inflammatory response followed by reepithelialization with subsequent dermal reorganization, it is imperative to look at the wound at 90 days to evaluate the middermis.

REFERENCES

1. Montagna W, Kirchner S, Carlisle K: Histology of sun-damaged human skin, *J Am Acad Dermatol* 21:907-918, 1989.
2. Glogau RG: Chemical peel preparation. American Academy of Dermatology Chemical Peel Symposium, 1991.
3. Brody HJ: Variations and comparisons in medium depth chemical peeling, *J Dermatol Surg Oncol* 15:953-963, 1989.
4. Van Scott EJ: Alpha hydroxy acids: procedures for use in clinical practice, *Cutis* 43:222-228, 1989.
5. Moy LS, Murad H, Moy RL: Glycolic acid peels for the treatment of wrinkles and photoaging, *J Dermatol Surg Oncol* 19:243-246, 1993.
6. Moy L, Peace S, Moy R: Comparison of the effect of various chemical peeling agents in a mini-pig model, *Dermatol Surg* 22:429-434, 1996.
7. Moy L, Howe K, Moy RL: Glycolic acid modulation of collagen production in human skin fibroblast cultures, in vitro, *Dermatol Surg* 22:439-442, 1996.
8. Becker FF, Langford FPJ, Rubin MG, et al: A histological comparison of 50% and 70% glycolic acid peels using solutions with various pHs, *Dermatol Surg* 22:463-468, 1996.
9. DiNardo JC, Grove GL, Moy LS: Clinical and histological effects of glycolic acid at different concentrations and pH levels, *Dermatol Surg* 22:421-428, 1996.
10. Ditre CM, Griffin TD, Murphy GF, et al: The effects of alpha hydroxy acids on photoaged skin: a pilot clinical, histological and ultrastructural study, *J Am Acad Dermatol* 34:187-195, 1996.
11. Griffin TD, Murphy GF, Sueki H, et al: Increased factor XIIIa transglutaminase expression in dermal dendrocytes after treatment with alpha hydroxy acids: potential physiologic significance, *J Am Acad Dermatol* 34:196-203, 1996.
12. Weiss JS, Ellis CN, Headington JT, et al: Topical tretinoin improves photoaged skin: a double-blind, vehicle-controlled study, *JAMA* 259:527-532, 1988.
13. Kligman AM, Grove GL, Hirose R, et al: Topical tretinoin for photoaged skin, *J Am Acad Dermatol* 15:836-859, 1986.
14. Bhawan J, Palko MJ, Lee J, et al: Reversible histologic effects of tretinoin on photodamaged skin, *J Geriatr Dermatol* 3(3):62-67, 1995.
15. Griffiths CEM, Russman AN, Majmudar G, Restoration of collagen formation in photodamaged human skin by tretinoin (retinoic acid), *N Engl J Med* 329:530-535, 1993.
16. Griffiths CEM, Kang S, Ellis CN, et al: Two concentrations of topical tretinoin (retinoic acid) cause similar improvement of photoaging but different degrees of irritation, *Arch Dermatol* 131:1037-1044, 1995.
17. Stegman SJ: A comparative histologic study of the effects of three peeling agents and dermabrasion on normal and sundamaged skin, *Aesthetic Plast Surg* 6:123-135, 1982.
18. Brody HJ, Hailey CW: Medium-depth chemical peeling of the skin: a variation of superficial chemosurgery, *J Dermatol Surg Oncol* 12:1268-1275, 1986.

19. Brody HJ: Unpublished observations.
20. Nelson BR, Fader DJ, Gillard M, et al: Pilot histologic and ultrastructural study of the effects of medium-depth chemical facial peels on dermal collagen in patients with actinically damaged skin, *J Am Acad Dermatol* 32:475-476, 1995.
21. Brodland DG, Cullimore KC, Roenigk RK, et al: Depths of chemexfoliation induced by various concentrations and applications of trichloroacetic acid in a porcine model, *J Dermatol Surg Oncol* 15:967-971, 1989.
22. Coleman WP, Futrell JM: The glycolic acid + trichloroacetic acid peel, *J Dermatol Surg Oncol* 20:76-80, 1994.
23. Tse Y, Ostad A, Lee H, et al: Medium depth chemical peels: the glycolic acid–trichloroacetic acid peel vs. the Jessner's–trichloroacetic acid peel. Presented at the American Society for Dermatologic Surgery, Hilton Head, SC, May, 1995.
24. Peikert JM, Kaye VN, Zachary CB: A reevaluation of the effect of occlusion on the trichloroacetic acid peel, *J Dermatol Surg Oncol* 20:660-665, 1994.
25. Griffin TD, Van Scott EJ, Maddin S: The use of pyruvic acid as a chemical peeling agent, *J Dermatol Surg Oncol* 15:1316, 1989 (abstract).
26. Stegman SJ: A study of dermabrasion and chemical peeling in an animal model, *J Dermatol Surg Oncol* 6:490-497, 1980.
27. MacKee GM, Karp FL: The treatment of postacne scars with phenol, *Br J Dermatol* 64:456, 1952.
28. Ayres S: Dermal changes following application of chemical cauterants to aging skin, *Arch Dermatol* 82:578-585, 1960.
29. Brown AM, Kaplan LM, Brown ME: Cutaneous alterations induced by phenol, A histologic bioassay, *J Int Coll Surg* 34:602, 1960.
30. Litton C: Chemical face lifting, *Plast Reconstr Surg* 29:371, 1962.
31. Spira M, Dahl C, Freeman R, et al: Chemosurgery: a histologic study, *Plast Reconstr Surg* 45:247, 1970.
32. Baker TJ, Gordon HL, Mosienko P, et al: Long-term histological study of skin after chemical face peeling, *Plast Reconstr Surg* 53:522, 1974.
33. Baker TJ, Gordon HL: Chemical face peeling and dermabrasion, *Surg Clin North Am* 51:387-401, 1971.
34. Behin F, Feuerstein SS, Marovitz WF: Comparative histological study of minipig skin after chemical peel and dermabrasion, *Arch Otolaryngol* 103:271-277, 1977.
35. Kligman AM, Baker TJ, Gordon HL: Long-term histologic follow-up of phenol face peels, *Plast Reconstr Surg* 75:652-659, 1985.
36. Brown AM, Kaplan LM, Brown ME: Phenol-induced histologic skin changes: hazards, technique and uses, *Br J Plast Surg* 13:158-169, 1960.
37. Zukowski ML, Mossie RD, Roth SI, et al: Pilot study analysis of the histologic and bacteriologic effects of occlusive dressings in chemosurgical peel using a minipig model. *Aesthetic Plast Surg* 17:53-59, 1993.
38. Hayes DK, Berkland ME, Stambaugh KI: Dermal healing after local skin flaps and chemical peel, *Arch Otolaryngol Head Neck Surg* 116:794-797, 1990.
39. Davies B, Guyuron B, Husami T: The role of lidocaine, epinephrine, and flap elevation in wound healing after chemical peel, *Ann Plast Surg* 26:273-278, 1991.
40. Cotton J, Hood A, Gonin R, et al: Histologic evaluation of pre- and postauricular human skin after high energy, short-pulse carbon dioxide (CO_2) laser, *Arch Dermatol* 132:425-428, 1996.
41. Adrian RM: Concepts in ultrapulse laser resurfacing. In Trends in Cosmetic Dermatologic Surgery course, American Academy of Dermatology, 1996, Washington, DC.
42. Fitzpatrick RE, Tope WD, Goldman MP, et al: Pulsed carbon dioxide laser, trichloroacetic acid, Baker-Gordon phenol and dermabrasion: a comparative clinical and histologic study of cutaneous resurfacing in a porcine model, *Arch Dermatol* 132:469-471, 1996.
43. Litton C: Observations after chemosurgery of the face, *Plast Reconstr Surg* 32:554-556, 1963.

3 Wound Healing

Controlled wounding with chemical agents produces, in strict terminology, a partial-thickness wound that heals by secondary intention. These wounds heal with minor modification by the same rules and regulations as wounds induced with cold steel, the laser, or cryosurgery. The dermatologic surgeon should recognize the conditions leading to proper reepithelialization and wound reorganization and minimize the risk factors that may impede proper healing. The preparation of the skin with tretinoin before peeling predicates an understanding of the basic principles involved.

Goslen[1] defines wound healing as the interaction of a series of complex events that leads to the resurfacing, reconstitution, and proportionate restoration of tensile strength of wounded skin. Partial-thickness wounds penetrate partially but not completely into the dermis. These defects heal by reepithelialization from residual adnexal epithelium or epithelium derived from adjacent uninjured skin. Healing is rapid, and scarring is clinically imperceptible because contraction does not generally occur. (See box below for stages of wound healing after peeling.)

The initial phases of wound healing in cold steel surgery, coagulation and inflammation, are intimately related and practically instantaneous in chemical peeling. Soluble factors are elaborated in clotting that activate the kinin and complement inflammatory pathways. Inflammatory mediators derived from these pathways function as chemoattractants for neutrophils, macrophages, and lymphocytes. Chemotactic factors such as C5a, leukotriene B_4, kallikrein, and fibrin lysis products attract both neutrophils and monocytes to the injury site.[2] Neutrophils enter the wound at the time of injury and are present for 3 to 5 days or longer. Macrophages are present from 3 to 10 days after injury. They direct the subsequent development of granulation tissue. The lymphocyte is present later at days 6 to 7 after injury and may augment fibroblast accumulation and proliferation.[1]

Our knowledge of the actual alteration of the inflammatory pathways by agents such as croton oil is limited. The inclusion of additional compounds to our traditional wounding agents to increase inflammation may impede or

Stages of Wound Healing after Chemical Peeling

- Coagulation and inflammation
- Reepithelialization
- Granulation tissue formation
- Angiogenesis
- Collagen remodeling

alter reepithelialization and produce complications. They may also serve to improve reepithelialization as well. This avenue has not been explored scientifically at present.

REEPITHELIALIZATION

An important factor in dermal wounding by chemical peeling after the initial epidermal necrosis from applying the chemical is the initial migration of undamaged keratinocytes from the wound margins and from residual adnexal epithelia at the base of the wound.[3-6]

This process of reepithelialization begins within 24 hours of wounding and is a directed event that does not require an initial increase in cellular proliferation (Fig. 3-1). Certain mediators released during inflammation, such as fibronectin, laminin, and platelet-derived growth factor, may stimulate keratinocyte cell movement. Migrating keratinocytes rely on a matrix at the wound bed on which to spread. This matrix consists of fibronectin, which is cross-linked to fibrin, collagen, and elastin. Fibronectin is a dimer that allows adhesion simultaneously to fibrin, collagen, and a variety of cells. After migration begins, cell proliferation at the wound margins increases to provide additional cells for wound coverage.

The water content of the wound bed is a major factor in the speed of epithelial cell migration. Maibach and Rovee[7] have shown that occluded wounds reepithelialize faster than open, desiccated wounds. This occurs partially because the epidermis does not need to grow as deeply into the dermis. After inducing partial-thickness epidermal wounds with resorcinol, many physicians allow the epidermis to desiccate for 24 hours, allegedly to promote separation. However, wound healing mechanisms are not activated with these very superficial peeling agents. Medium-depth and deep wounding agents heal best with maximum hydration applied to the skin. In the original descriptions of deep peeling from the 1960s, thymol iodide powder application 48 hours after peeling formed a crust, and the migrating epidermal cells moved beneath this crust to seek a plane of hydration. This is a route of delayed wound resurfacing. Wounds treated with topical ointments achieve a wound surface migration plane that results in more rapid epithelialization (Fig. 3-2).

The use of the newer **biosynthetic occlusive dressings** to decrease pain and speed healing (see the section on after-peel care in Chapter 7) has more application after dermabrasion than after peeling because the epidermis, although perhaps ineffective, is still intact immediately after the peel. These dressings may be valuable after deep peeling, however, when the entire necrotic epidermis is stripped off with occlusive tape removal. They are valuable in the management of delayed healing complications. (See Chapter 8.) Two major applicable varieties are available, but their actual value in peeling is uncertain at present. Whether dermal quality is enhanced or lessened with more rapid epithelialization is unknown. Both oxygen-permeable and impermeable dressings stimulate increased collagen synthesis in the dermis. Tensile strength, however, is related to maturity and intermolecular cross-linking, not to the amount of collagen synthesized. Any beneficial effects from increased collagen synthesis are unknown. The exact relationship between the rate of epidermal resurfacing and collagen synthesis remains to be determined.[8]

The **hydrogel membrane** prototype is Vigilon (Hermal Labs, Delmar, New York), a layer of hydrogel between two pieces of polyethylene oxide. It absorbs

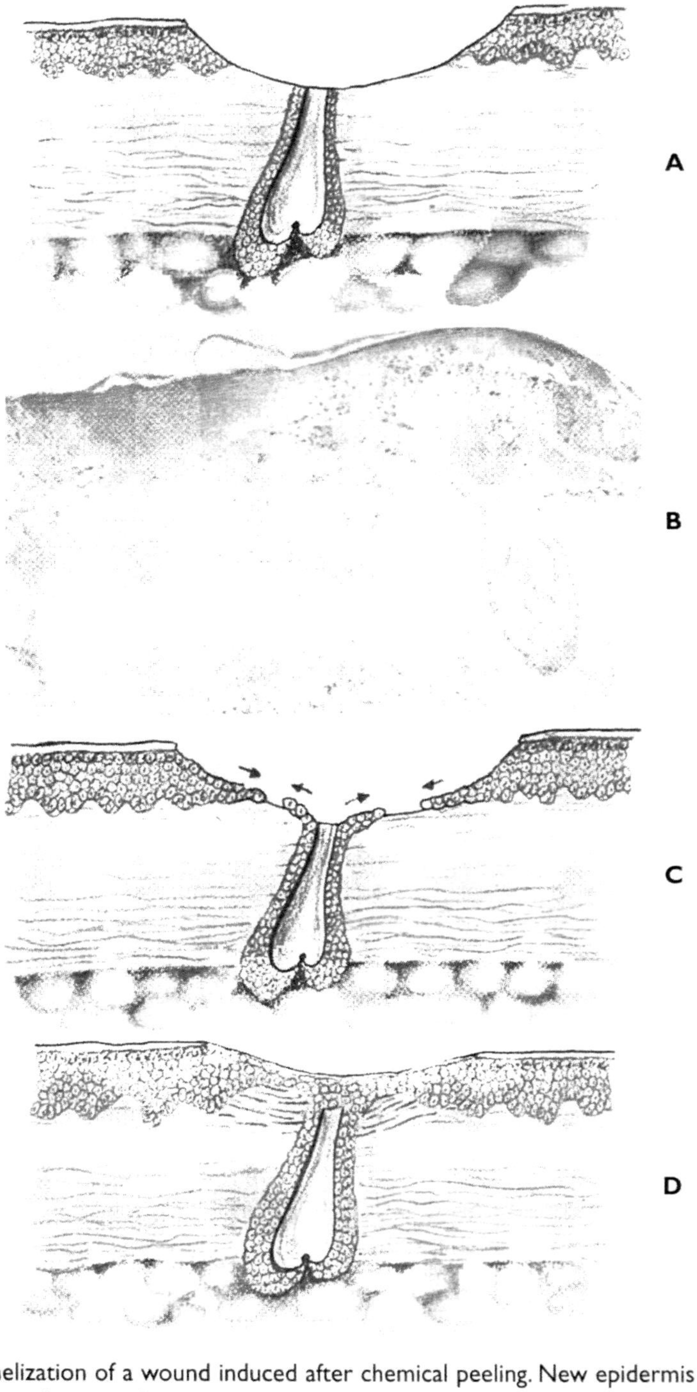

FIG. 3-1. Reepithelization of a wound induced after chemical peeling. New epidermis is derived from both the epidermis at the wound margin and adnexal structures. A hair follicle is shown. **A,** Epidermal and dermal wound. **B,** Migration of cells from the follicle with overlying necrotic epidermis, 10 x. *(Courtesy of Dr. Marian Finan.)* **C,** Epidermal migration from a hair follicle and adjacent epidermis. **D,** Healed wound. *(**A**, **C**, and **D** from Bennett RG: Fundamentals of cutaneous surgery, St Louis, 1988, Mosby.)*

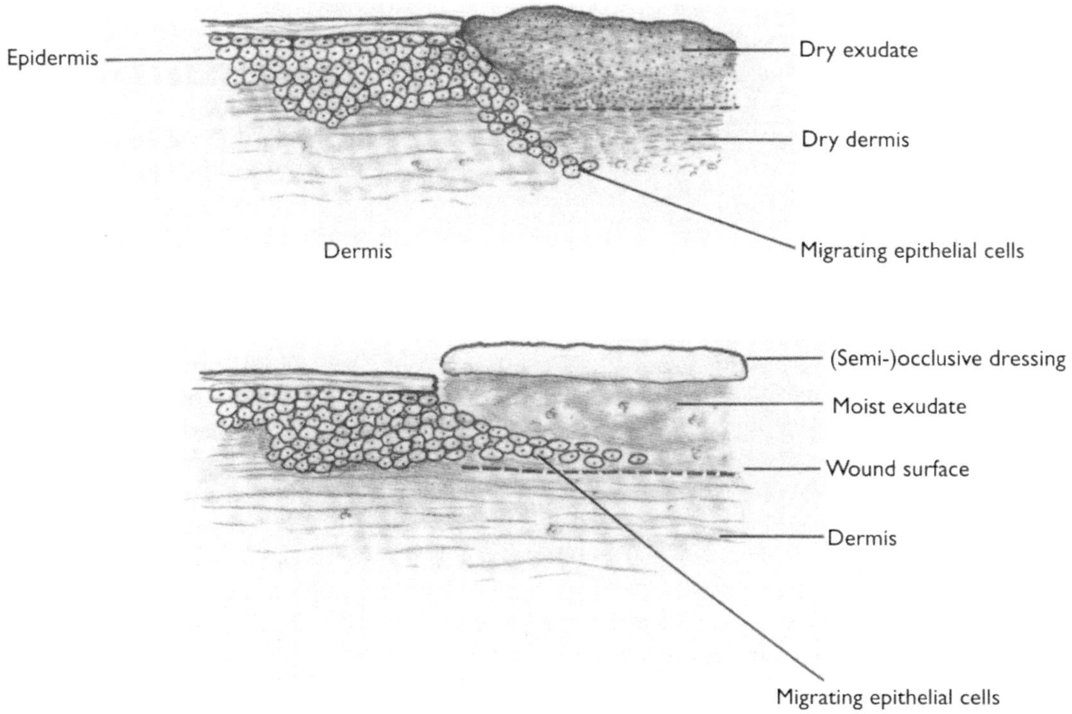

Fig. 3-2. Deeper migration of epidermis under the scab in a dry wound (A) vs. a moist (occluded) wound (B) that prevents scab formation. *(From Bennett RG: Fundamentals of cutaneous surgery, St Louis, 1988, Mosby.)*

exudative material and is occlusive to water while still transmitting oxygen. Because fungal infection may result after 48 hours, the dressings are used only for the first 2 days after the tape is removed and are changed daily.[9] Difficulty can be encountered in attaching the nonadherent dressings because peels are feathered into the hairline. They might be best for localized peels or repeat peel areas only. Not used in chemical peeling except in delayed healing (see Chapter 8), Duoderm (ConvaTec, Bristol Meyers-Squibb, Princeton, New Jersey) is a hydrocolloid dressing that is occlusive and oxygen impermeable.

The second variety is the **polyurethane membrane,** the prototype being Meshed Omiderm (Doak Dermatologics, Fairfield, New Jersey). These membranes are permeable to water, gases, and topical antimicrobials and are left in place until complete wound healing has transpired. They do not stick to the wound itself but are adherent to surrounding tissue. Op-site (Smith and Nephew Research, England) is an occlusive yet oxygen-permeable polyurethane film dressing also used in delayed healing management.

A third variety, a **silicone membrane** bonded to knitted nylon, is also available. Semipermeable and coated on one surface with collagen peptides, the dressing decreases water vapor loss from the wound.[10] Silicone and polytetrafluoroethylene interpenetrating polymer network dressings have a high rate of patient and nursing staff compliance (Silon II, BioMed Inc., Bethlehem, Pennsylvania).[11]

GRANULATION TISSUE FORMATION

Granulation tissue is a loose collection of cellular components including fibroblasts, inflammatory cells, fibronectin, glycosaminoglycans (GAGs), and collagen. Formation of granulation tissue begins on the second or third day after peeling and is maintained until reepithelialization is complete.[2,12-14] The chief cell in the formation of granulation tissue is the fibroblast. It produces fibrillar collagen and elastin, fibronectin, GAGs, and proteases such as collagenase. Collagenase is important in dermal remodeling. GAGs help maintain wound hydration and may assist in cellular migration and proliferation within the wound.

ANGIOGENESIS

After peeling the resumption of blood flow is essential to supply oxygen and nutrients to the healing wound.[15,16] Endothelial cells migrate directly into the wound and travel along the fibronectin matrix. Interference with this matrix formation may delay wound healing. Angiogenic growth factors may be important in this directed migration. They are released from in situ fibroblasts, macrophages, and endothelial cells themselves. The capillary ingrowth with the granulation tissue may explain persistent erythema after chemical peeling.

COLLAGEN REMODELING

Collagen and matrix remodeling begin at the advent of granulation tissue formation and continue for months after reepithelialization.[1,17] This remodeling is responsible for the texture of the skin after peeling. As collagen is laid down, fibronectin gradually disappears. Water is resorbed, and collagen fibers, particularly fibers of collagen types I and III, lie closer together. They reorient in a parallel fashion to the skin surface. There is a progressive digestion of collagen by collagenase and other locally produced proteases. The neovasculature gradually regresses and leaves a less vascular dermis. This remodeling does not manifest itself in medium-depth or deep peeling until well after 60 days, usually 90 days after peeling (Fig. 3-3). (See also the section on classification of wounding agents and techniques in Chapter 2.) See the preceding discussion on biosynthetic occlusive dressings for collagen deposition discussion.

MEDICATIONS AFFECTING REEPITHELIALIZATION

Local wound care in the form of topical creams or ointments or a simple vehicle may affect epithelial cell migration[1,18-21] (Table 3-1). The zinc moiety in bacitracin may stimulate reepithelialization directly. Even certain antiseptics such as 1% povidone-iodine, 0.5% chlorhexidine, or 3% hydrogen peroxide have been shown to delay the development of granulation tissue formation in pig skin.[20,21] However, in our experience, the use of a more dilute surgical scrub rather than the direct application of antiseptic solution may divert infection and not delay healing after peeling. A solution of 0.1% iodine is bactericidal.[22] We prefer to lather 1 tbsp of 7.5% povidone-iodine scrub solution, *United States Pharmacopeia (USP)*, in a basin of water. Polysporin ointment contains both polymyxin sulfate and zinc bacitracin but lacks the sensitizer

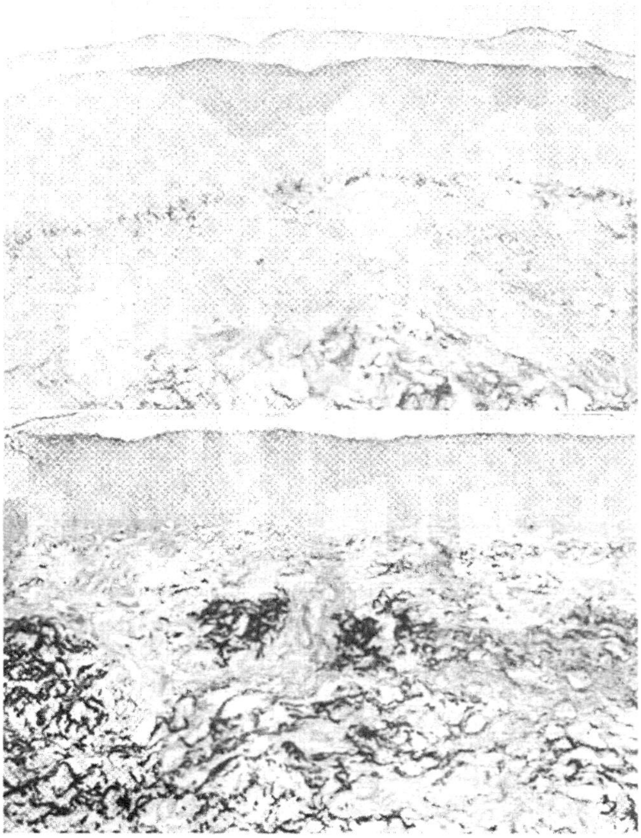

FIG. 3-3. Elastic stain of medium-depth wounding after 45 days shows **(A)** collagen remodeling and incomplete organization of elastotic dermal band formation. The band is not well organized until nearly 90 days after dermal peeling **(B)**.

neomycin. It seems to promote wound healing with minimal complications in our experience. We prefer the use of a petrolatum-based shark liver oil and phenylephrine HCl ointment (Preparation H, Whitehall) as the soothing ointment to promote reepithelialization in medium-depth peeling. The original formulation acted to increase oxygen consumption of dermal fibroblasts. Therefore collagen formation was increased, and wound healing rates were increased.[23,24] (See the section on aftercare in Chapter 6)

Petrolatum, a mixture of long-chain aliphatic hydrocarbons, is effective in treating dry skin with damaged stratum corneum by permeating throughout the horny layer interstices, accelerating normal barrier recovery despite its occlusive properties.[25] In an open, randomized study, petroleum jelly did not seem to retard healing after TCA chemical peeling and may hasten healing time.[26] The petrolatum vehicle of Neosporin ointment has a lower melting point than petroleum jelly and therefore an improved healing rate.[19] The use of petrolatum-based moisturizers without the low molecular weight hydrocarbons that are associated with grease and oil (e.g., Theraplex emollient, Medicis, New York; personal correspondence, Medicis Pharmaceuticals, New York, September, 1991) may be well tolerated by most patients after healing if petrolatum application is desired. Recent studies suggest that there is no difference in healing time or infection rate between petrolatum (Vaseline, Aquaphor) and the antibacterial ointments in wound healing.[27]

TABLE 3-1.
Topical Agents That Affect Epidermal Migration*

AGENT	RELATIVE HEALING RATE† (%)
Neosporin ointment‡	+25
Silvadene cream§	+28
Eucerin cream	+5
Petrolatum, USP (see text)	−8
Triamcinolone acetonide oinment, 0.1%	−34

*Adapted from Geronemus RG, Mertz PM, Eaglstein WH: *Arch Dermatol* 115:1311, 1979.
†Guinea pig skin.
‡Contains neomycin sulfate, polymyxin B sulfate, and bacitracin zinc.
§Contains 1% sulfadiazine silver.

Aloe vera gel in a patented formula with a polyethylene oxide-water gel dressing (Second Skin) has been reported to reduce wound healing time after dermabrasion in a human model.[28] Previously, the scientific results documenting its benefits have been unsatisfactory, perhaps because of a destabilized product or poor penetration of the aloe. Its usage and mechanism in chemical peeling are undetermined. Severe contact dermatitis to aloe vera juice applied after a Baker's solution peel has been reported.[29]

Retinoids

The use of topical **tretinoin** before chemical peeling is accepted as part of a routine photoaging prophylaxis program. The daily application of 0.1% tretinoin cream for 2 weeks before a 35% trichloroacetic acid (TCA) peel enhanced healing of the face, forearms, and hand in a double-blind, placebo study.[30] (See the section on Tretinoin in Chapter 5.) This confirms previous studies.[31,32] Tretinoin application before and after TCA does not significantly enhance the efficacy of the peel.[33]

In guinea pig skin that was pretreated with tretinoin before 50% phenol application and dermabrasion, the tretinoin group showed 1.5 times more epidermal regeneration histologically than the control group 1 week after wounding and twice the amount of epidermal hyperplasia at 2 weeks. At 6 weeks, the thickness of the epidermis was four to five cell layers in controls and seven to eight layers in the tretinoin group. Collagen regeneration appeared to be faster in the tretinoin group. The acceleration of epidermal regeneration may be the mechanism to speed healing.[34]

In contrast to the forearm or hand, in which no distinctive healing pattern is observed, facial healing always proceeds from the central portion of the face to the outer margins. This may occur because of the increased concentration of sebaceous glands in the central facial area. Because tretinoin alters the epidermal actinic damage, TCA frosting occurs more quickly after pretreatment with the drug. The actual peel depth depends on the amount of TCA applied and the degree of rubbing. Less TCA would be necessary, however, to produce the same wound in nonactinically damaged skin.

Systemic retinoids increase collagen synthesis and decrease collagenase production, thereby inhibiting the enzyme that degrades collagen.[35-38] A defect in collagen degradation could allow excess accumulation of collagen and resultant hypertrophic scarring. Fibronectin synthesis is increased by retinoids.[39] Retinoids may stimulate fibroblasts and epidermal migration, perhaps by decreasing the tonofilaments and desmosomal attachments, the events that begin reepithelialization.[40-42] Tretinoin increases mitosis in epidermal cells.[43,44]

Systemic **isotretinoin** administration may affect healing during chemical peeling. (See Chapter 8.)

Corticosteroids

Short-acting **corticosteroids** in the form of betamethasone are sometimes used to minimize edema in the immediate postpeel period. Although clinically morbidity is decreased, an inhibitory effect of moderate- to high-dose corticosteroids on early wound healing has been reported in the rat model. Cortisone delays the appearance of monocytes and lymphocytes as well as ground substance, fibroblasts, collagen, regenerating capillaries, and epithelial migration in the wound. By preventing the obligatory inflammation that is essential to successive phases, healing may be delayed. Long-term use of high-dose steroids retards wound healing by interfering with lysosome function in macrophages and inflammatory cells. High-dose vitamin A or β-carotene will reverse the effects of glucocorticoids on wound healing in rats.

Many systemic medications, such as corticosteroids and antineoplastic agents, may alter healing times in animal models but do not produce clinically noticeable adverse effects on healing in humans. The usage of cortisone after controlled wounding in humans is poorly understood, and its effect on dermal quality is uncertain. The actual time of administration before, during, or immediately after the peel, the drug dose given, the sustained duration of the drug, and the individual's predisposition to infection are all unknown factors at this time.[44,45]

Aging

Most older patients are in good health when they seek chemexfoliation and are not taking immunocompromising drugs. Naturally, the aging process itself affects all stages of wound healing. Older patients should be expected to reepithelialize at a slower rate, and their resultant erythema may take longer to resolve. Fibroblasts proliferate more slowly in vitro and synthesize less collagen.[47,48] Arteriosclerotic vascular occlusion may be present to some extent.

SUMMARY

Wound healing after chemical peeling obeys most of the same principles as healing after cold steel surgery. By understanding the phases of wound repair and the effects of medications, dressings, and systemic agents on the skin, we are able to optimize the environment for the stages of wound healing and provide better clinical results.

The clinical appearance following the stages of reepithelialization and successful collagen remodeling is the hallmark of a successful chemical peel. The wound healing stages may be affected by skin location and thickness because of varying numbers of adnexal structures present for reepithelialization. The character of dermal pathology—both the degree of histologic elastotic damage and the degree of scarring already present—may also affect the healing phases. Most important, the **inflammatory response** that is produced during healing depends on the skin location and the quality of elastotic damage as well as the inherent properties of the wounding agent. This inflammatory response of varying intensity may be an important factor in the clinical appearances of wound healing stages and may be a major factor in the evolution of complications (personal communication, Richard G. Glogau, 1991). (See also the sections on classification of wounding agents and techniques in Chapter 2, and histology and classification and scarring in Chapter 8, and complications of chemical peels for additional discussion.)

REFERENCES

1. Goslen JB: Wound healing after cosmetic surgery. In Coleman WP, Hanke CW, Alt TH, et al, editors: *Cosmetic surgery of the skin,* Philadelphia, 1991,BC Decker, pp. 47-63.
2. Clark RAF: Cutaneous tissue repair: basic biologic considerations, *J Am Acad Dermatol* 13:701, 1985.
3. Krawczyk WS: The pattern of epidermal cell migration during wound healing, *J Cell Biol* 49:247, 1971.
4. Martinet N, Harne LA, Grotendorst GR: Identification and characterization of chemoattractants for epidermal cells, *J Invest Dermatol* 90:122, 1988.
5. Hebda PA, Alstadt SP, Hileman WT, et al: Support and stimulation of epidermal cell outgrowth from porcine skin explants by platelet factors, *Br J Dermatol* 115:529, 1986.
6. O'Keefe EJ, Payne RE, Russell N, et al: Spreading and enhanced motility of human keratinocytes on fibronectin, *J Invest Dermatol* 85:125, 1985.
7. Maibach HF, Rovee DT: *Epidermal wound healing,* St Louis, 1972, Mosby.
8. Alvarez OM, Mertz PM, Eaglestein WH: The effect of occlusive dressings on collagen synthesis and reepithelialization in superfical wounds, *J Surg Res* 35:142-148, 1983.
9. Eaglstein WH, Davis SC, Mehle AL, et al: Optimal use of an occlusive dressing to enhance healing. Effect of delayed application and early removal on wound healing, *Arch Dermatol* 124:392, 1988.
10. Wheeland RG: New surgical dressings aid postoperative healing, *Dermatol Perspect* 7:1-5, 1991.
11. Weiss RA, Weiss MA: New interpenetrating polymer network. *Cosmet Dermatol* 8:31-32, 1995.
12. Van Winkle W: The fibroblast in wound healing, *Surg Gynecol Obstet* 124:369, 1967.
13. Folkman J, Klagsbrun M: A family of angiogenic peptides, *Nature* 329:671, 1987.
14. Folkman J, Klagsbrun M: Angiogenic factors, *Science* 235:442, 1987.
15. Folkman J: Angiogenesis: initiation and control, *Ann N Y Acad Sci* 401:212,1982.
16. Sholley MM, Gimbrone MA Jr, Cotran RS: The effects of leukocyte depletion on corneal neovascularization, *Lab Invest* 38:32, 1978.
17. Doillon CJ, Dunn MG, Bender E, et al: Collagen fiber formation in repair tissue: development of strength and toughness, *Collagen Rel Res* 5:481, 1985.
18. Eaglstein WH, Mertz PM: "Inert" vehicles do affect wound healing, *J Invest Dermatol* 74:90, 1980.
19. Geronemus RG, Mertz PM, Eaglstein WH: Wound healing: the effects of topical antimicrobial agents, *Arch Dermatol* 115:1311, 1979.
20. Lineaweaver W, McMorris S, Soucy D, et al: Cellular and bacterial toxicities of topical antimicrobials, *Plast Reconstr Surg* 75:394, 1985.
21. Nieder R, Schopf E: Inhibition of wound healing by antiseptics, *Br J Dermatol* 115(suppl 31):41, 1986.
22. Goodman LS, Gillman AG: *The pharmacological basis of therapeutics,* New York, 1980, MacMillan, p. 973.
23. Goodson W, Hohn D, Hunt T, et al: Augmentation of some aspects of wound healing by "skin respiratory factor," *J Surg Res* 21:125-129,1976.
24. Kaplan JZ: Acceleration of wound healing by a live yeast cell derivative, *Arch Surg* 119:1005-1008, 1984.
25. Ghadially R, Halkier-Sorensen L, Elias PM: Effects of petrolatum on stratum corneum structure and function, *J Am Acad Dermatol* 26:387-396, 1992.

26. Elson ML: Effects of petroleum jelly on the healing of skin following cosmetic surgical procedures, *Cosmet Dermatol* 6:18-22, 1993.
27. Smack DP: Bacitracin ointment vs. white petrolatum USP; comparison of post-procedural infection incidence and wound healing in dermatologic surgery patients. *Dermatol Times* 17(7):24-29, 1996.
28. Fulton JE: The stimulation of postdermabrasion wound healing with stabilized aloe vera gel-polyethylene oxide dressing, *J Dermatol Surg Oncol* 16:460-466, 1990.
29. Hunter D, Frumkin A: Adverse reactions to vitamin E and aloe vera preparations after dermabrasion and chemical peel, *Cutis* 47:193-197, 1991.
30. Hevia O, Nemeth AJ, Taylor JR: Tretinoin accelerates healing after trichloroacetic acid chemical peel, *Arch Dermatol* 127:678-682, 1991.
31. Mandy SH: Tretinoin in the preoperative and postoperative management of dermabrasion, *J Am Acad Dermatol* 15:878-879, 1986.
32. Hung VC, Lee JY, Zitelli JA, et al: Topical tretinoin and epithelial wound healing, *Arch Dermatol* 125:65-69, 1989.
33. Humphreys TR, Werth V, Dzubow L, et al: Treatment of photodamaged skin with trichloroacetic acid and topical tretinoin, *J Am Acad Dermatol* 34:638-44, 1996.
34. Vagotis FL, Brundage SR: Histologic study of dermabrasion and chemical peel in an animal model after pretreatment with Retin-A, *Aesthetic Plast Surg*19:243-246, 1995.
35. Beach RS, Kenney MC: Vitamin A augments collagen production by corneal endothelial cells, *Biochem Biophys Res Commun* 114:395, 1983.
36. Forest N, Boy-Letevre ML, Duprey P, et al: Collagen synthesis in mouse embryonal carcinoma cells: effect of retinoic acid, *Differentiation* 23:153-163, 1982.
37. Lee KH: Studies on the mechanism of action of salicylates III: effect of vitamin A on the wound healing retardation action of aspirin, *J Pharm Sci* 57:1238-1240, 1968.
38. Abergel RP, Meeker CA, Oikarinen H, et al: Retinoid modulation of connective tissue metabolism in keloid fibroblast cultures, *Arch Dermatol* 121:632-635, 1985.
39. Kenney MC, Shih LM, Labermeir U, et al: Modulation of rabbit keratocyte production of collagen, sulfated glycosaminoglycans and fibronectin by retinol and retinoic acid, *Biochim Biophys Acta* 889:156-162, 1986.
40. Jetten MA: Retinoids specifically enhance the number of epidermal growth factor receptors, *Nature* 284:626-629, 1980.
41. Williams ML, Elias PM: Nature of skin fragility in patients receiving retinoids for systemic effect, *Arch Dermatol* 117:611-619, 1981.
42. Clark RAF: Cutaneous tissue repair: basic biologic considerations I, *J Am Acad Dermatol* 13:701-725,1985.
43. Lee KH, Cherny-Chyi Fu, Spencer MR, et al: Mechanism of action of retinyl compounds on wound healing III: effect of retinoic acid homologs on granuloma formation, *J Pharm Sci* 62:896-899, 1973.
44. Zil JS: Vitamin A acid effects on epidermal mitotic activity, thickness, and cellularity on the hairless mouse, *J Invest Dermatol* 59:228-232, 1972.
45. Bennett RG: Fundamentals of cutaneous surgery, St Louis, 1988, Mosby, pp. 78-87.
46. Ehrlich HP, Hunt TK: Effects of cortisone and vitamin A on wound healing, *Ann Surg* 167:324, 1968.
47. Goodson WH, Hunt TK: Wound healing and aging, *J Invest Dermatol* 78:88, 1979.
48. Chvapil M, Koopmann CF: Age and other factors regulating wound healing, *Otolaryngol Clin North Am* 15:259, 1982.

4 General Peeling Concepts

Observation of the basic tenets and rules in this chapter can facilitate simple and straightforward chemical peeling evaluation. After the physician has assessed the **indications,** knows the **factors in patient selection,** the proper **rejuvenation regimen,** and the **methods to quantitate and apply peeling techniques,** the physician is prepared to obtain **informed consent** and **select the proper peeling technique** for the desired indication.

INDICATIONS FOR CHEMICAL PEELING

The boxed material below and Tables 4-1 and 4-2 list the indications for chemical peeling with the depth of peel necessary for improvement of each condition. In reality no defect treated with chemical peels except superficial melasma is purely epidermal. The basal cell layer must be eliminated to eradicate freckles or lentigines (see Fig. 2-3 in Chapter 2). Otherwise, they are only lightened or partially eradicated. It is best to choose the agent necessary to wound to a depth under the histologic defect with the exception of pigmentary disorders. Superficial peels may improve pigmentary disorders that are deeper than the wounding agent by allowing bleaches applied between peels to penetrate deeper. Minimal papillary dermal collagen reorganization may or may not be induced. These tables are to be used as general guidelines and not as dogma. If every defect that is observed in a cosmetic unit is within normal epidermis except for one growth, for example a seborrheic keratosis, a nevus or an actinic keratosis, then that lesion can be removed by traditional dermatologic surgery techniques such as cryosurgery, electrosurgery, or curettage immediately before peeling. A superficial peel as indicated for epidermal peeling may be performed simultaneously, avoiding the lesion. One should not forget that chemical peeling is only one tool in the surgical armamentarium of skin care.

Indications for Chemical Peeling

Actinic keratoses
Actinic rhytides
Pigmentary dyschromias
Superficial scarring
Radiation dermatitis
Acne vulgaris and rosacea

TABLE 4-1.
Peel-Responsive Skin Defects

UPPER EPIDERMAL DEFECTS	EPIDERMAL AND DERMAL DEFECTS	DERMAL DEFECTS
Ephelides (freckles)—basal layer	Lentigines	
Superficial melasma	Combined melasma	
	Postinflammatory hyperpigmentation	
	Actinic keratoses with mucinous dermis	
	Superficial wrinkles	Deep wrinkles
	Acne	Scarring
	Radiation dermatitis	

Actinically Induced Keratoses and Actinic Rhytides

Peeling can be effective for actinic keratoses, epidermal Bowen's disease, and sun-induced rhytides.[1] Deep peels are most effective, the effects being sustained for as long as 15 years,[2] and medium-depth peels are adequate in many cases, especially for men who cannot wear makeup. Because the photodamaged solar elastotic histology may extend below the peel depth, regeneration of the actinic damage may occur and necessitate repeat medium-depth peels after several years. Superficial peeling is less effective, especially because injury to a depth of just below the epidermis is necessary on the initial peel for destruction of epidermal growths. Repetitive superficial peeling is not effective for severe sun damage. (See the section on Jessner's solution in Chapter 5.)

Pigmentary Dyschromias

Pigment in the skin from melasma or after inflammation will respond to peeling of all varieties, especially if the majority of the melanocytic pigment is within the peel depth. (See Tables 4-1 and 4-2.) Melanocytes, the melanin pigment producing cells, are present in the basal cell layer of the epidermis. **Freckles (ephelides)** consist of hypertrophied, dopa-positive melanocytes with increased melanin granules in the epidermal basal cell layer. **Actinic lentigines** have elongation of epidermal rete ridges with focal increases in the number of melanocytes with increased melanin production. (See Fig. 2-3 in Chapter 2) Complete elimination of freckles and lentigines requires total epidermal replacement. Superficial peeling may only fade these lesions. If epidermal pigment is accompanied by deep dermal melanocytes as in postinflammatory hyperpigmentation, pigment may still be present after peeling. However, the regeneration of a less-pigmented epidermis or upper dermis after a peel may result in a lighter-appearing skin irrespective of residual dermal pigment.

Use of the Wood's Light

The pigment of **melasma** may be variable in depth and may therefore respond inconsistently.[3] Examination of patients using both visible light and Wood's light, a mercury lamp with a nickel oxide filter emitting 320 to 400 nm, may be useful in classifying the type of melasma in correlation with the localization of pigment granules (melanosomes) in the epidermis and dermis.[4] When the melasma skin of types I to III is examined with natural solar radiation, three types of melasma are described: an epidermal type (usually light brown), (Fig. 4-1); a dermal type (usually deep brown, ashen gray); and a mixed type

TABLE 4-2.
Indications and Peel Depth

INDICATION	PEEL DEPTH FOR BEST RESPONSE*	SEE FIG.
Actinic keratoses	Medium	5-3; 6-6; 11-10
	or deep	—
Actinic rhytides,		
Very mild	Superficial or medium	5-20
Mild	Medium	6-13, *C-D*
Moderate	Medium or deep	6-9; 6-10; 6-15
Severe	Deep	7-11; 7-12; 11-2; 11-13
Pigmentary dyschromias		
Melasma—superficial	Superficial or	5-10
	medium	—
Melasma—combined	Superficial, medium, or	6-11; 5-19; 6-14; 11-6; 11-7
	deep	—
Postinflammatory hyperpigmentation	Superficial, medium, or deep	5-8;11-11
Ephelides (freckles)—basal cell layer	Superficial or	5-9
	medium	6-13; 11-3
Lentigines—basal cell layer	Superficial or	—
and upper dermis	medium	11-5; 6-9; 6-11; 11-17
Scarring	Medium or other resurfacing modality	6-7; 11-14
Acne	Superficial when active; medium after clear	5-2; 5-14; 5-18
Radiation dermatitis	Medium or deep	—

*See text discussion of individual entities.

(usually dark brown). When examined with the Wood's light, pigmentary abnormalities primarily of epidermal origin selectively exhibit enhancement of lesional color. Melasma of mixed type or dermal type exhibits no enhancement of dark color and does not increase in contrast. A fourth type of melasma, a Wood's light–inapparent type, exists in dark-complected patients of Fitzpatrick skin types V and VI (e.g., Asians and Blacks)[5] because the epidermal and dermal pigment is so dense that dermal melanophages block the reemission of ultraviolet and blue light.

Examination with the Wood's lamp does not predict clinical response to peels as clearly as anticipated. The combined epidermal-dermal melasma variety is actually more common than previously reported. In those patients with mixed-depth melasma, the dermal pigmentation may obscure the epidermal melasma. If there is a large component of epidermal melasma, the patient may respond better than if the component is minimal.[6] Patients with dermal melasma may respond to superficial peels because the peels may make the skin more receptive to topical bleaching regimens; therefore the evaluation with the Wood's light is less helpful. (See Chapter 11, Fig. 11-6 for illustration of the **serial repetitive increasing strength peels** to treat melasma.)

Depressed Scarring

Depressed scarring is improved variably by chemical peeling. Dermabrasion or the resurfacing laser are generally more effective, but properly performed

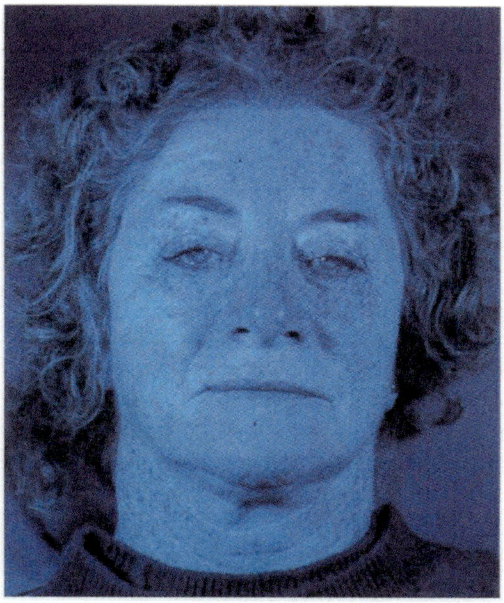

FIG. 4-1. Wood's lamp examination of a Fitzpatrick type I patient illustrating epidermal hyperpigmentation accentuated by the lamp. *(Photo courtesy of Dr. Seth L. Matarasso.)*

peeling can be beneficial. Phenol peeling has been reported in the last 40 years with variable but generally disappointing results.[7,8] Medium-depth peeling with solid carbon dioxide (CO_2) to efface the rims or the edges of depressed scars with the immediate repetitive application of 35% to 50% trichloroacetic acid (TCA) afterward to these rims has resulted in substantial improvement because the CO_2 is a physical modality followed by the acid.[9]

Pitted scars will not respond to peeling, nor will deep scars with severe atrophy of both the dermis and fat. These are best removed by punch grafting or excision 4 to 6 weeks before dermabrasion, peeling, or the laser. Improvement of scarring with multiple solid carbon dioxide slushes has been reported and refuted on the basis that patients forget how their scarring looked before peeling or that scarring improves with time alone. Older reports, moreover, did not always differentiate between pitted or depressed scarring. Multiple superficial peels may improve depressed scarring minimally, but the actual degree of improvement is variable and may be due to temporary edema in many instances. Even the most unsightly scars may have a normal epidermis.

Radiation Dermatitis

Superficial x-irradiation of 80 to 120 kV became a standard for dermatology in 1934. Before this time, the amount of radiation delivered to the face for acne treatment was highly unpredictable. In conjunction with natural solar radiation, the doses of carcinogenic radiation delivered were substantial. Lay electrologists were administering superficial radiation until the late 1940s to destroy facial hair. These individuals sustained extensive radiodermatitis of the face (personal communication, Sturm HM, Hardin F, Atlanta, April, 1991).

Changes in skin from superficial radiation and from therapeutic radiation may be variably helped with chemical peeling if the adnexal structures are intact to provide epidermal regeneration.[10] A skin biopsy as well as the presence of vellus hairs may assist the physician in this decision.[11,12] Both medium-depth and deep peels have been performed to treat radiation dermatitis and poikiloderma. The telangiectasias should be either electrodessicated or removed by laser before or after peeling. Telangiectasias frequently recur and may need to be treated repetitively with either modality.

Acne Vulgaris and Rosacea

Acne vulgaris may be improved by superficial chemical peeling. In actively scarring acne, an additional benefit may be a more rapid resolution with a lower probability of scarring.[13]

It is generally helpful but not imperative for acne to be treated and quiescent before aggressive medium-depth peeling is performed. The patient is more comfortable and any scarring can be more easily evaluated without the presence of pustulation or tender cysts. Moreover, with acne rosacea comprised of erythema with or without pustules, it is best to properly treat and control the rosacea before proceeding with medium peels, especially if scarring or dyschromia is present. In rosacea the existing erythema of the disease makes medium peeling more risky for persistent tenderness or erythema. Medium peeling can aggravate acne or produce acne of any morphology. (See the section on acne in Chapter 8.)

Application of 50% TCA directly to comedones has been reported to produce comedolysis. In a study of 30 patients 50% TCA was carefully applied with a 23-gauge needle without excess solution to 1 to 2 mm comedones without manual extraction. Comedones cleared with no recurrence at 6 months of follow up in almost all patients. Only 5% of patients required reapplication of the acid.[14] This technique is not really a chemical peel but rather local comedone destruction.

PATIENT SELECTION

From the aforementioned indications, every face must be scrutinized carefully to ascertain which peeling agent or agents would give the greatest improvement with the least morbidity based on the patient's lifestyle, the depths of the defects to be corrected, and the composite characteristics of the skin to be treated. For example, one may choose to use a deep-peeling agent on the upper lip only and a medium-depth agent on the remainder of the face. If the elastotic changes in the forms of wrinkling and actinic keratoses in the skin are properly assessed, the pigmentary discrepancy between areas after the procedure will be practically undetectable. Before peeling, the factors listed in the box on p. 44 must be evaluated.

Fitzpatrick Skin Type

Fitzpatrick's classification[5] gives a measure of pigmentary responsiveness of the skin to ultraviolet light and many times a background of ethnic origin (Table 4-3). Patients can be asked if they might sunburn on initial sun exposure of about 45 to 60 minutes at noon after an interval of no sun exposure in

TABLE 4-3.
Fitzpatrick's Classification of Sun-Reactive Skin Types

SKIN TYPE	COLOR	REACTION TO FIRST SUMMER EXPOSURE
I	White	Always burn, never tan
II	White	Usually burn, tan with difficulty
III	White	Sometimes mild burn, tan average
IV	Moderate brown	Rarely burn, tan with ease
V	Dark brown*	Very rarely burn, tan very easily
VI	Black	No burn, tan very easily

*Asian Indian, Asian, Hispanic, or light African descent, for example.

early summer. When the skin type is combined with the eye color in chemical peeling evaluation, the outcome of the peel as well as the choice of wounding agent will be more predictable. Some people with dark brown hair and blue or green eyes may have types I or II sun-reactive skin. Types I to III are ideal for peeling of all varieties, but the white line of demarcation between peeled and unpeeled skin is most prominent in the very actinically damaged type I skin with severe neck poikiloderma. (See Chapter 8 and earlier in this chapter for evaluation of melasma.) Type IV skin can be peeled with all peeling agents, but if the patient has an eye color other than brown, for example, green, light brown, or blue, the likelihood of postinflammatory pigmentation is less. Types V and VI can also be peeled with all peeling agents, but the risk of unwanted pigmentation is greater. (See the section on pigmentary changes in Chapter 8). We perform test spots at the hairline on patients who are at greatest risk, types V and VI, but this is no assurance that the remainder of the face will respond identically.[15]

Actinic Damage and Degree of Photoaging

Assessment of the degree of sun damage is essential to the examination and evaluation prior to peeling in order to choose the most appropriate wounding

Factors to Assess in Patient Evaluation for Subsequent Relative Contraindications

Physical findings
- Fitzpatrick skin type
- Degree of actinic damage and photaging

History
- Philosophy of sun exposure
- Philosophy of cosmetic usage
- Present and past sebaceous gland density—previous isotretinoin or radiation
- Prior cosmetic surgery
- Philosophy of smoking
- General state of physical and mental health
- Medications
- Pregnancy history
- History of herpes simplex
- History of hypertrophic scarring
- Realistic expecations

agents and to plan future peels, if indicated. Specifically, one must document the number of actual keratoses, the degree of actinically induced rhytides, and the presence or absence of poikiloderma because the latter change is more difficult to eradicate completely. Sometimes the patient's sun damage can be eradicated with one procedure in the form of a medium or deep peel. Because of lifestyle or work scheduling, several superficial or medium peels may be a better long-term goal. **Men** may never be satisfied with the inevitable but sometimes minimal hypopigmentation that occurs after deep peeling, and medium-depth procedures are a better choice for them. If their actinic damage is severe enough and they are good peel candidates with respect to skin type and low sebaceous density, a decrease in the number of new actinic keratoses may warrant the appearance of slight hypopigmentation. Some physicians have noted that thick male skin does not respond as well to deep phenolic wounding agents. We have not found thick male skin to be less responsive to medium-depth wounding agents if the skin is properly prepared and if the actinic keratoses are adequately coated with TCA.

It is important to note whether the appearance of the skin has already been altered by topical medications such as tretinoin, in use as a single agent for the treatment of photoaging by many patients since the mid-1980s. The α-hydroxy acids available in cream or gel form may alter epidermal permeability. (See the section α-hydroxy acids in Chapter 5 as well as the regimen section in this chapter.) These may alter wounding agent quantitation (see the separate section in this chapter).

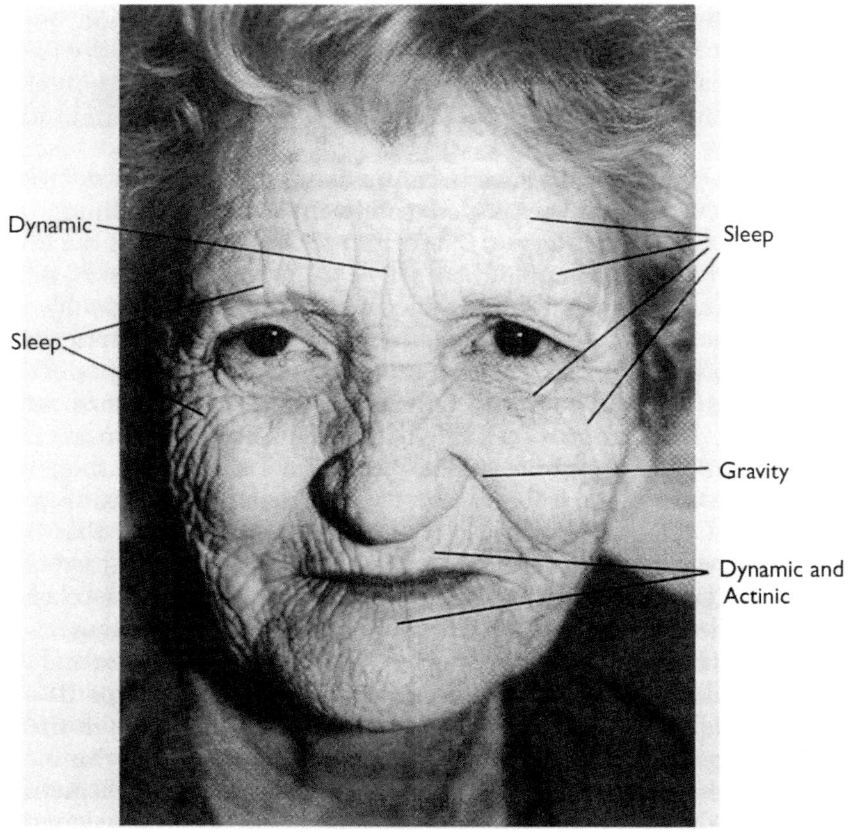

FIG. 4-2. Nasolabial furrows are worsened by gravity and dynamics, perioal wrinkles are both dynamic and actinic, and vertical lateral forehead wrinkles are sleep induced.

Photoaging Groups—Glogau's Classification*†

Group I—Mild (usually age 28-35 yr)
No keratoses
Little wrinkling
No scarring
Little or no makeup
Group II—Moderate (usually age 35-50 yr)
Early actinic keratoses—slight yellow skin discoloration
Early wrinkling—parallel smile lines
Mild scarring
Little makeup
Group III—Advanced (usually age 50-65 yr)
Actinic keratoses—obvious yellow skin discoloration with telangiectasia
Wrinkling—present at rest
Moderate acne scarring
Wears makeup always
Group IV—Severe (usually age 60-75 yr)
Actinic keratoses and skin cancers have occured
Wrinkling—much cutis laxa of actinic, gravitational, and dynamic origin
Severe acne scarring
Wears makeup that does not cover, but cakes on

*Adapted from J Geriatr Dermatol 2(1):30-35, 1994.
†See Fig. 4-3.

It is imperative to distinguish between rhytides associated with sun exposure and dynamic, motion-associated wrinkles of expression (Fig. 4-2). The wrinkles, creases, and furrows associated with movement[16] will not be permanently altered by peeling and are best improved by soft-tissue filling agents such as collagen, Fibrel (Mentor Corp., Santa Barbara, California), or autologous fat. Silicone was an excellent filling substance used in earlier years, and patients who have been previously treated with microdroplet silicone injections may be peeled safely. Injectable Botulinum A exotoxin (Botox-Allergan, Inc., Irvine, California) for the muscles of the brow or forehead provides considerable therapeutic value for the creases and furrows of these areas. Gravitational folds and furrows must be surgically ameliorated by rhytidectomy, coronal lift, or blepharoplasty in conjunction with a peel, but at a different time. (See Chapter 8 and the section on periorbital peeling techniques later in this chapter.) Sleep creases usually respond best to a change of sleep patterns or filling agents, but repetitive superficial peels and medium or deep peels may "blunt," "ease," or even remove these wrinkles for variable time periods if they are not yet permanently etched into the skin.

Glogau[17] has developed a classification of photoaging that is helpful in assessing sun damage in patients with and without a history of sebaceous gland activity or acne (Fig. 4-3). (See the box above.) This classification is comparable to four groups within a photonumeric scale range, with 2 being mild and 8 being severe sun damage.[18] One cannot generalize and treat groups I and II with superficial or medium-depth peels and groups III and IV with medium-depth or deep peels. Some patients have scarring in the absence of sun damage or sun damage in the absence of scarring, and this may affect the choice of the type of medium-depth peel procedure. Every cosmetic unit of the skin from the perioral, periorbital, cheek, forehead, and nasal areas should be *individually assessed* to determine which peeling agent or procedure is necessary for best correction of the area without undue risk.

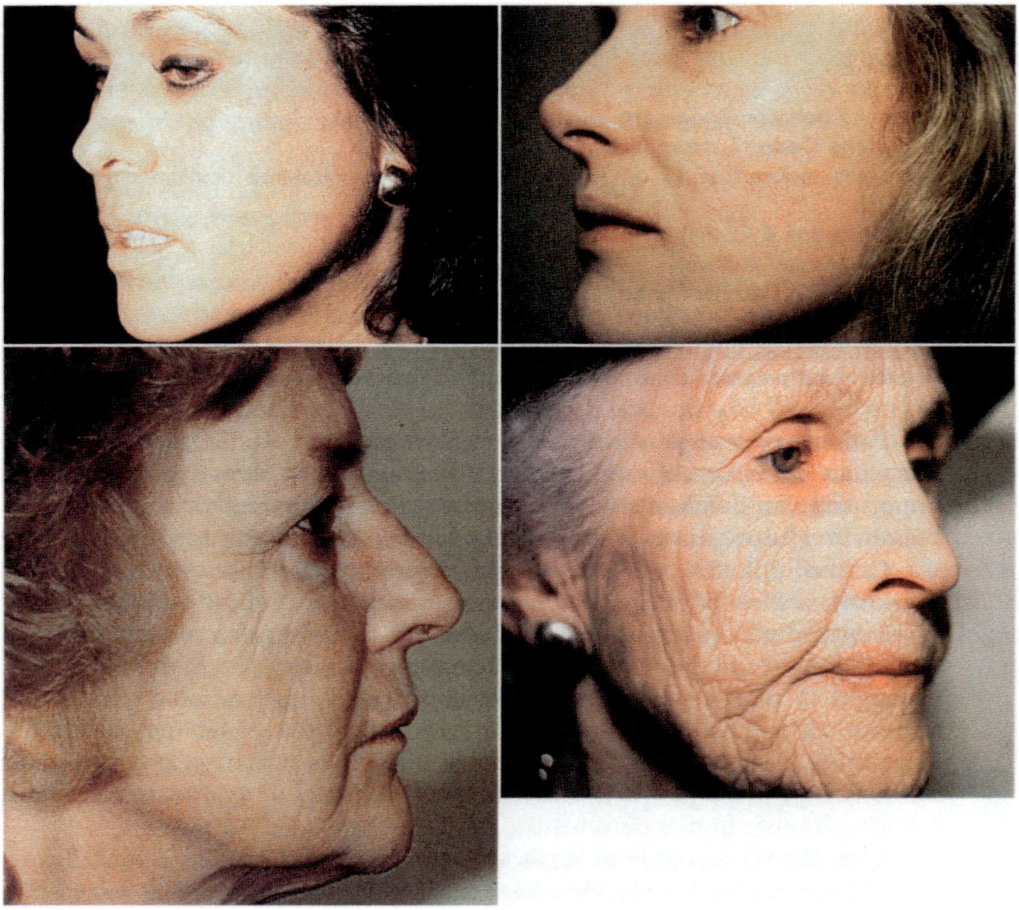

FIG. 4-3. Four photaging groups. See box on p. 46. *(Courtesy of Dr. Richard G. Glogau.)*

Actinic telangiectasias occur as a response to sunlight and should be treated before peeling with electrodessication, sclerotherapy, or laser surgery. Excellent review articles are available.[19] The patient should realize that improvement is limited with peeling alone.

Patients must decide to change their lifestyle and philosophy to minimize future **sun exposure**. Sunscreens must be used while outside. Some patients with outdoor occupations or those who participate in daily outdoor sports are negligent in using wide-brimmed hats or daily sunscreen moisturizers or aftershaves. It is unwise to perform a deep peel on them or to suggest that one procedure will be the total solution to their problem. Only 10 minutes in the sun may be enough to induce splotchy pigmentation in sensitive individuals and to defeat the purpose of peeling for freckling or sun-aggravated melasma.

To protect patients from the sun a product with a sun protection factor (SPF) of 15 is adequate for use as a moisturizer for a woman or an aftershave for a man on a daily basis. (See the box on p. 48.) If outdoors, patients with light-colored skin may need to apply SPF-30 sunscreens. These have a greater risk of producing acne either on a grease-induced or a sun-induced basis. This is a nuisance before or after peeling, and a simpler solution is to persuade patients to keep their face protected from the sun with visors and umbrellas. (See the section on rejuvenation regimen later in this chapter for further discussion of sunscreens.)

Selected Examples of Easily Available Sunscreens with Minimum SPF 15 for Daily Use*

Purpose 15 (Johnson & Johnson)
Coppertone Shade 15 cream (Schering) or gel for oily skin
Neutrogena moisturizer 15 or 30 (Neutrogena) or chemical-free titanium dioxide 17 block
DML 15 (Person & Covey)
Solbar 30 (Person & Covey)
TiScreen 15 (T/I Pharmaceuticals)
Olay 15 (Olay Co.)

*A nonexclusive list of products that are well tolerated in clinical practice—cosmetic companies not included.

Patients may require the use of heavier makeup after a deep peel because they may not tan evenly and because they may have to cover hypopigmented but improved scars. Patients who are averse to using **cosmetics** at all times or to restricting future sun exposure are not good candidates for deep chemical peels.

Currently many sunscreens and cosmetics contain **vitamin E (tocopherol),** which is alleged to decrease ultraviolet radiation–induced oxygen free radical generation in the skin, which is thought to be responsible for the formation of erythema and epidermal cytotoxicity. Free radical stress is thought to play a principal role in skin photoaging and skin cancer. Tocopherol sorbate as an antioxidant or free radical scavenger may be useful in providing significant protection against ultraviolet radiation as a new generation skin protectant.[20] It is limited by its tendency to aggravate acne and its production of contact dermatitis.

Vitamin C (ascorbic acid) in topical products (Cellex-C, Dallas, Texas) is capable of protecting the skin against damage from ultraviolet A and B and may be helpful after sun exposure to reduce redness and inflammation.[21] It does not act as a sunscreen by absorbing ultraviolet light but rather acts as an antioxidant to protect the skin against free radicals produced by light that may cause damage. It may have a cosmetic effect to improve wrinkles. Animal studies and preliminary human studies indicate some reversal of sun damage with cream application perhaps through collagen stimulation. Irritant reactions are rare. For a discussion of ascorbic acid derivatives as bleaching agents see the section in this chapter on the rejuvenation regimen.

Past and Present Sebaceous Gland Activity

Noting the type of scars is crucial in predicting the efficacy of peeling. (See the section under indications in this chapter.) Residual seborrhea or oiliness in a patient with or without scarring will make obtaining an even peel difficult and underscores the importance of defatting the skin before peeling. (See the section on defatting the skin later in this chapter) Peeling does not alter after-peel oiliness, which causes caking of makeup late in the day to reveal hypopigmented skin after some, but not all, deep peels. Patients should be forewarned if the physician expects them to wear makeup for life. The oiliness thus defines the ease and permanence of makeup application and the degree of satisfaction that the patient will sustain after peeling.

The **past and present use of systemic isotretinoin** must be ascertained because its usage may be associated with a greater risk of scarring after peeling. (See the section on scarring in Chapter 8.) If the patient has a **past history of superficial x-ray** treatment for acne, the adnexal structures should be assessed by observing the presence of vellus hairs or by punch biopsy to ensure adequate, albeit delayed reepithelialization.

Prior Cosmetic Surgery

If the patient has had prior rhytidectomy, a coronal brow lift, or blepharoplasty, the patient is a good candidate for peeling from the standpoint that he or she is accustomed to the evaluation for cosmetic surgery and may in fact relish the procedure. Cosmetic surgery "junkies" exist who wish to be peeled aggressively on a monthly or bimonthly basis and who like the postpeel edema and erythema after reepithelialization. If the patient has had a previous peel, it is important to ascertain the type that it was and how long ago it was performed to ensure that proper and adequate dermal collagen remodeling has been completed. A time interval of 4 to 12 weeks is recommended between peeling and procedures involving undermining. (See the section on scarring in Chapter 8.) It is important to notice whether subclinical ectropion with minimal loss of apposition of the lid to the sclera exists before peeling. This may indicate a risk of even worse ectropion after peeling or possibly the appearance of scarring.

Smoking

If the patient is a candidate for deep peeling, it should be pointed out to smokers that the dynamic action of puffing and squinting has contributed to their wrinkles and that these wrinkles will likely return within 6 months after peeling. In addition, because excessive mouth movement in the immediate after-peel period may contribute to perioral scarring, this may be a minor factor to consider. Smoking may multiply the wrinkling effects of sunlight, and the compounds in the smoke may activate enzymes that damage elastin and collagen.[22] Collagen and elastin may be damaged either by generation of free radicals or by direct induction of microvascular changes. Broken blood vessels on the face may be accentuated also. Certainly smokers have undergone peeling without complication, and they are usually grateful for the improvement that is sustained, but discussing this limitation with them before peeling may allay unrealistic expectations.

General State of Physical and Mental Health

There are few absolute contraindications to the entire spectrum of chemical peeling because superficial peeling may be tolerated with little risk in almost all patients of all skin types regardless of their general state of health. If a deep phenol peel is being considered for more than one cosmetic unit, the patient must have adequate hepatorenal status to ensure renal clearance of phenol and should have a recent electrocardiogram and blood studies to serve as a baseline because cardiotoxicity in the form of arrhythmias is a possibility. (See Chapter 7, Deep Peeling.) Vegetarians may have a higher risk of scarring after peeling. (See Chapter 8, Scarring.)

Systemic **medications** should be noted. The use of hormones in the form of postmenopausal estrogens by mouth or patch and oral contraceptives may sensitize the skin to the sun or may produce postinflammatory splotching. (See the section on pigmentary changes in Chapter 8.) Whether the patient developed melasma with every preceding **pregnancy** may help predict pigmentation after peeling. Ideally, the use of warfarin (Coumadin) anticoagulants is relatively contraindicated in deep peels, but patients have been peeled while taking aspirin or nonsteroidal antiinflammatory agents without difficulty because there is instant coagulation with chemical application.

Patients receiving intermittent or recent **chemotherapy** or some patients infected with human immunodeficiency virus **(HIV)** may experience delayed healing or be at risk for secondary infection after peeling. The immediate postoperative healing phase with blistering and crusting is a theoretical time for transmission of HIV, although very unlikely because no blood is present, and aftercare is performed by the patient. If CD4 helper-inducer lymphocyte counts are high, usually over 500 cells per cubic millimeter, peeling can be performed with little risk of complications. We have performed medium-depth peeling on HIV-positive patients for extensive molluscum contagiosum without complication. (See the section on solid carbon dioxide and trichloroacetic acid in Chapter 6.)

If the patient has a **history of recurrent herpes simplex,** prophylactic acyclovir, valacyclovir, or famciclovir may be given during medium-depth or deep peeling. (See the section on Infections in Chapter 8.) A dose of 400 mg of acyclovir three times daily during the healing period should be adequate for most patients and can be instituted on the day of the peel.

True **hypertrophic scar or keloid formers** are at greater risk to scar with deep as opposed to medium-depth peeling. A test area can be performed, which may reassure the physician and the patient without a guarantee of similar response on the rest of the face.

Complete assessment of the patient ensures that the physician and the patient have an excellent relationship and that the patient is not saddled with **unrealistic expectations** that may impede a healthy postoperative course.

The key to documentation of the evaluation before peeling is the mapping and detailing of the defects on a diagram to provide further insight into the individual's potential for future repeat peeling[23] (Fig. 4-4). This also justifies

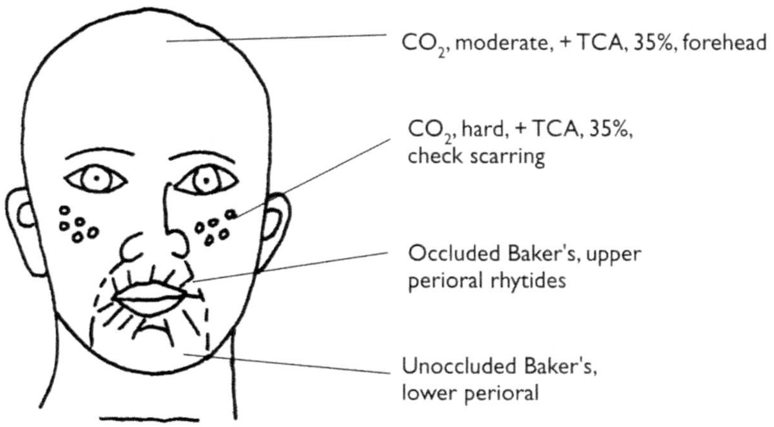

FIG. 4-4. Example of rubber stamp diagram mapping the defects and types of peels performed on a given patient.

peeling in the event of litigation. For example, if a patient is peeled with several strengths of TCA on different portions of the face and scarring occurs where the weakest strength was applied, the diagram would illustrate this and support the contention that the physician's choice of peeling agent was not the chief factor in scarring. Also, there may be a lapse of time between the consultation and the scheduling for the peel, and the map gives the physician instant recall on the chart.

Photodocumentation before and after peeling displays the changing progression of all these factors. At least five systematic views of the face before peeling are useful: right profile, right one quarter, left profile, left one quarter, and full front (Fig. 4-5). Optional close perioral or periorbital views are sometimes helpful.

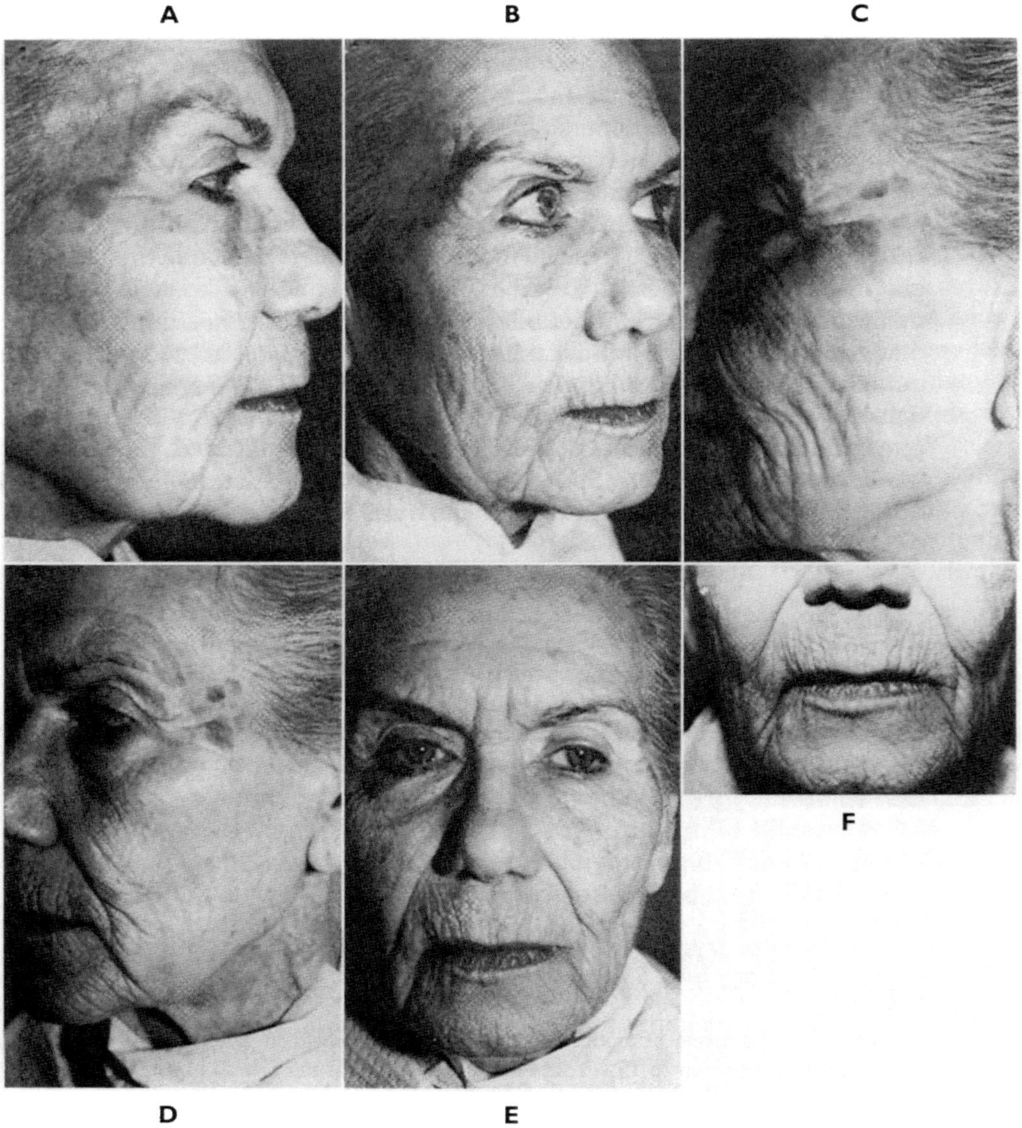

FIG. 4-5. Proper photodocumentation with six views.

REJUVENATION REGIMEN FOR THE SKIN BEFORE AND AFTER PEELING

Immediately after evaluation the patient should be informed that strict sun avoidance and the **daily morning use of a sunscreen** with a sun protection factor of 15 or greater as a moisturizer or aftershave is imperative on an indefinite basis. Practically speaking, this is not always feasible in a mobile and outdoor society. Sunscreens in makeup bases are generally not as effective and are of lower protective value than are moisturizers rubbed in before foundation application. The majority of sunscreens contain octyl-dimethyl PABA (padimate O) as the main ultraviolet B (UVB) absorber.[24] The cinnamate UVB-absorbing derivative, octyl methoxycinnamate (parsol MCX) is also used. Most sunscreens that contain more than one ingredient have oxybenzone as the additional additive with an absorption peak partially in the ultraviolet A range as well as in the UVB spectrum. Sunscreens are available that are non-stinging, waterproof, PABA-free for PABA-allergic patients, fragrance-free for perfume-sensitive patients, oil-free in gels for seborrheic patients, and non-chemical for patients who are unable to tolerate most protectives. Subjective sensory irritation or contact urticaria may warrant discontinuing use because of discomfort. The patient should be comfortable using a product before peeling to minimize the chances of intolerance on newly peeled skin when the product is reinstituted. (See the box on p. 48.)

Most patients who can tolerate the application of **tretinoin (all-trans-retinoic acid)** nightly to the face including the periorbital area up to the lower cilial margin[25] will benefit from its antiaging effects in reducing solar pigmentation as well as from its abilities to promote faster healing in the immediate postpeel period. Topical tretinoin also potentiates the action of hydroquinone.[26] Tretinoin application before and after TCA does not significantly enhance the efficacy of the peel.[27] Its role in prepeel treatment in the actual prevention of pigment return after peeling is unsubstantiated. (See Chapter 3, wound healing, for information; tretinoin in Chapter 5, superficial peeling, for dosage; and Chapter 2, histology for the basis for usage.)

Bleaching Formula for Darker Skin Types: Bleach-eze.

The initial concentration of hydroquinone is 6%. This may be increased if pigmentation returns after peeling. Ascorbic acid prevents the hydroquinone from oxidizing. Hytone (hydrocortisone) cream (Dermik) is paraben free. Creams with high concentrations of hydroquinone should be discontinued as soon as the appropriate amount of pigment loss is achieved to avoid paradoxic hyperpigmentation.

Hydroquinone 6%-10%*
Ascorbic acid 0.05%*
Retinoic acid 0.1%*
Propylene glycol 4%
Dissolve the three crystals* in propylene glycol and mix with Hytone cream 2.5% (Dermik), 30g or may use 2.5% hydroscortisone powder in a vanishing cream.
Sig: apply b.i.d.

This cream may be locally compounded or ordered for individual patients by prescription in concentrations up to 15% from Medical Center Pharmacy, 4600 N. Habana Ave., Tampa, FL 33614 at 1-800-226-7094; fax: 813-876-9095. Its potency decreases if not used in 2 months.

FIG. 4-6. HYDROQUINONE

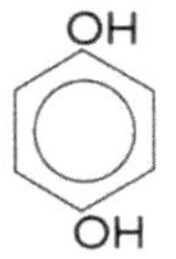

Hydroquinone (HQ), which has chemical characteristics similar to phenol (Fig. 4-6), has a role in the treatment of pigmentary disorders and in chemical peeling. It affects the melanocyte system by decreasing the formation and increasing the degradation of melanosomes by causing structural changes in the membranous organelles of the melanocyte. It also inhibits tyrosinase.[28] Depigmentation is not immediate because hydroquinone interferes only with the formation of new melanin. The production of melanin is resumed when treatment with the drug is discontinued. Any skin type III to VI may benefit especially from the prior use of 4% hydroquinone gel (Solaquin Forte gel, ICN Pharmaceuticals, Costa Mesa, California) twice daily for at least a month before peeling to begin bleaching of epidermal pigment. Four percent hydroquinone in a combination with 12% glycolic acid cream or gel (Viquin Forte, ICN Pharmaceuticals) is a useful product but may cause irritation in some patients because of a pH of 2.5. Alcohol-based hydroquinone tinctures may sting too much for many patients, and the creams are less effective in our clinical experience. Intolerance of the gel requires reassurance and temporary discontinuation for several days. Gel application may be alternated with the cream in frequency of application. Resumption of usage as soon as tolerable after reepithelialization for at least 3 months or indefinitely on a twice-weekly maintenance regimen will retard the appearance or reappearance of hyperpigmentation after peeling. Its role in prepeel treatment in the prevention of pigment return after peeling is unsubstantiated.

There is evidence that hydroquinone in concentrations between 3% and 6% improves both epidermal and dermal hyperpigmentation to some degree after 3 months of use.[29] However, compared with placebo, there was a statistically significant difference induced by 6% compared with 3%. Because clinicians strive for complete dyschromic elimination rather than only improvement, potentiating agents such as tretinoin, an α-hydroxy acid, or a series of superficial partial epidermal peels may increase dermal hydroquinone activity and therefore eliminate more pigment than hydroquinone alone.

In peeling Fitzpatrick types V and VI skin or recalcitrant I-IV skin, hydroquinone concentrations of 6% to 8% in the Bleach Eze formula should be used, beginning with 6%. (See the box to the left.) There will be resistant cases of pigmentation in Asian, Hispanic, Asian-Indian, or Black skin. The pigment may disappear with TCA peeling but may promptly return even darker within 5 to 30 days. If this occurs or is anticipated, the concentration can be increased to 10% to 15%. This may be tried for a week before peeling and if partially successful may be applied for *1 week only* after the peel to stabilize pigment resolution and to prevent pigment return. The hydroquinone can then be rapidly tapered from 10% to 4% or the patient can be given different doses of hydroquinone on alternate days. Close weekly follow-up is necessary. Some patients, particularly **Asian** patients or patients with minimal sun damage and dry atopic skin but extensive melasma, will find these high concentrations of bleach very difficult to use. They may hyperpigment from the irritation of the bleaching agents or their oxidative products or from any peel greater than Jessner's solution or low-strength glycolic acid. (See Case 11-6.)

These patients need exceptional follow-up and patience with strict adherence to the regimen that they can tolerate. Peeling may commence and end with superfical peels of Jessner's solution or low-strength 20% to 50% glycolic acid.

High concentrations of hydroquinone for long periods of time may paradoxically produce **ochronosis**. This exogenous sooty blue-black pigmentation can result from the application of hydroquinone in concentrations of less than 4% in unpeeled Fitzpatrick type VI patients. The etiology of the hydroquinone-induced exogenous ochronosis is not clear, and it can appear in type V patients, especially Asian or Asian-Indian persons. (Richard G. Glogau, personal communication, 1991). It is much more common in South African black skin than in the United States. Perhaps its rarity in the United States may be due to the fact that both hydrocortisone and/or tretinoin are often combined with the hydroquinone.[3,30] Treatment with dermabrasion or an appropriate laser may be effective in some patients.[31]

Kojic acid (KA) is related to hydroquinone chemically, has a similar tyrosinase-suppressive mechanism, and is a metabolic by-product of an *Aspergillus* species fungus that grows on corn in Japan.[32,33] It is water and alcohol soluble, has antibacterial properties, and has a role in chelating iron to prevent free radical generation.[34] Immune system stimulation through leukocyte activity enhancement[35] is purported to occur when KA is taken internally as in the Japanese diet. It has been used in Japan in skin care products since 1988 as a skin lightening agent. Its addition directly to peeling solutions in the United States and its marketing as a bleaching agent with few published efficacy studies make unbiased objective evaluation difficult. Garcia and Fulton[36] performed a clinical comparison in 39 patients with chiefly epidermal melasma of the lightening effects of 5% glycolic acid with 2% HQ vs. 5% glycolic acid with 2% KA for 3 months. Both were equally efficacious, but the HQ was less irritating and less expensive.[36] Comparison of 4% HQ and 12% glycolic acid (Viquin Forte, ICN Pharmaceuticals) with KA and glycolic acid has not been performed, but the former may be faster and more efficacious for melasma. A study using 1% and 2.5% KA cream on a variety of hyperpigmented disorders found no difference in the two strengths when treating a variety of hyperpigmented disorders of all histologic depth (melasma, lentigines, and postinflammatory hyperpigmentation).[37] The range of improvement for each type of pigmentation is uncertain.

Hydroquinone intolerance or sensitization may occur more frequently in Asian populations, but it is less common in the United States in lighter skin types. Kojic acid is better tolerated than higher-strength hydroquinone in Asians. However, kojic acid has been reported to have a high sensitizing potential for inducing contact dermatitis in Asians.[38] The exact concentration of kojic acid to produce effective results with minimal sensitization is unknown.

Kojic acid is presently marketed as an alternative to hydroquinone for the treatment of pigmentation, but the depth and type of pigmentation for response are not clear. More double-blind studies are needed comparing kojic acid with other bleaching agents with and without other additives in different strengths for specific indications. Glycolic acid is more stable in solutions with kojic acid than with hydroquinone (personal communication, Lawrence S. Moy, M.D., February, 1996).

The additional application of an **α-hydroxy acid** in the morning with or without hydroquinone may also improve epidermal quality. (See the section on α-hydroxy acids in Chapter 5.) Perhaps their induction of corneocyte detachments facilitates hydroquinone penetration (See Chapter 2). Preliminary uncontrolled studies suggest that the combination of the application of glycolic acid in the morning and tretinoin at night causes more significant epidermal thickening and increased mucin than the application of tretinoin alone.[39,40]

Azelaic acid 20% cream (Azelex, Allergan Herbert, Inc. Irvine, California) added to the regimen for 6 to 12 months at minimum may be beneficial in fading hyperpigmentation, though its benefits are slow and variable. Azelaic acid is a naturally occurring, straight-chained, saturated dicarboxylic acid. Its bleaching effect on the skin is attributed to inhibition of the energy-producing property or DNA synthesis of the benign hyperactive melanocyte and the inhibition of tyrosinase. Azelaic acid is reported to have a cytotoxic effect on the hyperactive or proliferating human malignant melanocyte. Its effect on malignant rather than benign melanocytes may be either due to the superpharmacologic concentrations that seem necessary for action or due to the drug's increased ability to penetrate through the cell membrane of malignant-pigment cells.[41,42] It may have a role in the treatment of lentigo maligna.[43] Twice-daily application of 15% to 20% azelaic acid creams are used to treat acne as well as pigmentary skin changes.[44]

Topical 20% azelaic acid has been shown to be as effective as but not superior to 4% hydroquinone and is well tolerated in the treatment of melasma after application for 6 months.[45] Studies show variability in efficacy,[46] but the drug may be useful as an addendum to or perhaps a substitute for hydroquinone in the treatment of hyperpigmentation. Tretinoin augments its effect. Azelaic acid does not depigment ephelides or lentigines in uncontrolled trials perhaps because the melanosomes in the melanocytes are full but melanogenically quiescent.[47] Allergic sensitization, phototoxic reactions, burning, pruritis, erythema, and scaling are rare. Irritant side effects from azelaic acid are more prevelant in atopic or some Asian nonoily skin types. A mild inflammatory response with minimal scaling accompanies slow improvement in 6 months. Addition of the cream to a peel regimen for either resistant melasma or hydroquinone intolerance in Asian or dark-skinned patients does not benefit all patients. After future research, azelaic acid may prove to be used as frequently as hydroquinone in treating pigmentary disturbances occurring after chemical peels.

Topical **hydrocortisone** lotion (Hytone 2½%—Dermik) may be useful twice daily as an addition if erythema with bleaching or after peeling is persistent. Fluorinated glucocorticoid creams should not be used on the face after chemical peeling because of their potential to produce telangiectasias. (See the section on pigmentary changes and prolonged erythema or pruritus in Chapter 8.)

The judicious use of epidermabrasive scrubbing pads, which may facilitate peeling by stratum corneum sloughing and may efface wrinkles and remove comedones, is easy to tolerate daily if part of this regimen. Polyester fiber sponges (Buf-Puf, 3M, St. Paul, Minnesota) when used on a daily basis are effective in stimulating epidermal cell renewal by 25% to 40%, and cytomorphologic examination shows that corneocyte size is reduced by 9%, similar to but perhaps less effective than the AHAs, although a different mechanism.[48,49] The patient may regulate the pressure to his or her skin type. Cream absorption will be increased by prior manual **epidermabrasion**.

Shaving the skin on a daily basis can be beneficial to men as well as women[50] and will efface superficial stratum corneum cells and follicular orifices, providing women with additional benefits of easier makeup application

Regimens for Use with Peeling

For pigmentary dyschromias especially in darker skin types, the regimen should be instituted preferably before but certainly after peeling (see text and also discussion of pigmentation in Chapter 8.)

For Fitzpatrick types I and II:

AM:	PM:
Shave, buf, or both	
Sunscreen moisturizer or gel	Moisturizer (optional)
Bleach gel	Bleach gel
α-Hydroxy acid	tretinoin

For Fitzpatrick types III through VI:

AM:	PM:
Shave, buf, or both	
Sunscreen	α-hydroxy acid
Bleach-eze*	Bleach-eze*
Azelaic acid (optional)	Azelaic acid (optional)
Kojic acid (optional)	Kojic acid (optional)
Ascorbic acid derivative (evolving)	Hydrocortisone cream (optional)

*The formula for Bleach-eze is given earlier in this chapter on p. 52 and repeated in Chapter 8.

and less superficial wrinkles and comedones by exfoliation. The aesthetic barrier to shaving by women in western civilization is cultural. There is no associated increase in the hair growth rate or density.

Any patient who is to benefit from peeling will also benefit from this program outlined on p. 56. The regimen is imperative after peeling for pigmentary dyschromias to prevent reappearance of pigment, especially in the darker skin types. In the lighter skin types the regimen retards the spontaneous reappearance of physiologic or mild actinic freckles. The formula for Bleach-Eze is given in the box on p. 52 and is repeated in Chapter 8 in the section on pigmentation. The chief advantage in using it before peeling is to sensitize the patient to using products with ease and to ensure that the patient's tolerance to the compounds and their concentrations is stable for the more important use *after* peeling. As with tretinoin, the use of hydroquinone before peeling in the treatment of pigmentary disorders has not been critically studied to establish its necessity.[51] Its use is acceptable for 1 week or longer before peeling to test the patient's reactivity to the product.

Although bleaches can be used indefinitely, the frequency of application may be gradually tapered or the bleach may be applied on weekends only, for example, in patients at risk for repigmenting. If the tretinoin alone or when compounded with the bleaches produces too much irritation, less frequent application may be indicated, such as on an every-other-day basis, but it must not be applied so seldom that repigmentation occurs. The amount of sun

Factors Slowing Wounding Agent and Peel Regimen Absorption

Actinic damage and epidermal thickness
Dermal scarring
Location
Skin sebaceousness

damage regardless of skin color is the chief limiting factor in the toleration of the irritancy of the regimen. (See the box below for other factors in the toleration potential of the regimen.)

Vitamin C or E creams as discussed above in the section on actinic damage may someday be integrated into this regimen either as bleaching agents, wrinkle-softeners, or sunscreens. **Ascorbic acid** (vitamin C) is added to hydroquinone in concentrations of less than 1% at this time to prevent oxidation. In larger concentrations it is quickly oxidized and decomposed in aqueous solution and is not generally useful as a depigmenting agent. Magnesium L-ascorbyl-2–phosphate **(VC-PMG)**, a stable derivative of ascorbic acid, has some efficacy in Japan as a depigmenting agent.[52] A lightening effect was significant in treating melasma and ephelides in some patients. Refinements in the chemistry of new derivatives may produce new bleaching agents best suited for darker Fitzpatrick skin types.

The nonsteroidal antiandrogen ethoxyhexyl bicyclooctanone (Ethocyn) is marketed as a cosmetic and is promoted as an agent that increases elastin in the dermis with twice daily application. In the future, cosmetics such as these may supplement the benefits of chemical peels. The comparative evaluation to other existing cosmetics to ascertain superiority will eventually produce a priority of agents to apply.

WOUNDING AGENT QUANTITATION AND APPLICATION

More severe actinic damage requires techniques to increase the peel depth. The physician may vary the peel depth by varying the defatting of the skin, the method of wounding agent application, the avoidance of inadvertent dilution of the wounding agent, and the use of tape or occlusive ointments. (See the box below.)

Defatting the Skin

The ideal skin degreaser should be a solvent or a detergent with high lipid solubility, and it should be nontoxic, nonflammable, easily usable, and residue free. All of these qualities are difficult to find in a single agent. Acetone continues to be the preferred and the most commonly used degreaser with TCA peels in spite of its flammability. However, a study comparing acetone with

Factors during the Peel to Quantitate Wounding Agents and Determine Peel Depth

- Skin defatting technique
  - Agent used with time and mode of scrub
- Mode of application
  - Number of cotton appilcators, gauze sponges, sable brush
  - How wet and for how long
- Dilution documentation
  - If performed—when and how long
- Occlusion
  - Tape variety, location, and when removed

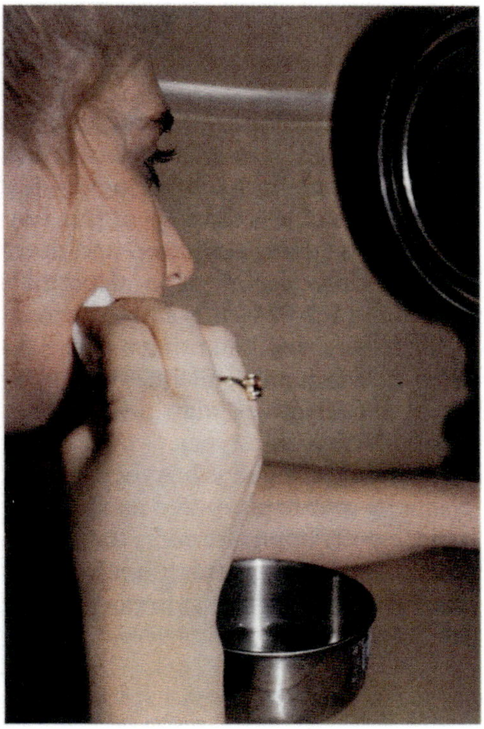

FIG. 4-7. Patient self-scrubbing with acetone for 3 minutes before peeling.

rubbing alcohol (isopropyl alcohol, acetone, and lipid-soluble ketone) trifluorotrichloroethane, and Hibiclens (chlorhexidine gluconate, Zeneca Pharmaceuticals, Wilmington, Delaware) showed no greater TCA, 35% penetration in the acetone-treated scalps of six sun-damaged males.[53] This may have been a reflection of the physiologic atrophic epidermis in this location.

Before the application of all wounding agents, the skin is prepared by cleansing with alcohol or acetone-soaked sponges to remove cutaneous oils. It is generally accepted that this cleansing promotes more even penetration of the wounding agent. Certainly removal of the stratum corneum facilitates penetration of the wounding agent. Optimally, the patient removes makeup, washes the face with an antiseptic skin cleanser (e.g., povidone-iodine or chlorhexidine), and then self-scrubs with acetone on gauze for 3 to 5 minutes. Patients will always underscrub themselves (Fig. 4-7). The physician or nurse then wipes the skin with isopropyl alcohol and vigorously scrubs the skin with acetone for 2 minutes to strip the stratum corneum. A small handheld fan is used to disperse acetone fumes during the scrub. Aggressive scrubbing to the point of bleeding implies dermal penetration and is not warranted or appreciated by the nonsedated patient. Unless scrupulous attention is paid to defatting, thick sebaceous skin of male or female patients with a history of severe acne may not respond as well to peeling. Excessive defatting before 70% glycolic acid peels may cause untoward peeling erythema or pigmentation.

Mode of Application and Choice of Applicator

The amount of wounding agent applied, the degree of rubbing, and the duration of skin contact must be carefully monitored to ensure good results.

A 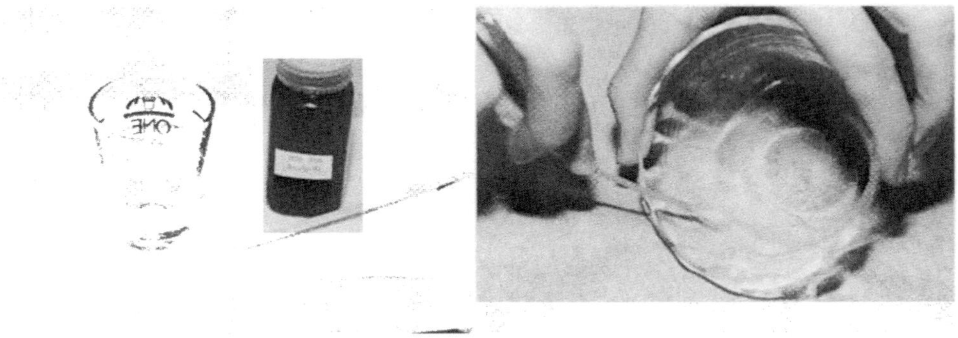 B

FIG. 4-8. A, Pouring the wounding agent into a glass cup before application eliminates contamination from the neck of the master bottle, prevents cotton-tipped applicator disintegration, and conserves solution. **B,** Nonmiscible Baker's solution should be stirred before application, and the cotton-tipped applicator should be semidry.

Pouring a selected amount of wounding agent, for example, Jessner's solution or TCA, into a glass cup or shot glass will ensure uncontaminated application (Fig. 4-8, *A*). (See the section on inherent errors within the peel procedure in Chapter 8.) Whether applying with one or two **cotton-tipped applicators** and whether they were wrung out, damp, or wet should be noted. A 4 × 4–inch. **gauze sponge** similarly utilized for aggressive application should be described in the patient's record. One moist cotton-tipped applicator rubbed with moderate pressure delivers more solution than a single, lightly applied, slightly damp cotton-tipped applicator. Two wet cotton-tipped applicators with hard-pressure rubbing deliver wounding agent more rapidly than does a slightly damp cotton-tipped applicator with light pressure.

In superficial peeling with Jessner's solution, the number of coats applied with **sable brushes** will increase penetration and consistent reproducibility. A damp 1-inch sable brush will deliver more wounding agent to a wider area than will a 4 × 4–inch wrung-out damp gauze sponge or two wrung-out cotton-tipped applicators. Homemade large cotton-tipped applicators similar to proctology swabs can be used for superficial peeling agents, and these swabs act as a reservoir for the peeling agent.[54] Streaking with uneven application is eliminated, but a great deal of the wounding agent is soaked up and wasted in the proctology swab. They are not optimal with phenol mixtures because they deliver too much phenol to the skin too rapidly. The phenol solution should be mixed fresh and applied with a maximum of one or two small cotton-tipped applicators (Fig. 4-8, *B*). (See the section on application of wounding agents in Chapter 7 for specific phenol application techniques.)

Actinically damaged skin wounds in a similar fashion to nonactinically damaged skin, but the application of more wounding agent may be necessary for sun-damaged skin to produce the same wound depth.[55] Portions of thick sebaceous skin may require more rigorous defatting before peeling and may also require more wounding agent to cause an adequate frost. The nose area and glabellar complex may frost slower than the central portion of the cheek if they are not properly defatted. If adequately defatted, they may frost at exactly the same rate. Factors affecting wounding agent absorption are listed in the bottom box on p. 56.)

A 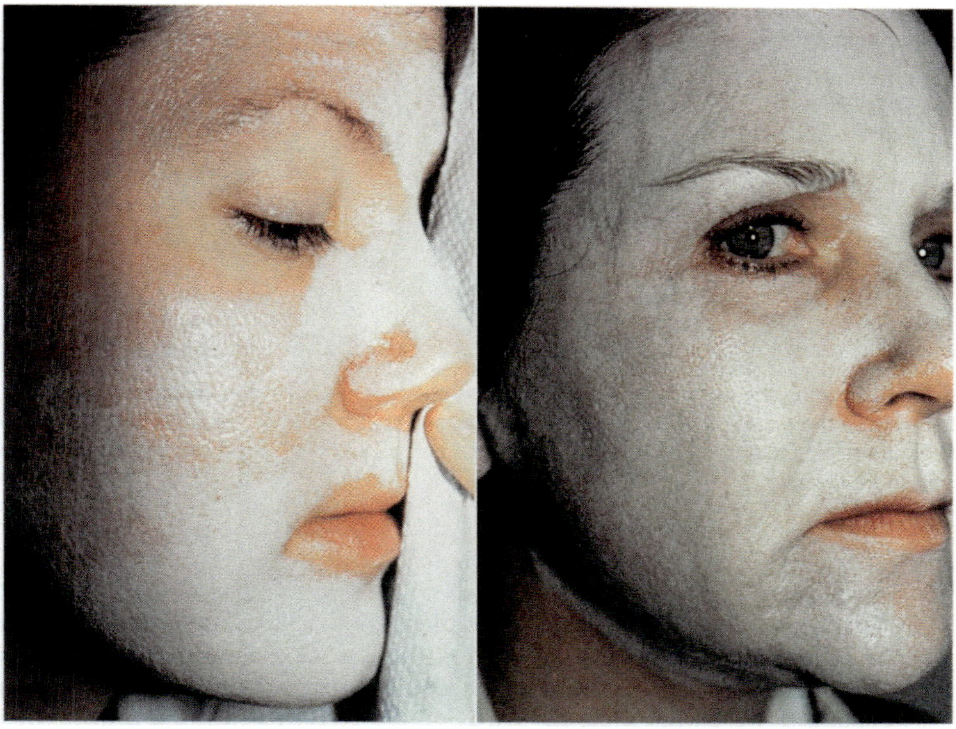 B

FIG. 4-9. A, Different frosting with a single 25% TCA application. The temple frosts very lightly with one semidry cotton-tipped applicator, the cheeks frost lightly with two moist cotton-tipped applicators, and the chin frosts heavily with gauze sponge application. **B,** Heavy, even frosting with gauze sponge application of TCA, 35%, preceded by CO_2 application.

Frosting

Frosting with different wounding agents is variable in rate and appearance and depends on the preexisting photodamaged status of the skin, the choice of applicator, and the adequacy of defatting. Observation of the frost itself as a measure of depth is not as valuable as the actual selection of proper wounding technique or wounding agent (Fig. 4-9). The appearance of the frost does give an index of how evenly the agent has been applied. If the skin is treated first with tretinoin or AHAs, or if the corneal layer has been stripped with acetone or alcohol, the frosting and uniformity of application will be faster. If not, the frosting or penetration will be slower and more variable. Either way, absorption will occur because photodamage itself is not a barrier to wounding agents.

The application of all solutions results in penetration of the chemical and a resultant frost based on the all-or-none inherent quality of wounding agent. Jessner's solution, TCA, and Baker's phenol exhibit slow, medium, and rapid evolutions, respectively, resulting in distinctive white frosts unique to each chemical, assuming similar epidermal control photodamage. If the skin is very sun damaged or insufficiently degreased with insufficient stratum corneum stripping, these frost comparisons are less obvious. Glycolic acid does not produce a perceptible frost of the same nature (Table 4-4).

The frost demonstrates evenness of penetration and may represent protein agglutination. Continual application or overcoating of solution after the color end point has been reached will result in deeper penetration and increased risk of complications. Cessation of application before the frosting end point is

TABLE 4-4.
Skin Frosting Color End Points for Peeling Agents If Peel in Cosmetic Unit Is Pushed to End Point*

AGENT	COLOR	SPEED OF FROSTING
Jessner's solution	Thin pale white	Slow evolution
TCA greater than 30%	Solid white	Medium evolution
Baker's phenol	Gray white	Rapid evolution

*Evolution of frost assumes mildly photodamaged skin that has not been overtreated with tretinoin before peeling.

reached is acceptable and may be desired, especially if a "freshening peel" concept is desired with superficial or medium-depth agents.

Application of Jessner's solution is easily accomplished by rapid brushing of one coat of solution liberally on the desired area. Jessner's solution will produce an even but light white frost when applied with a sable brush, but a very weak, slower, and uneven frost occurs with two cotton-tipped applicators. There is always some evaporation of alcohol in the vehicle, leaving some microcrystallization of ingredients on the skin at the conclusion of application. After waiting 3 to 4 minutes to see the extent of frosting, if any, a second coat is brushed on, and the process may be continued until the end point color is reached. This produces a 5-day peel beginning with a lifting of the epidermis and a darkening of facial pigment on day 1 progressing to a nonvesicular but significant peeling on days 2 through 4. If a patient desires less aggressive peeling, fewer coats are applied without reaching the end point.

Application of TCA, 35%,[56] can be accomplished with a single 4 × 4 gauze pad (Fig. 4-10). The end point (solid white frost) is associated histologically with penetration into the papillary dermis. For full face peeling with TCA alone or in combination with another peeling agent (see Chapter 6), the TCA can be applied with a single moist cotton–tipped applicator under the eyes while the patient is temporarily looking up. The physician then switches to a moist gauze pad and rapidly applies TCA to the remaining cosmetic units. (The order of areas to be peeled is discussed later in the chapter.) Gel ice packs are applied after the skin begins to turn white. The skin turns progressively *thin pale white, white, and solid white*. A predictable exact estimation of depth cannot be appreciated from the color or from palpation, although the progression to stronger colors may certainly indicate increasing penetration. If

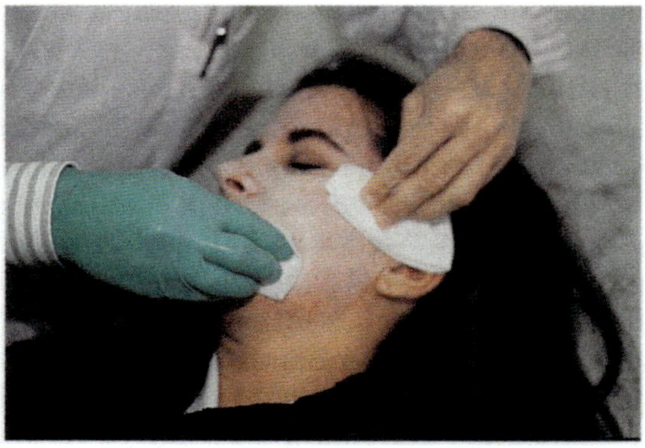

FIG. 4-10. Application of TCA with a saturated single 4 × 4 gauze pad in a gloved hand for more liberal application. The other hand holds a dry gauze pad to avoid inadvertent application.

this exact judgment were possible, scarring might be reduced or eliminated. If several colors of white remain in the skin after 5 or 10 minutes, the decision may be made to return to the light white areas and reapply TCA. This results in increased protein coagulation and wounding. If the assumption is made that initial solution application did occur in these lighter areas, reapplication is usually not necessary, and the clinical result will be typically even and excellent, as expected for this generally safe wounding agent. Forcing uptake by continued reapplication in an area of increased photodamage is acceptable in the treatment of actinic keratoses or scarring, for example, but for photopigmentation or rhytides, reapplication may engender greater risk for complications. As a general rule, the production of the typical very white frost of 35% TCA is not associated with long-term complications.

The technique of application of 50% TCA is the same as for 35% except that, because TCA is concentration dependent, the stronger agent will cause more rapid coagulation and penetration immediately to the reticular dermis. The thin pale white color rarely occurs, and frost development is more rapid. The margin of safety is much narrower, and the risk of complication is much higher. If 50% TCA is forced into the deep dermis to attempt to remove severe rhytides and the whitest frost is produced, the result is more unpredictable, as is inherent with the concentration of the agent. Some wrinkles may disappear, whereas others may not. Texture changes may result, and scarring may occur with 50% TCA in spite of the appearance of the frost, the preexisiting status of the skin, the method of application, the method of TCA preparation, and other factors. Application of 50% TCA should be performed judiciously by only those surgeons with significant experience in chemexfoliation and on patients that understand the increased risk of scarring. Pretreatment of the skin with solid CO_2, JS, or glycolic acid allows deeper safe penetration of 35% TCA and makes the use of 50% TCA as a single peeling agent less necessary. (See Chapter 6.)

Additives to TCA have been utilized to change the ability of TCA to penetrate and allegedly to cause more uniform distribution, less patient irritation, and better frost observation.[57-59] The addition of emulsifiers such as glycerin, surfactants such as polysorbate 20 (Tween 20), and other additives to 50% TCA in the hope of slowing penetration may change the ability of the chemical to penetrate but does not alter the capability of 50% TCA to produce scarring because the additives do not significantly alter the final concentration of TCA. Additives may even increase the penetration of TCA to the lower dermis,[60] giving a false sense of security to the physician and thus leading to overcoating and the production of contractile scarring due to deep dermal penetration. However, 35% TCA does not seem to inherently possess as great a risk of scarring and even without additives can deliver excellent results alone or in combinations (see Chapter 6) for all photoaging indications except severe rhytides. The risk of overcoating is minimal. Trichloroacetic acid in any concentration is not superior to phenol in the amelioration of significant coarse rhytides, so full face 50% TCA peels are less necessary and more risky. Clinical results with and without additives are similar.[61] If additives are used with TCA, safety should be the paramount concern since there are no proven advantages to their use.

Although the application of **phenol** produces a deeper white frost more quickly, this may not be the end point of the peel. Severely actinically damaged wrinkles may require an additional 15 seconds of repeated rubbing of Baker's solution past the initial white to a gray end point to effectively remove wrinkles, even with occlusion.[16]

Reapplication of TCA or Baker's phenol 10 minutes after frosting will substantially increase the wound depth.[62] (See the section on multiple frosting in Chapter 2.) This concept of multiple frosts is especially helpful in selected sun-damaged areas with impaired penetration such as in areas with actinic keratoses or in areas where increased penetration is desired with less risk of skin texture change.

Nonfacial frosting with TCA may vary considerably with location, possibly based on skin metabolism. Frosting is invariably slower on nonfacial areas. The rate is a function of the degree of actinic damage or scarring present as well as location. (See the section on this topic in Chapter 5.)

α-Hydroxy acids do not produce a frost, and their mode of application is outlined in the section on AHAs in Chapter 5.

Dilution

Dilution of peeling solution on the skin before frosting, if performed as described in the old superficial peeling techniques (see the section on TCA in Chapter 5), should be documented. The old concept of "neutralization" of TCA with alcohol or water immediately after frosting is useless to reverse the immediate effect of the application of the wounding agent. The term originated in 1926 when Dr. H. Leslie Roberts in England gave his clinical opinion on "neutralizing" TCA with water after application to avoid patient stinging.[63] The term has remained in dermatology since then and been misconstrued over the decades. Once frosting has occurred, penetration is already achieved. Adding water to an aqueous wounding agent on the skin before frosting is actually dilution and will affect the concentration and reproducibility of the peel. We do not "neutralize" TCA and consider the technique outdated and the term a misnomer.

α-Hydroxy acids do not frost in the same fashion as TCA, and they slowly induce erythema from the time of application. Their penetration is dependent on the contact time with the skin, and washing them from the skin after a given amount of time is important.

Occlusion

Occlusion and wound depth of phenol peels but not TCA peels are thought to be affected by the porosity of different tapes. The most porous tape is the least occlusive, zinc oxide tape being less porous than silk or paper tape. Noting the brand and type of tape used in deep peeling is important for evaluating peel results and for proper selection of adequate wounding techniques for future peels. Tape can be applied selectively to the areas with the most severe problems, and an entire face mask is not imperative. A mechanical tape barrier is more effective than the immediate application of an occlusive ointment in increasing absorption and penetration of phenol. The occlusive tape by maceration immediately after peeling causes deeper penetration. Clinically the result may be the same with or without the tape as long as the elastotic damage present is penetrated and altered. (See the section on taping the mask in Chapter 7.)

In an attempt to standardize terminology, *unoccluded* and *occluded* will be used in lieu of the old terms *open* and *closed*.

WOUNDING AGENT APPLICATION CONCEPTS

Order of Areas to Be Peeled in Superficial and Medium-Depth Peeling

With superficial and medium-depth peeling, we like to begin with the most sensitive lower eyelash area first because the patient is unsedated and alert. Moving in rapid succession to the upper eyelids, nose, cheeks, perioral area, and the least sensitive forehead area affords greatest ease for the physician to safely peel the periorbital area, and best tolerance for the patient because of inevitable progressive squirming for 1 to 2 minutes while frosting is occurring. Peeling does not affect hair follicles or hair growth. Careful feathering of the solution into the hairline and around the angle of the mandible conceals the line of demarcation between nonpeeled and peeled skin. Earlobes should be peeled to maximize visual results. Specific cosmetic unit area techniques are listed in the following. The deep-peeling technique is generally in the reverse order to that described earlier with the eyes being peeled last, but the patient is usually sedated. (See Chapter 7 for specific technique differences; see the section on trichloroacetic acid 50% peel in Chapter 6 for further discussion.)

Periorbital Peeling Techniques

Infraorbital skin darkening may be caused by dermal melanin, postinflammatory hyperpigmentation, superficial dermal blood vessels, excessive lower eyelid skin shadowing, and the translucence of thinned eyelid skin allowing the underlying muscle color to be visible through it.[64] Peeling with Baker's phenol solution becomes necessary in darker skin types in order to lighten the skin color if it is due to pigment deposition. (See Fig. 11-11) Blepharoplasty may be the treatment of choice if the appearance of the blood vessels is the origin of the discoloration.

Careful peeling of the eyelash skin with various wounding agents will allow peeling of the entire periorbital complex. Irrespective of the use of one or two cotton-tipped applicators, they should be wrung out and semidry so that dripping cannot occur. Generally, the entire complex except for the crow's feet has thin skin, and using one applicator is reasonable for better control. Care is taken not to pass the applicator over the eyes during the procedure. An assistant should be prepared with a syringe of saline for flushing if the wounding agent is accidentally introduced into the eye, although tears will aid dilution.

The head of the patient should be elevated to 30 degrees. Tears should be wiped away during peeling with a cotton-tipped applicator at the medial and lateral canthus while holding the eye open to avoid pulling solution into the eye by capillary action. On the lower lid, the patient's eyes should be open and looking superiorly. The chemical should be applied to within a millimeter of the eyelash margin by moving from the lateral crow's feet to the medial canthal area. The upper lid can be peeled with the eyes closed by proceeding similarly from the crow's feet below the eyebrow border to the inner canthal area. Upper eyelid skin can be peeled only to the superior border of the tarsal plate to minimize edema. However, if sun damage is extensive enough to warrant peeling down to within a millimeter of the upper eyelashes, this may be performed by using a superficial peeling agent no stronger than 35% TCA. Local ice packs are helpful for 5 to 10 minutes after TCA application and for 6 to 8 hours after phenol application.[65] Cardiac monitoring is not necessary for application of phenol to one cosmetic unit because of the small amount of chemical applied. (See Chapter 7 for a discussion of specific periorbital wounding agents; the section on scarring in Chapter 8 for a discussion of

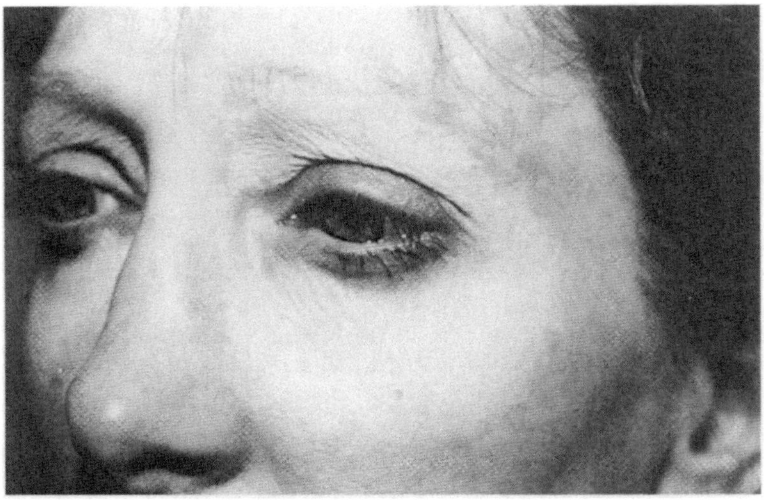

FIG. 4-11. Selective periorbital peeling should extend at least to the orbital rim.

ectropion; and the section on inherent errors in Chapter 8 for spilling of solutions into the eye.)

A bland protective ophthalmic ointment containing petrolatum (Lacrilube, Allergan Pharmaceuticals, Irvine, California) is utilized by some physicians as ophthalmic protection, but if the cotton-tipped applicator is well wrung out, this is not necessary,[16] and the ointment may promote excessive tearing and blinking. We do not use it.

If performing a periorbital peel only, always peel to the orbital rims to avoid a line of demarcation (Fig. 4-11). However, a more superficial agent beyond these areas will never be detrimental and will assist in blending the demarcated areas. Thirty-five percent TCA is always acceptable as a peeling agent for the entire periorbital unit (Fig. 4-12). Progressing to full-strength phenol or Baker's phenol solution for severe sun damage or hyperpigmentation in darker skin types is acceptable in thick and medium periorbital skin unless ectropion is present or blepharoplasties have been performed previously.

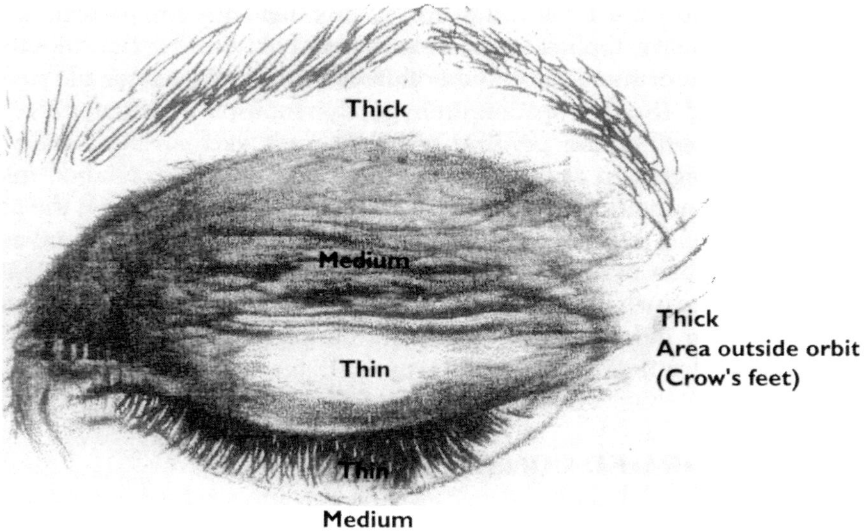

FIG. 4-12. Dermal thicknesses of the eye. *(Adapted from Morrow DM: J Dermatol Surg Oncol 18:108, 1992.)*

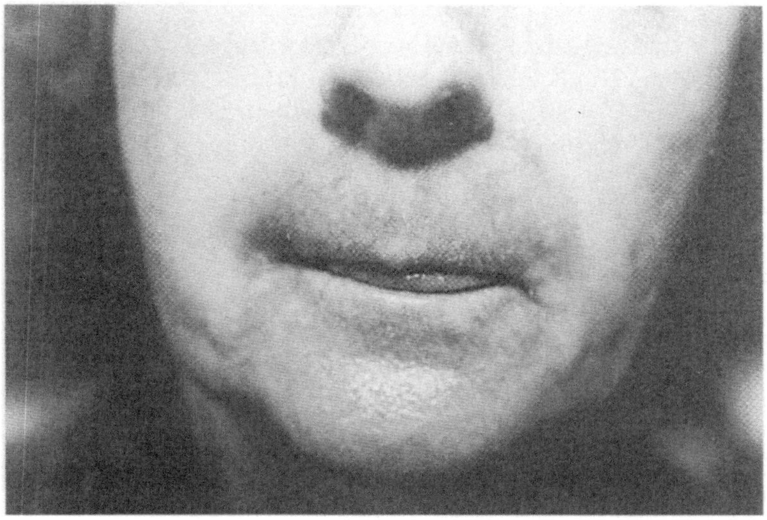

FIG. 4-13. Six days after a selective deep perioral peel extending immediately beyond the nasolabial fold and into the vermilion.

Perioral Peeling Techniques

The perioral area is an important area to most patients because both actinic and dynamic motion-related rhytides may intensify here. Wounding agents should be applied at least 3 mm onto the vermilion to eradicate wrinkles. Manually stretching the skin will allow deeper and more even penetration. Rubbing the wounding agent into thick, actinically damaged local rhytides will increase penetration. The wooden portion of a broken cotton-tipped applicator may serve to apply solution to an individual rhytid, especially on a repeat peel. McCollough and Langsdon[12,66] advocate heavier application with exceptionally aggressive prepeel defatting of this area. (See the section on application of wounding agent in Chapter 7.) Our impression is that the extremely deep wrinkles of the very severely actinically damaged individual respond most favorably with heavy application under selective occlusion of this area. This application and occlusion vary according to the degree of actinic rhytides present. Aesthetically, the most natural result is not the smooth, porcelain lip of the extremely heavy application of Baker's phenol but rather the smoother lip with preservation of some color and architecture, even if every single rhytid has not disappeared. (See the section on hypopigmentation in Chapter 8.)

When peeling the perioral cosmetic unit exclusively, always apply the wounding agent to at least immediately beyond the nasolabial fold to avoid lines of demarcation (Fig. 4-13). Feathering or peeling below the angle of the mandible and the remainder of the face with a more superficial agent either simultaneously or at a later time will blur this demarcation line. This is important if there will be a visible difference in pigmentation after peeling, for example, in either a very actinically damaged Fitzpatrick type I or a very tanned and sun-damaged type IV patient.

OBTAINING INFORMED CONSENT

Before a wounding agent or technique is selected, patients should be given an instruction sheet and sign a consent form (Figs. 4-14 and 4-15). Informed con-

Chemical Peels–What They Can and Cannot Do

Dermatologic surgeons have been using peeling agents for the last 50 years. Light peels to correct mild defects, medium-depth peels to correct moderate defects, and deep peels to correct severe defects can be used over the entire face and neck area uniformly or in combining light, medium-depth, and deep peels on the same face to correct different skin problems. Today with rejuvenation of the skin and reversal of the aging process paramount in the minds of many, chemical peeling has emerged as an exciting supplement to a total skin care program.

Most chemical peels today are supplemented by the peeling effects of creams such as retinoic acid (Retin-A or RENOVA) on a daily basis, which give a constant turnover of the top layers of the skin, further improving the integrity. 5-Fluorouracil cream can also be used in a limited fashion to eradicate superficial sun damage.

What Chemical Peels Can Do

1. Correct sun damage (actinic degeneration)
2. Flatten mild scarring
3. Remove rhytides (wrinkles)
4. Improve irregular hyperpigmentation

The mild and moderate peels are called freshening peels because they improve the quality of the skin without altering its normal architecture. The ability of the skin to tan again and return to the same color after peeling or sunlight exposure is unchanged.

With deeper peels usually involving phenol, the color of the skin is lighter after peeling and may not ever tan again; instead it may freckle.

What Chemical Peels Cannot Do

1. Chemical peels cannot change pore size, if anything, they might increase pore size temporarily.
2. Chemical peels cannot improve lax skin; removal of fine wrinkling and cross-hatching may not make any difference if there is profound lax skin that needs a face-lift.
3. Chemical peels cannot improve deep scarring. Dermabrasion, the laser, punch grafting, punch elevation, or excision of scarring is much more effective.
4. Chemical peels cannot always totally remove hyperpigmentation in dark-skinned whites, Asians, or blacks and may not be indicated.
5. Chemical peels cannot remove broken blood vessels on the face.

FIG. 4-14. Patient instruction sheet.

CHEMICAL PEEL CONSENT

I, ________________________,consent to the treatment known as a chemical peel. The treatment has been explained to me, and I have had an opportunity to ask questions. The procedure will cause swelling of my face that may be uncomfortable. The skin will turn red, blister, and crust, and look like a very bad sunburn before it heals. The peeling usually lasts about 1 to 2 weeks, although it may last longer.

I understand that there is a risk of developing a temporary or permanent pigment (color) change in the skin. There is a small incidence of the reactivation of "cold sores" (herpes infection) in patients with a prior history of herpes. Bacterial infection (impetigo) or the appearance of acne can occur during or after the peel.

Wind and sun sensitivity can be persistent. There is also a rare incidence of allergy to the creams used after the peel. There is a rare incidence of scarring. I also consent to the taking of medical photographs.

The actual degree of improvement cannot be predicted or guaranteed.

________________________	________________________
Patient's Signature (or Guardian)	Date
________________________	________________________
Witness	Date

FIG. 4-15. Peel consent form.

Perspective How to Peel

From the boxed material in Chapter 2 on p. 26, the boxed material in this chapter on p. 39 and Tables 4-1 and 4-2 the reader can select peeling techniques and indications with alternative possibilities for peeling on each cosmetic unit. Illustrative examples are given throughout this book. The following principles must be observed.

1. Be certain that the proper indications for peeling are actually present on the skin.
2. Perform a proper history and physical to evaluate for contraindications (See the boxed material on p. 44)
3. Choose the proper peel for individual cosmetic unit photodamage. Be sure that the entire face does warrant the same process on each unit. (See Table 4-2 on p. 41.) If not, perform a combined peel with varying techniques on different cosmetic units.[68]
4. Observe and record factors during peeling that quantitate the wounding agent and determine the peel depth (See the boxed material on p. 57)
5. Be thoroughly familiar with complications and their treatment. (See Table 8-1 and the box at the top of p. 56.)
6. Be sure the patient is confident that he or she will be certain to receive priority attention during and after the recovery period.
7. Treat facial broken blood vessels first with electrosurgery, sclerotherapy, or laser surgery prior to peeling if possible. Any resulting post inflammatory pigmentation can be treated with subsequent peeling.

sent rests on good communication and joint decision making between physician and patient.[67] This consent form is adequate for all medium and deep peels and is used in concert with a postpeel instruction sheet found at the end of each chapter on the respective peel type. If a consent form is desired for superficial peels this one can be used, but there are no expected permanent sequelae from superficial peels, and complications are extremely rare. The postpeel instruction sheet is self-explanatory (See Fig. 5-21.)

WOUNDING TECHNIQUE OR AGENT SELECTION

The selection of the proper wounding agent or wounding technique (see the box on p. 26) is based on the experience of the physician, the depth and location of the problem to be corrected in each cosmetic unit of the face (See Tables 4-1 and 4-2 and the above sections on indications and patient selection), the duration of healing time anticipated by the patient, and the patient's tolerance of the procedure, assuming adequate skin health for reepithelialization and collagen remodeling. Varying morbidity may be a factor in wounding agent selection. Some patients who cannot afford time away from occupations to heal may benefit from a series of nonvesiculating superficial peels to treat pigmentation. Scar correction will require the application of a medium-depth peeling agent and 7 to 10 days of healing or alternately evaluation for dermabrasion or laser resurfacing. Mild to moderate rhytides may benefit from superficial peels, allowing the patient to continue to work, followed eventually by a medium-depth peel based on the patient's schedule. Very severe actinic rhytides improve most with a deep peel, but a medium-depth peel may be performed first with less morbidity and less dramatic results until time permits.

Final results achieved with different superficial, medium, or deep peeling agents within the same category may be similar. With the foundation of knowledge of the peels in the following chapters, the histology and characteristics of the patient's defects, and the evaluation of the patient's wound healing status, a variety of different peels in different sequence can achieve effective results.

REFERENCES

1. Collins PS: The chemical peel, *Clin Dermatol* 5:57-74, 1987.
2. Kligman AM, Baker TJ, Gordon HI: Long-term histologic follow-up of phenol face peels, *Plast Reconstr Surg* 75:652-659, 1985.
3. Grimes PE: Melasma: etiologic and therapeutic considerations, *Arch Dermatol* 131:1453-1457, 1995.
4. Sanchez NP, Pathak MB, Sato S, et al: Melasma: a clinical, light microscopic, ultrastructural, and immunofluorescence study, *J Am Acad Dermatol* 4:698-710, 1981.
5. Fitzpatrick TB: The validity and practicality of sun-reactive skin types I through VI, *Arch Dermatol* 124:869-871, 1988.
6. Lawrence NL, Cox SE, Brody HJ: A comparison of Jessner's solution and glycolic acid in the treament of melasma in dark skinned patients: a double blind study, *J Am Acad Dermatol* 36:589-593, 1997.
7. MacKee GM, Karp FL: The treatment of post-acne scars with phenol, *Br J Dermatol* 64:456-459, 1952.
8. Stegman SJ, Tromovitch TA: Chemical peeling. In *Cosmetic dermatologic surgery,* St Louis, 1984, Mosby, pp. 27-46.
9. Brody HJ, Hailey CW: Medium-depth chemical peeling of the skin: a variation of superficial chemosurgery, *J Dermatol Surg Oncol* 12:1268-1275, 1986.
10. Wolfe SA: Chemical face peeling following therapeutic irradiation, *Plast Reconstr Surg* 69:859-862, 1982.
11. Baker TJ, Gordon HL: Chemical peel with phenol. In Epstein E, Epstein E Jr, editors: *Skin surgery,* ed 6, Philadelphia, 1987, Saunders, pp. 423-438.
12. McCollough EG, Langsdon PR: Dermabrasion and chemical peel, a guide for facial plastic surgery, New York, 1988, Thieme Medical, pp. 53-112.
13. Stagnone JJ: Superficial peeling, *J Dermatol Surg Oncol* 15:924-930, 1989.
14. Thappa DM: Comedone extraction with trichloroacetic acid, *J Dermatol* 21:61, 1994 (letter).
15. Swinehart JM: Test spots in dermabrasion and chemical peeling, *J Dermatol Surg Oncol* 16:557-563, 1990.
16. Stegman SJ, Tromovitch TA, Glogau RG: *Cosmetic dermatologic surgery,* St Louis, 1990, Mosby, pp 35-58.
17. Glogau RG: Chemical peeling and aging skin, *J Geriatr Dermatol* 2(1):30-35, 1994.
18. Griffiths CEM, Wang TS, Hamilton TA, et al: A photonumeric scale for the assessment of cutaneous photodamage, *Arch Dermatol* 128:347-351, 1992.
19. Goldman MP, Weiss RA, Brody HJ, et al: Treatment of facial telangiectasia with sclerotherapy, laser surgery, and/or electrodessication: a review, *J Dermatol Surg Oncol* 19:899-906, 1993.
20. Jurkiewicz BA, Bissett DL, Buettner GR: Effect of topically applied tocopherol on ultraviolet radiation–mediated free radical damage in skin, *J Invest Dermatol* 104:484-488, 1995.
21. Pinnell SR: Vitamin C shields skin from UV light, presented at the American Academy of Dermatology, February, 1995.
22. Kadunce DP, Burr R, Gress R, et al: Cigarette smoking: risk factor for premature facial wrinkling, *Ann Intern Med* 114:840-844, 1991.
23. Brody HJ: The art of chemical peeling, *J Dermatol Surg Oncol* 15:918-921, 1989.
24. Funk JO, Dromgoole SH, Maibach HI: Sunscreen intolerance, *Dermatol Clin* 13(2):473-481, 1995.
25. Stagnone JJ: Skin rejuvenation program in chemical peeling and chemabrasion. In Epstein E, Epstein E Jr, editors: *Skin surgery,* Philadelphia, 1987, Saunders, pp. 413-420.
26. Kligman AM, Willis I: A new formula for depigmenting human skin, *Arch Dermatol* 111:40, 1975.
27. Humphreys TR, Werth V, Dzubow L, et al: Treatment of photodamaged skin with trichloroacetic acid and topical tretinoin, *J Am Acad Dermatol* 34:638-44, 1996.
28. Goodman LS, Gilman AG: *The pharmacological basis of therapeutics,* New York, 1980, MacMillan, p. 959.

29. Glenn MJ, Grimes PE, Chalet M, et al: Evaluation of clinical and light microscopic effects of various concentrations of hydroquinone, *Clin Res* 39:83A, 1991 (abstract).
30. Weiss RM, del Fabbro E, Kolisang P: Cosmetic ochronosis caused by bleaching creams containing 2% hydroquinone, *S Afr Med J* 77:373, 1990.
31. Diven DG, Smith EB, Pupo RA, et al: Hydroquinone-induced localized exogenous ochronosis treated with dermabrasion and CO_2 laser, *J Dermatol Surg Oncol* 16:1018-1022, 1990.
32. Bollman M: Kojic acid, *Advanced Dermatologics News*. 4(4):1-8, 1995.
33. Kim S, Suh K, Chae Y, et al: The effect of arbutin, glycolic acid, kojic acid and pentadecenoic acid on the in vitro and in vivo pigmentary system after ultraviolet irradiation, *Korean J Dermatol* 32(6):977-989, 1994.
34. Molenda J, Basinger M, Hanusa T, et al: Synthesis and iron binding properties of 3-hydroxypyrid-4-ones derived from kojic acid, *J Inorgan Biochem* 55(2):131-146, 1994.
35. Akamatsu H: Kojic acid scavenges free radicals while potentiating leukocyte functions including free radical generation, *Inflammation* 15(4):303-315, 1991.
36. Garcia A, Fulton JE: The combination of glycolic acid and hydroquinone or kojic acid for the treatment of melasma and related conditions, *Dermatol Surg* 22:443-448, 1996.
37. Mishima Y, Ohyama Y, Shibata T, et al: Inhibitory action of kojic acid on melanogenesis and its therapeutic effect for various human hyperpigmentation disorders, *Skin Res* 36(2):134-150, 1994.
38. Nakagawa M, Kawai K: Contact allergy to kojic acid in skin care products, *Contact Dermatitis* 32(1):9-13, 1995.
39. Rubin MG: Conference on AHAs, Orlando, Fla, December 1994.
40. Kligman AM: The compatibility of combinations of glycolic acid and tretinoin in acne and in photoaged facial skin, *J Geriatr Dermatol* 3(suppl A)(3):25A-28A, 1995.
41. Cunliff WJ: International symposium on acne and related diseases, Cardiff, Wales, 1988.
42. Nazzaro-Porro M: The depigmenting effect of azelaic acid. *Arch Dermatol* 126:1649-1653, 1990 (letter).
43. Prieto MAR, Lopez PM, Gonzalez IR, et al: Treatment of lentigo maligna with azelaic acid, *Int J Dermatol* 32(5):363-364, 1993.
44. Nazzaro-Porro M: Beneficial effect of 15% azelaic acid cream on acne vulgaris, *Br J Dermatol* 109:45,1983.
45. Nguyen QH,Bui TP: Azelaic acid: pharmacokinetic and pharmacodynamic properties and its therapeutic role in hyperpigmentary disorders and acne, *Int J Dermatol* 34(2):75-84, 1995.
46. Grimes PE. Melasma: etiologic and therapeutic considerations, *Arch Dermatol* 131:1453-1457, 1995.
47. Breathnach AS. Melanin hyperpigmentation of skin: melasma, topical treatment with azelaic acid, and other therapies, *Cutis* 57:36-45, 1996.
48. Grove GL, Lutz JB, Maass KC, et al: Effect of daily cleansing with a polyester fiber sponge on epidermal cell renewal, 3M Company research, St Paul MN 55144-1000.
49. Bergfeld W, Tung R, Vidimos A: Improving the cosmetic appearance of photoaged skin using glycolic acid, *J Am Acad Dermatol* 36:XX, 1997 (in press).
50. Merrill K: The bearded ladies, *Allure* p. 80, November 1995 .
51. Glogau RG, Matarasso SL: Chemical peels, *Dermatol Clin* 13(2):263-276, 1995.
52. Kameyama K, Sakai C, Kondoh S, et al: Inhibitory effect of magnesium L-ascorbyl-2-phosphate (VC-PMG) on melanogenesis in vitro and in vivo, *J Am Acad Dermatol* 34:29-33, 1996.
53. Peikert JM, Krywonis NA, Rest EB, et al: The efficacy of various degreasing agents used in trichloroacetic acid peels, *J Dermatol Surg Oncol* 20:724-728, 1994.
54. Gross BG, Maschek E: Phenol chemosurgery and removal of deep facial wrinkles, *Int J Dermatol* 19:159-164,1980.
55. Stegman SJ: A comparative histologic study of the effects of three peeling agents and dermabrasion on normal and sun damaged skin, *Aesthetic Plast Surg* 6:123-135, 1982.
56. Brody HJ: Trichloroacetic acid application in chemical peeling, *Operative Techniques Plast Reconstr Surg* 2(2):127-128, 1995.
57. Dinner MI, Artz JF: Chemical peel—what's in the formula? *Plast Reconsr Surg* 94:406-407, 1994.
58. Johnson JB, Ichinose H, Obagi ZE, et al: Obagi's modified trichloroacetic acid (TCA)–controlled variable-depth peel: a study of clinical signs correlating with histological findings, *Ann Plast Surg* 36:225-237, 1996.
59. Glogau R, et al: Letter to the editor re Obagi's modified trichloroacetic acid–controlled variable-depth peel. *Ann Plast Surg* 38:298-302, 1997.

60. Laub DR: Polysorbate as an adjunctive chemical in the TCA peel, *Plast Reconstr Surg* 95:425, 1995.
61. Clinical Discussions, Joint Meeting of Florida Society of Dermatologic Surgery and Florida Society of Plastic and Reconstructive Surgery, Miami, Fla, Sept 15, 1990, and American Academy of Facial Plastic and Reconstructive Surgery, Indianapolis, Ind, March 3-4, 1993.
62. Brody HJ: Variations and comparisons in medium-depth chemical peeling, *J Dermatol Surg Oncol* 15:953-963, 1989.
63. Roberts HL: The chloracetic acids: a biochemical study, *Br J Dermatol* 38:323-391, 1926.
64. Lowe NJ, Wieder JM, Shorr N, et al: Infraorbital pigmented skin: preliminary observations of laser therapy, *Dermatol Surg* 21:767-770, 1995.
65. Morrow DM: Chemical peeling of eyelids and periorbital area, *J Dermatol Surg Oncol* 18:102-110, 1992.
66. McCollough EG, Langsdon PR: Chemical peeling with phenol. In Roenigk H, Roenigk R, editors: *Dermatologic surgery: principles and practice*, New York, 1989, Marcel Dekker, pp. 997-1016.
67. Hirsh BD: The ethical and legal status involving informed consent, *Cosmet Dermatol* 7(8):25-28, 1994.
68. Monheit GD: The Jessner's–trichloroacetic acid peel, *Dermatol Clin* 13(2):277-283,1995.

5 Superficial Peeling

Perspective on Superficial Peeling

Superficial peeling agents have been marketed more than any other agent because when used alone they have a high safety record with little risk of complication. (See the top box on page 74.) They have little effect when applied once and generally require multiple weekly or monthly applications for effectiveness. Multiple superficial peels do not produce the same effects as one medium peel unless the defects treated were originally extremely superficial. The peels are generally epidermal and therefore pose little risk of scarring. They are not meant to be forced deeply into the dermis to produce the effects of dermal peels. They do not vesiculate, and patients generally continue normal activities. They can be used on all Fitzpatrick skin types and skin colors. These agents may amplify 5-fluorouracil (5-FU) (see JS section) and are therefore preparatory agents for papillary dermal peeling agents (e.g., TCA, 35%) to penetrate deeper.

For decades the theory has been that all superficial peeling agents induce upper dermal "changes" by repeated epidermal sloughs. These changes range from mild edema to marginal increased collagen production to marginal increased elastin production to increased mucin in the papillary dermis. With the emergence of the AHAs these beliefs are again examined. Realistically there are no unbiased studies that compare AHAs with the other preexisting peeling agents. Because the appearance of new upper dermal collagen does not presuppose the production of persistent supportive cross-linked collagen later it is too premature to think that these agents can be used to improve significant dermal pathology. There has been no evidence to suggest that anything other than dermal penetration by peeling solutions or physical modalities such as dermabrasion or laser can alter dermal pathology such as scarring, actinic damage with advanced inflammatory mucinous changes, or rhytides other than the most superficial.

After the application of 70% glycolic acid alone or 35% TCA alone to the volar non–sun-damaged forearm of a single patient (upper epidermal penetration) without any application of sunscreens, tretinoin, and AHAs, the skin biopsy will return to a state of prepeel condition in the span of 2 years.[1] The limitations of superficial peels must be accepted. Marketing hype that raises the expectations of patients and physicians alike must be punctuated with reality.

Qualities Common to Superficial Peeling Agents

Require multiple applications for effectiveness
Penetrate epidermis only with little risk of complication
Do not vesiculate
Can be used on all skin colors and Fitzpatrick skin types
May amplify 5-FU or deeper peeling agents

PEELING TECHNIQUES

Superficial peeling is defined as the application of wounding agents sufficient to wound the epidermis and the papillary dermis, in whole or in part. (See Chapter 2 for details on wounding.) These peels are sometimes called "freshening peels" or "light peels."[2] They are generally performed multiple times to achieve the desired result. By peeling the epidermis weekly, biweekly, or monthly, the appearance of skin may be improved. All Fitzpatrick skin types I to VI may be superficially peeled. The choice of superficial agent depends on the schedule of the patient and the expertise of the physician. Although the ease of application and healing times vary, the net improvement in clinical appearance and epidermal quality is potentially equivalent with most of the modalities mentioned in the box below. The time required to achieve maximal improvement, however, varies considerably between agents.

The slow frost or erythema occurring after application of superficial agents can be minimal because of the wide areas rapidly treated and the varying amounts of epidermal sun damage and sebaceous hyperplasia that impair initial penetration of wounding agents. The addition of sodium fluorescein in a 1:15 ratio to the peeling agents can be helpful in delineating skip areas of epidermal application on viewing with a Wood's light.[3] (See the section on pigmentary dyschromias in Chapter 4.) Alternatively, a low nonpeeling strength of salicylic acid in a 1:5 ratio can be added. After application of TCA, Jessner's solution, or glycolic acid with the fluorescent marker added, a skip area can be easily ascertained as less enhancement with the light (Fig. 5-1). Salicylic acid fluoresces green, and sodium fluorescein fluoresces a yellow-orange. The skip area may be due simply to lack of chemical skin contact on application. Danger of overcoating with these superficial agents is minimal, and spot recoating with this group of compounds is easily performed with good visualization. Peeling agents with preadded fluorescent markers are available commercially. (See Chapter 12.)

Superficial Peeling Agents

Trichloroacetic acid, 10%-25%
Modified Unna's resorcinal paste
Jessner's resorcinol/salicyate/lactate solution
Salicylic acid
Solid carbon dioxide slush
α-Hydroxy acids
Tretinoin
Trichloroacetic acid, 35% (variable—may be epidermal or may enter the papillary dermis)

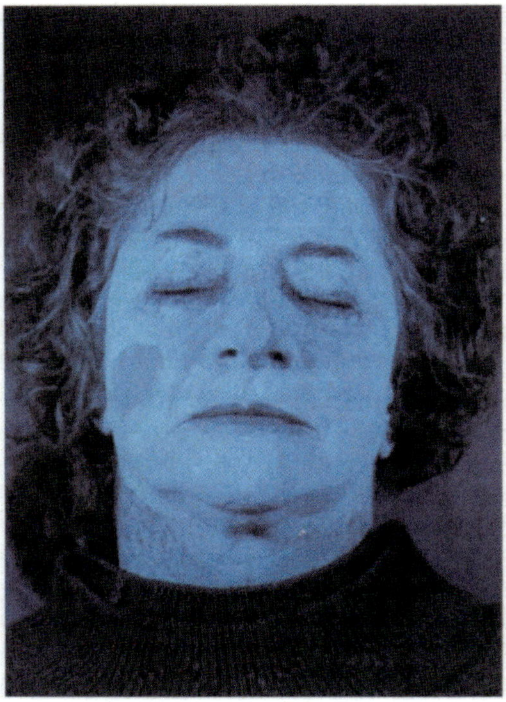

FIG. 5-1. Wood's light examination of the skin after application of Jessner's solution illustrating skip area on right cheek. *(Photo courtesy of Dr. Seth L. Matarasso.)*

Trichloroacetic Acid, 10% to 35%

Trichloroacetic acid (TCA) has been the prototype of chemical peeling since it was described in 1926 by Roberts[4] and used in acne scarring by Monash[5] in 1945. Reactions to and penetration of TCA vary with different regions of body skin. Roberts believed that differences in skin metabolism in different body areas accounted for this variability in reaction. The reaction is slower on the extensor surface than on the flexor surface of the arm, for example, and there is practically no reaction on the sides of the fingers or toes. The leg may require multiple applications or scrubbing with a gauze pad at 50% to 75% strength to acquire frosting, although these strengths may produce complications in this location. We know now that the amount of epidermal and dermal sun damage and the thickness of the epidermis affect the penetration of TCA. Nonfacial location, skin sebaceous units, and any scarring are also relative barriers to absorption. (See the box on the bottom of page 56 in Chapter 4.) Trichloroacetic acid precipitates epidermal proteins and causes necrosis and sloughing of normal and actinically damaged cells. Its acidity is neutralized by serum in the superficial dermal vessels after application, and it is nontoxic to internal body organs.

Preparation and Stability of Trichloroacetic Acid

Because alcoholic solutions of TCA do not penetrate skin, aqueous solutions must be prepared for dermatologic use. The solution should be pharmaceutically prepared by mixing the desired concentration in grams of *United States Pharmacopeia* (USP) TCA crystals with the appropriate volume of distilled water to make 100 cc.[6] For example, 15% TCA is mixed by diluting 15 g of TCA crystals in distilled water up to a total volume of 100 cc. This TCA preparation is expressed as the standard pharmaceutical term **weight-to-volume (wt/vol) method**. If other methods of TCA calculation are employed as in the past (Table 5-1), tremendous variation in concentration is found. Those erroneous methods include mixing grams of TCA with 100 ml of water, dissolving grams of TCA in enough water to make a total weight of 100 g (called the wt/wt method), and diluting fully saturated 100% TCA.

To avoid complications caused by concentration variation, the wt/vol method should be used.[7] Excellent commercial preparations of TCA are available for purchase through Delasco (800-831-6273) and Pharmatopix (800-445-2595).

The crystals are hygroscopic and deliquescent, but once in solution, they do not gather further moisture. Aqueous solutions of TCA are stable for at least 6 months unless contaminated.[8] Preparing fresh TCA solutions more frequently is unnecessary. Analysis has shown that Delasco TCA solutions retain their labeled strength for 24 months. (Delasco Laboratories, Council Bluffs, Iowa, personal communication.) The solution is stable both at room temperature and when refrigerated. Because there is no evidence that TCA is light sensitive, it may be stored in clear or amber glass bottles.[9] Avoid using a wax-covered paper seal or lining for the cap because the action of TCA on the paper can result in an imperfect seal.

TCA will destroy plastic containers made of polycarbonate or low-density polyethylene tetrathalate, which are the most common plastics found in pharmacies. TCA-resistant plastic containers with resistant caps and seals do exist but are not readily available in all pharmacies. The solution should be poured from the master bottle into a small container or shot glass or directly onto a gauze sponge for use.

Trichloroacetic acid is marketed as a paste mask application (ICN Pharmaceuticals, Cosa Mesa, California), but it is more expensive in this form and offers no clear therapeutic advantage over the aqueous application at this time. No clinical or histologic comparisons to other existing superficial peeling agents are available.

Use of Trichloroacetic Acid in Superficial Peeling

For the appearance of the frost in application of **35%** to **50% TCA,** see the section on frosting-application of TCA in Chapter 4.

Strengths of **TCA from 10% to 35%** are used to accomplish superficial chemical peeling. The TCA is applied with a wrung-out damp gauze sponge or two cotton-tipped applicators with smooth strokes. An even redness or slight whitish film is sought, and uneven or unresponsive areas are recoated.

There are two ways to perform superficial TCA peeling. When the solution is applied in the less frequently used traditional method, timing begins when the chemical is first applied to the skin. For the first treatment of 10% or 15%

TABLE 5-1.
Comparative TCA Strengths According to Mixing Methods (Ref. 7)

RANK	METHOD
1 (weakest)	Grams of TCA + 100 cc of water
2	Wt/vol* method
3	Wt/wt method
4 (strongest)	Dilution of saturated solution

*Best, most consistent method for use.

TCA, the treated areas may be sponged with cool water after 1 minute. Treatments are given weekly or biweekly, and the time is increased by 30 seconds each week, up to 2 minutes. After 2 minutes the water dilution is not effective, although it may be continued for patient comfort. The concentration may be increased by 5% if 2-minute peels at the lower strength do not produce the desired effect. Timing is reset at 1 minute again with each increase in concentration. Most patients reach their tolerance and maximum benefit with concentrations between 25% and 35% TCA. The patient monitors the extent and duration of exfoliation and decides with the physician whether to increase the concentration, whether to increase the rubbing or coating, or whether to decrease the interval between treatments.[10] (See the section on dilution in Chapter 4.)

A second method of application involves no water dilution after application. A single coat of 15% to 25% TCA without dilution produces erythema that may persist from 1 hour to 1 day. Several repeat applications at 3-minute intervals at the same sitting produce more erythema and the whitish film, or **frost,** that changes to red after an hour. The skin turns brown the following day. Light exfoliation without vesiculation equivalent to a mild sunburn begins about the second day and lasts from 3 to 6 days. Sunscreens, light moisturizers, and makeup may be applied, and care is minimal and nonrestrictive after peeling (Fig. 5-2).

These superficial peels may be repeated every 7 to 14 days and are relatively safe from complications of permanent depigmentation and scarring. Transient hyperpigmentation can occur. They do not have to be applied sym-

A B

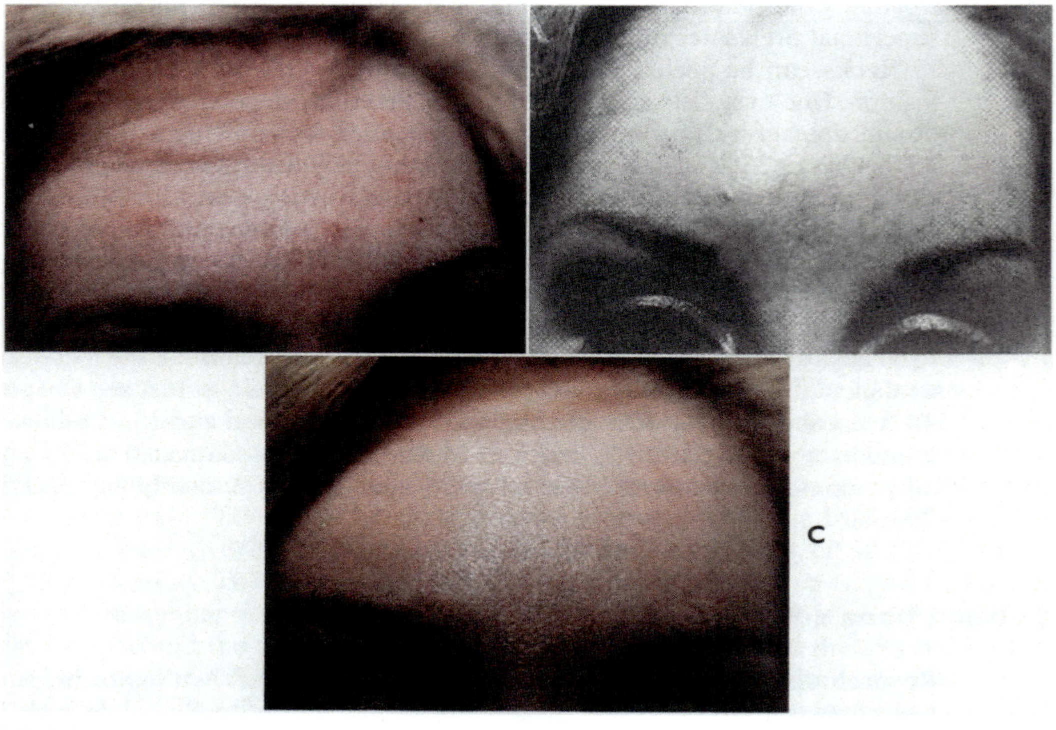

C

FIG. 5-2. A, Mild pigmentation and comedones, forehead. **B,** Resultant erythema 5 days after TCA, 20%. **C,** Clearing after two repeat peels biweekly.

metrically because eventually no line of demarcation is obvious on the skin. Repeeling with slight erythema still present is acceptable and may induce slight papillary dermal change producing a softening of superficial rhytides. This is in contrast to medium-depth dermal peels with which repeeling while postpeel erythema is still present may increase the risk of scarring.

Attempts to ease the discomfort after TCA peeling by pretreatment with topical lidocaine and prilocaine preparations or eutectic mixture of local anesthetics (EMLA) (lidocaine and prilocaine—Astra, Inc., Westborough, Massachuetts) have reduced discomfort but have resulted in skin that frosted more slowly, irregularly, and intensely, increasing the risk of overpeeling. EMLA should not be used especially in concentrations above 30% because the vasoconstriction induced may decrease the dermal fluid available to neutralize TCA, thereby allowing deeper penetration.[11,12] Rebound stinging may occur. Adequate relief of discomfort can usually be obtained with a fan or cool gel pack application.

Excellent results have been obtained in **treating hands and arms** by utilizing superficial repetitive chemosurgery with 20% to 25% TCA every 2 to 3 weeks.[13,14] Either 25% or 35% TCA is applied to individual keratoses until frosting appears, usually in 3 to 5 minutes. After the individual keratoses have been peeled, dropping the concentration 5% to 10% for a light 20% to 25% peel to the entire surface of the dorsal hand without frosting will give the skin a uniform appearance.

The hand or arm peel can be repeated in 14 to 21 days. If much erythema and peeling occur, monthly repetition is acceptable. Water and moisturizer applications to the hands are discouraged for 24 to 48 hours after the peel. The use of tretinoin to pretreat the dorsa of the hands for a minimum of 3 weeks makes this repetitive peeling technique easier for the physician because the frosting time may be reduced. (Fig. 5-3.) (See the section on aftercare for superficial peels later in this chapter.)

Necks can be peeled using low-strength TCA, 20% to 35%, in the same fashion. One may elect to test the area for reactivity depending on the degree of sun damage or previous tretinoin application by applying a tiny drop of 25%, 30%, or 35% TCA. The degree of frosting may determine the application technique and concentration. A lesser degree of frosting even with 30% or 35% TCA suggests that the agent can be applied with a gauze pad rather than a cotton-tipped applicator. (See Case 15 in Chapter 11.) Although a heavier frost with 35% TCA may remove pigmentation quicker than repeated 25% peels, one should always choose the low concentration and locally repeel again in 14 to 60 days after erythema has almost entirely receded because of the increased tendency of neck skin to scar. (For technique to apply 35% TCA see Chapter 4.) A combination of 70% glycolic acid without prepeel defatting followed immediately by TCA, 20%, can also be used for photodamaged necks and other nonfacial locations. (See glycolic acid and TCA combined peel in Chapter 6.)

Modified Unna's Resorcinol Paste

Resorcinol (*m*-dihydroxybenzene) (Fig. 5-4) is isomeric with catechol and hydroquinone.[15] It is structurally and chemically related to phenol. Soluble in water, alcohol, ether, and fats, it possesses, in alkaline solution, a strong affinity to oxygen and is a reducing agent. It has been shown to disrupt the

A 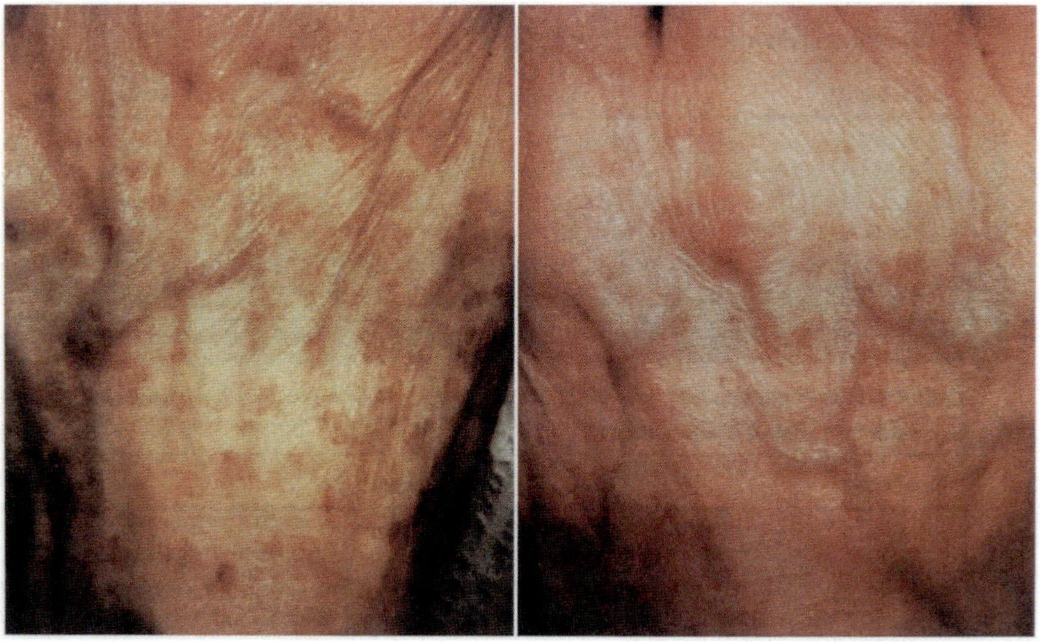 B

FIG. 5-3. A, Lentigos and actinic keratoses of the dorsum of the hand. **B,** Four months after two spot lesion 25% TCA treatments at a 14-day interval, followed by a final uniform peel of the hand for blending. *(From Collins PS: J Dermatol Surg Oncol 15:933-940, 1989. Used by permission.)*

FIG. 5-4. RESORCINOL

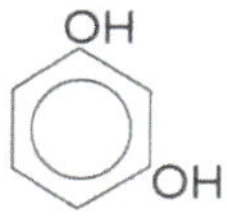

weak hydrogen bonds of keratin and is therefore a keratolytic in concentrations as low as 5%.[16] It can cause a nonspecific irritant reaction or rare contact allergic sensitivity.[17] As a bactericidal agent, resorcinol is one third as active as phenol,[18] which is bactericidal in a 1% dilution in 10 minutes.

Unna described the use of resorcinol paste as a peeling agent in concentrations of 10% to 30% in the late 1800s (Table 5-2). Letessier in France modified his formula to treat acne, melasma, and sun-damaged skin by using 50% resorcinol[19] (Table 5-3). Letessier avoided excessive erythema by using axungia, a derivative of pig fat or lard, added to a clay-bearing soil, ceyssatite, for homogeneity. The term *ceyssatite* is derived from the French town of its origin and is similar to kaolin in American compounding. A test site is performed on skin behind the ear. The paste is left on for 15 minutes, and the test site is evaluated in 4 days for erythema to detect contact sensitivity to resorcinol.

At the time of the peel the patient is placed in the supine position to avoid syncope. Alcohol or acetone may be employed as a degreasing agent. Warming the paste by immersing the plastic container in hot water for 2 to 3 minutes

TABLE 5-2.
Peeling Paste Formula*

INGREDIENT	AMOUNT (g)
Resorcinol	40
Zinc oxide	10
Kaolin	5
Olive oil	12
Wool fat	10
Petrolatum	10

*Adapted from Pascher F: *Dermatologic formulary, New York skin and cancer unit,* New York, 1957, Hoeber-Harper.

TABLE 5-3.
Letessier's Modified Unna's Paste*

INGREDIENT	AMOUNT (G)
Resorcin	40
Zinc oxide	10
Ceyssatite	2
Benzoin axungia	28

*Adapted from Letessier SM: Chemical peel with resorcin. In Roenigk RK, Roenigk HH, editors: *Dermatologic surgery: principles and practice,* New York, 1996, Marcel Dekker.

facilitates its application.[20] The paste is applied on the face with gloved fingers and left on for 25 minutes the first day (Fig. 5-5). The time is increased by 5 minutes each day for 3 days. If the **back** is treated for 3 days, the times should be increased to 50, 60, and 70 minutes, respectively. Less time may be appropriate for more sensitive patients. A burning sensation may increase in intensity during application and after removal of the paste, but it is transient and tolerable. As the paste dries, the skin is wiped with a tongue depressor and dry gauze to leave a gray "resorcin membrane" film. Avoidance of water or cream application to the face for at least 4 to 7 days is recommended to promote dessication. Micronized water sprays may soothe and prevent patients from picking the skin if necessary, however. (See the earlier discussion in the TCA section regarding dessication after superficial peeling.) The use of topical tretinoin by the patient for at least 21 days before this peel increases the reactivity of the skin and decreases the application times needed.[21]

Hernandez Perez[22] in El Salvador employs both a 24% superficial and a 53% medium-strength solution for epidermal peels (Table 5-4). The superficial solution is applied with a brush weekly for 2 or 3 weeks, allowed to remain on the skin for 10 minutes, and increased by 5-minute increments each week. The medium-strength solution is applied for 30 seconds and increased by 30-second increments. The frequency of sessions varies according to the patient's tolerance and schedule. They may be applied weekly for several months to produce varying degrees of epidermal wounding.[23] Eventually, these peels can be performed monthly or every 2 to 3 months. Water avoidance is not imperative, and moisturizers are not prohibited.

Complications of these peels include transient hyperpigmentation, which necessitates the judicious use of sunscreens and hydroquinone before and after peeling. (See the regimen section in Chapter 4.) There has been one

A 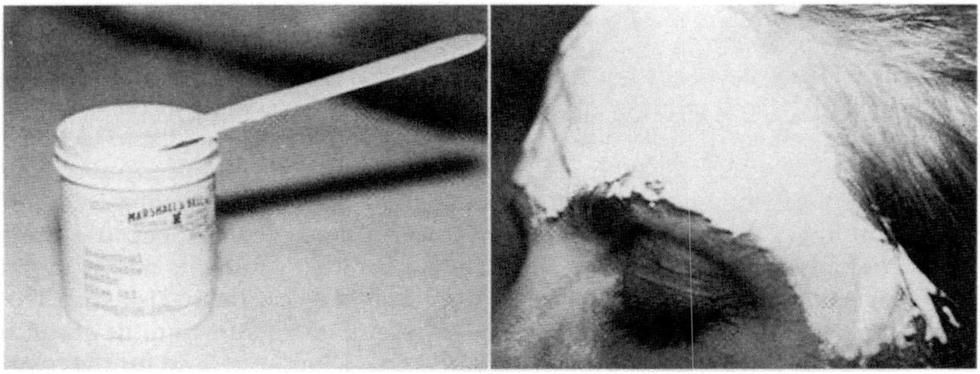 B

FIG. 5-5. A, Peeling paste applied with a tongue blade. **B,** Peeling paste application.

report of dizziness, pallor, cold sweat, tremors, and collapse on final application of a 40% peeling resorcinol paste applied daily for 3 weeks. A possible cause was hypothyroidism induced by the peeling agent.[24] Caution should be exercised in treating children with acne or patients with low body weight. Myxedema associated with ochronosis can be induced by repeated application of resorcinol paste to leg ulcers. Resorcinol in high concentrations exhibits antithyroid activity similar to that of methylthiouracil.[25]

Although methemoglobinemia has been reported with the application of resorcinol paste to open leg ulcers, this has not been reported in chemical peeling of any variety.[26]

These paste peels are not always practical in a dermatologist's busy office because of space or time constraints of both the physician and the patient. They do not, however, generally interrupt a patient's work schedule, and their results are acceptable although attainable by utilizing other equivalent superficial peeling modalities. Aestheticians have performed this type of procedure well for decades. The salons of the 1930s and 1940s were replete with this kind of chemical peel. Today there is a resurgence of their use in salons.

TABLE 5-4.

Epidermal Peeling Formulas*

INGREDIENT	CONTENT (%)
Superficial strength	
Sulfur	24
Resorcin	24
Carboxymethyl cellulose	0.5
Aluminum-magnesium silicate	1.0
Sorbitol	2.5
Glycerine	2.5
Deionized water	45.5
Medium strength	
Resorcin	53
Glyceril monstearate	5
Cetyl alcohol	5
Deionized water	37

*Adapted from Hernandez Perez E: *Am J Cosmet Surg* 7:67-70, 1990.

Jessner's Solution

In addition to peeling pastes, resorcinol has been used in concentrations of 10% to 50% in ether or alcohol to treat hyperkeratotic disorders and to promote peeling.[27] The combination of resorcinol, salicylic acid, and lactic acid in ethanol was formulated by Dr. Max Jessner to lower the concentration and toxicity of any one agent and to enhance the effects as a keratolytic (Table 5-5). Absolute *USP* ethanol is preferred to denatured alchohol because the latter contains ketones, gasoline, and other unknown ingredients added to prevent ingestion. (See Chapter 12 for chemical availability through Delasco.) The syncopal and thyroid-depressing effects of resorcinol and the tinnitus of salicylism can be avoided with this formula. The solution has been used for the treatment of comedones in acne and has been called both the "Combes' peel" after Dr. F.C. Combes and "Horvath's concoction" when used at Walter Reed Army Medical Center in the 1960s.[28,29] Unless the solution is stored in a dark bottle, it may turn a pink color on exposure to air and light and discolor the fingernails yellow-orange.[25]

Application can be light or heavy, varying with the mode of application or number of coats. (See the section on frosting with Jessner's solution in Chapter 4.) Less solution is applied with a wrung-out gauze sponge than with a 1-inch sable brush, which is the author's preference. Sable brushes are available at art supply stores and may be cleaned with povidone-iodine solution (Fig. 5-6). One application or coat of solution may be reapplied in 3 or 4 minutes. Increasing the number of coats applied, beginning with one coat the first week and advancing to three coats the third week, increases the reaction (Fig. 5-7.) Heavier pressure and quantity of solution increase the depth of penetration. A frost that is very white and even occurs and produces prolonged peeling and flaking for as long as 7 or 8 days. Permanent complications are extremely rare. The initial darkening of the skin with subsequent sloughing of portions of the epidermis in the first 2 or 3 days may interfere with the work schedule of some patients. The number of coats applied is determined by the patient's schedule and desire for rapid results. Jessner's solution application produces similar epidermal changes to tretinoin and may be useful in tretinoin-intolerant patients. It can be useful in treating postinflammatory hyperpigmentation, a condition that usually resolves spontaneously with time. The resolution can be accelerated with peeling. (Fig. 5-8). See Fig. 5-21 for patient instructions after peeling.

Contact dermatitis to resorcinol in Jessner's solution may occur and may appear as profound edema out of context to the peel. (See Fig. 11-12.) One week of oral prednisone in rapidly tapering doses is effective treatment.

TABLE 5-5.
Jessner's Solution or Combes' Formula

Resorcinol	14 g
Salicylic acid	14 g
Lactic acid (85%)	14 g
Ethanol (95%) q.s. ad*	100 cc

**q.s. ad,* Quantity sufficient to add up to.

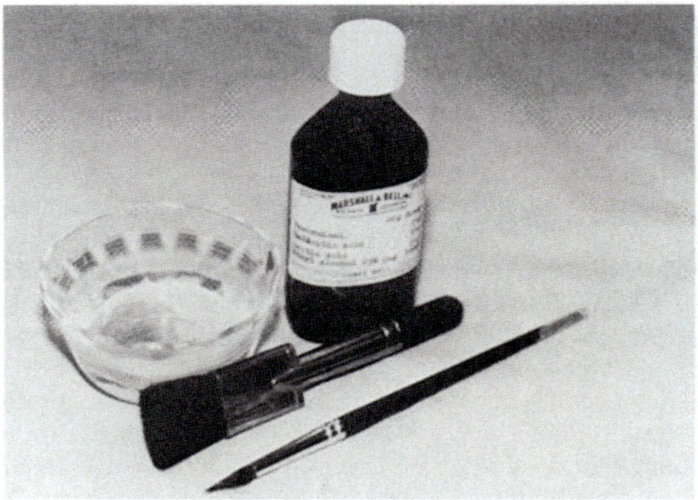

FIG. 5-6. Sable brush for general application or a squirrel brush for periorbital areas for application of Jessner's solution.

A 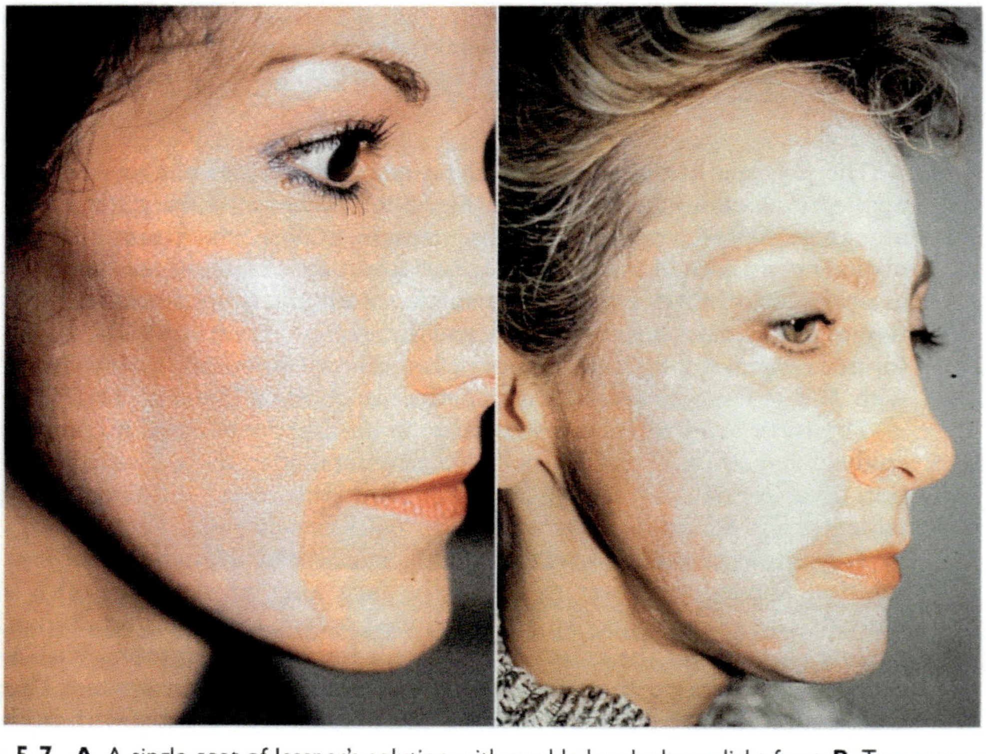 B

FIG. 5-7. A, A single coat of Jessner's solution with a sable brush shows light frost. **B,** Two coats of Jessner's solution after two previous biweekly applications show greater reactivity and frosting.

A 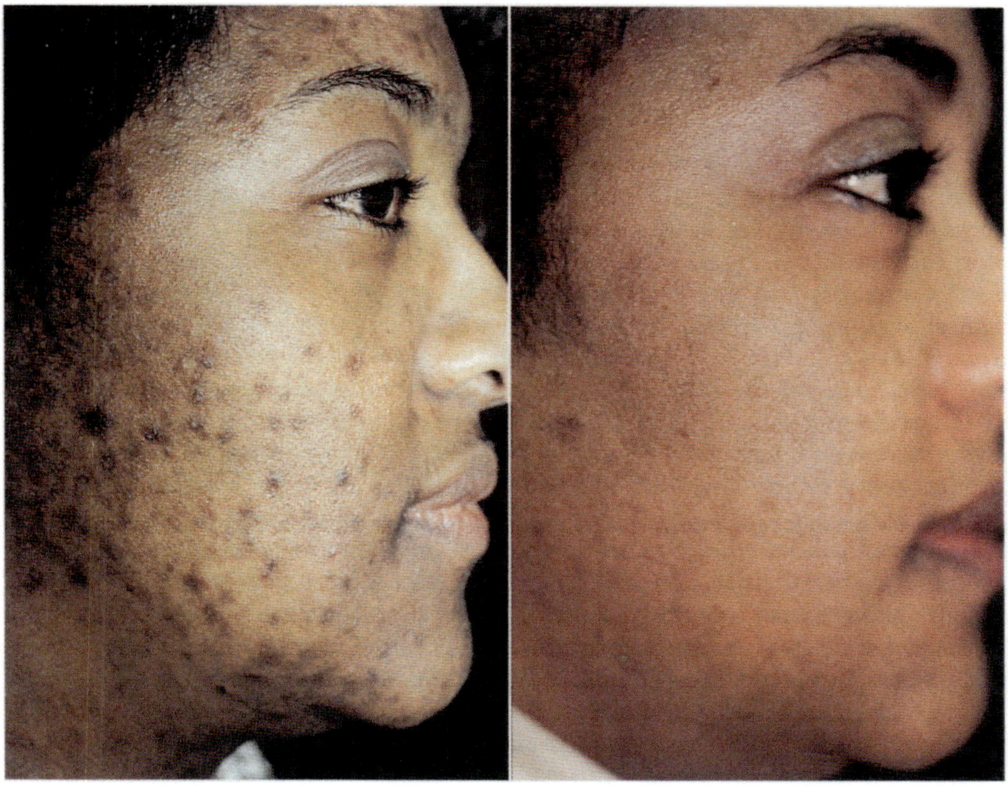 B

FIG. 5-8. A, Fitzpatrick skin type VI with postinflammatory hyperpigmentation of greater than 2 years' duration from acne vulgaris. **B,** After three monthly applications of two coats of Jessner's solution with a sable brush and concomitant use of the regimen outlined in Chapter 4, good response was achieved.

The pigment of the **neck and chest** responds well to one or two monthly applications of Jessner's solution (Fig. 5-9.) However, if the patient picks at any areas during reepithelialization, depigmentation may result and become obvious in an area of poikiloderma. The advantages of using Jessner's solution as opposed to TCA are that only a single solution is needed, timing the duration of application is unnecessary, and dilution or "neutralization" is not performed (Fig. 5-10). Efficacy in more photodamaged patients may be increased with TCA if Jessner's solution is not effective enough. (See Fig. 11-15.)

The lactic acid in Jessner's solution is an α-hydroxy acid. A comparative study of glycolic acid and Jessner's solution detailed in the α-hydroxy acid section later in this chapter revealed equivalent efficacy for melasma, but more patient comfort and predictability with Jessner's solution.

Treatment of actinic keratoses with eight weekly applications of Jessner's solution applied with wet gauze to the face after an acetone scrub in 20 patients was poorly effective and produced only a 15% clearing. Superficial peeling alone is not the treatment of choice for actinic keratoses. With a preceding acetone wipe the combination of Jessner's solution applied liberally with gauze followed immediately by the application directly with a gloved hand of 5% 5-fluorouracil (5-FU) solution to the face on a weekly basis for 8 weeks produced an average of 88% clearing of actinic keratoses. Using 70% buffered glycolic acid with skin contact for 2 minutes instead of JS produced

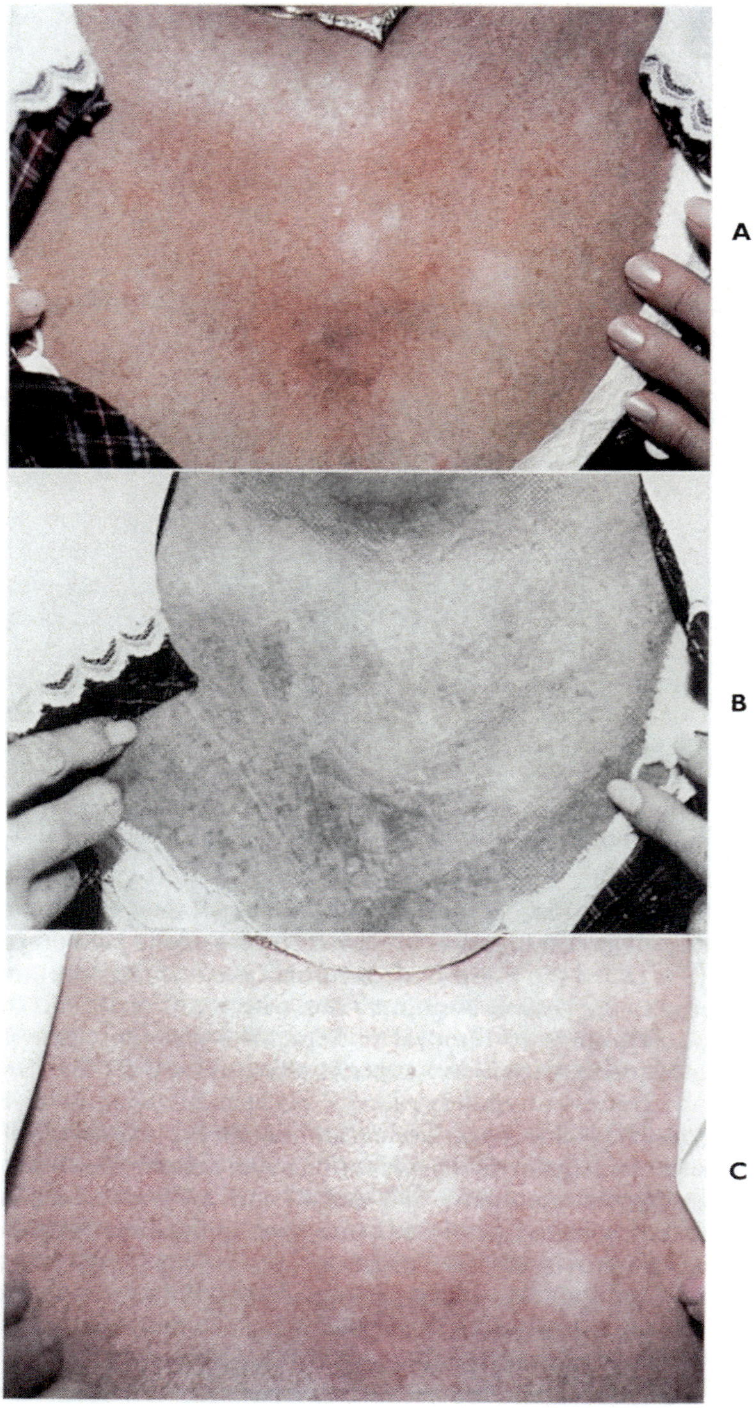

FIG. 5-9. A, Freckles and lentigines with hypopigmented macules from actinic damage and previous keratosis removal on the chest before sable brush application of two coats of Jessner's solution. **B,** Immediately after frosting. **C,** Two months after two monthly applications with resultant fading of freckling and lentigines.

A 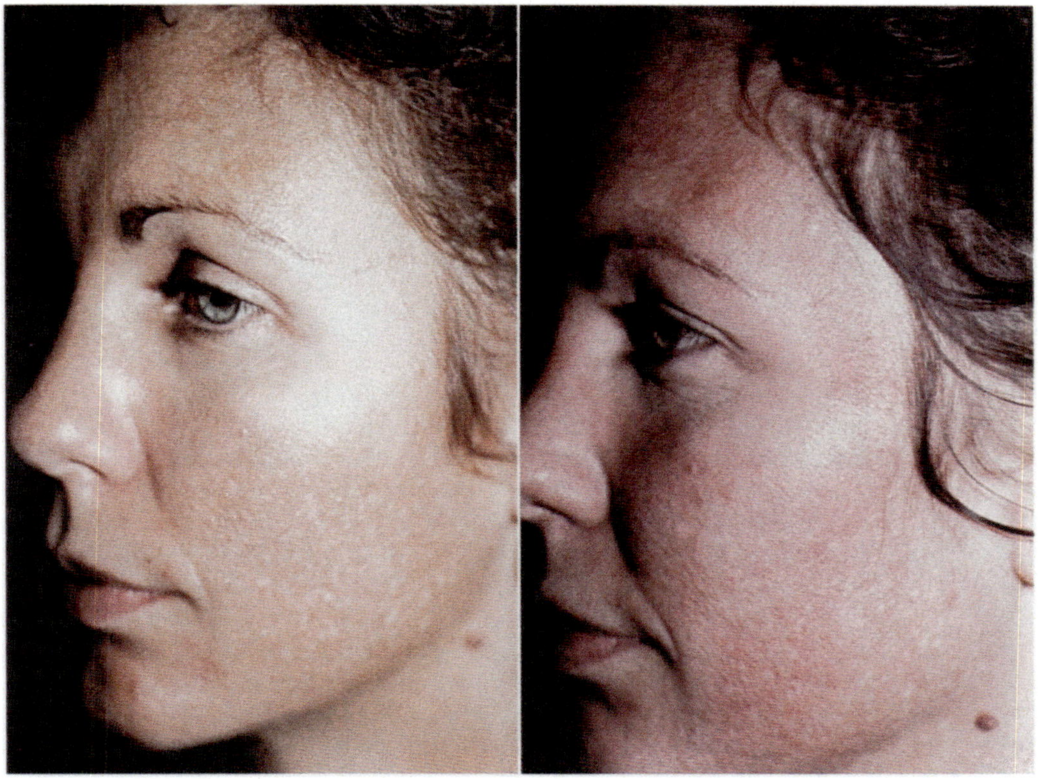 B

FIG. 5-10. A, Superficial variety of melasma responding to two monthly single sable brush applications of Jessner's solution. **B,** Erythema is persistent with chronic tretinoin therapy.

comparable results. The patients did not wash their faces until the following morning. This combination in which JS or glycolic acid amplifies the effects of 5-FU is called the **Fluor-hydroxy pulse peel.**[30] It has the advantages of little irritation to the patient by comparison with traditional 5-FU therapy, the therapeutic advantage of removal of keratoses, and the cosmetic advantage of easing of pigmentation and superficial wrinkles with the JS. The JS loosens the cohesiveness of epidermal cells, perhaps allowing the 5-FU to penetrate more deeply. 5-Fluorouracil is an antimetabolite that inhibits DNA and RNA synthesis and destroys hyperproliferative actinic keratoses. Studies comparing the combination of 5-FU and JS with 5-FU alone are in progress.

For the combination of 5-FU with spot application of pyruvic acid, see the section on pyruvic acid in Chapter 6.

Perspective on Jessner's Solution

Applications of Jessner's solution with a sable brush on a monthly basis for 3 months to the partial face or to the entire face will freshen the skin, improve melasma, slough comedones, and soften very fine rhytides. The frosting that results after each application of increasing coats depends on the amount of tretinoin the patient used before the peel or the success of previous applications of Jessner's solution. If frosting is intense, no further coats need be applied. Edema is minimal unless frosting is maximized, and even then it does not equal that of medium peels. This once-a-month for 3 months

Jessner's peel is the author's preferential superficial peel because it can provide the best results in the least amount of time in this peeling category. The patient may apply makeup at any time, but on the first day after the peel all pigmented lesions will appear darker in color. Peeling without vesiculation occurs in the ensuing 3 to 4 days, and flaking may persist for several more days. Moisturizer and makeup will camouflage changes, but not always completely. As long as the patient's occupation does not require perfection of the skin during healing, this peel of all the superficial peels delivers excellent results in the shortest time interval. (See Figs. 5-8 and 11-6).

Salicylic Acid

Salicylic acid (*ortho*-hydroxybenzoic acid) (Fig. 5-11), a β-hydroxy acid, has been a mainstay in dermatologic therapy for many decades. In concentrations of 3% to 5% it is a keratolytic and an enhancer for topical penetration of other agents. In Whitfield's ointment, 3% salicylic acid is mixed with benzoic acid and has mild potency as a topical fungicide.[31] Ordinarily, salicylic acid alone is not potent enough to act as an adequate wounding agent for chemical peeling.

Swinehart[32] described a method of using 50% salicylic acid ointment under occlusion to peel lentigines, pigmented keratoses, and actinically damaged skin from the dorsa of the hands and forearms of 11 patients. This method was based on 81 patients treated by Aronsohn in 1984.[33] Pretreating the patient's skin with tretinoin, 0.1%, thoroughly degreasing the skin with alcohol and acetone, and pretreating large keratoses with 20% TCA will enhance penetration of the salicylic acid formula. (See the box on page 88.) One or two drops of croton oil may be added to this formula as an option for enhanced effect (Fig. 5-12). The salicylic acid paste is applied to the affected areas with a tongue blade after cotton balls have been placed between the fingers to protect the palms. Plastic wrap followed by a gauze roll wrap secures the ointment in place on the arms. The dressing is kept dry for 48 hours and then removed. The resulting epidermal desquamation and maceration heal with the application of antibiotic ointment or biosynthetic dressing within 4 weeks. Ninety percent of the cutaneous lesions resolve, and no scarring has been noted.

Patients may experience excessive salicylate absorption resulting in ringing in the ears, muffled hearing, dizziness, or headache several hours after the dressing has been in place. Increased water intake or early bandage removal may ameliorate this mild salicylism. The bulky dressing is a disadvantage, and the hands and forearms may be treated separately.

A peeling solution of 35% salicylic acid in ethanol has been applied to the face with cotton-tipped applicators for improvement of comedones and fading of pigment.[34] Smoothing of the skin surface and reduction of fine rhytides has

FIG. 5-11. SALICYLIC ACID

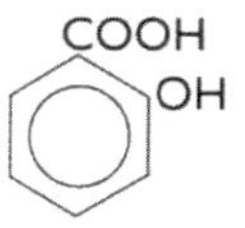

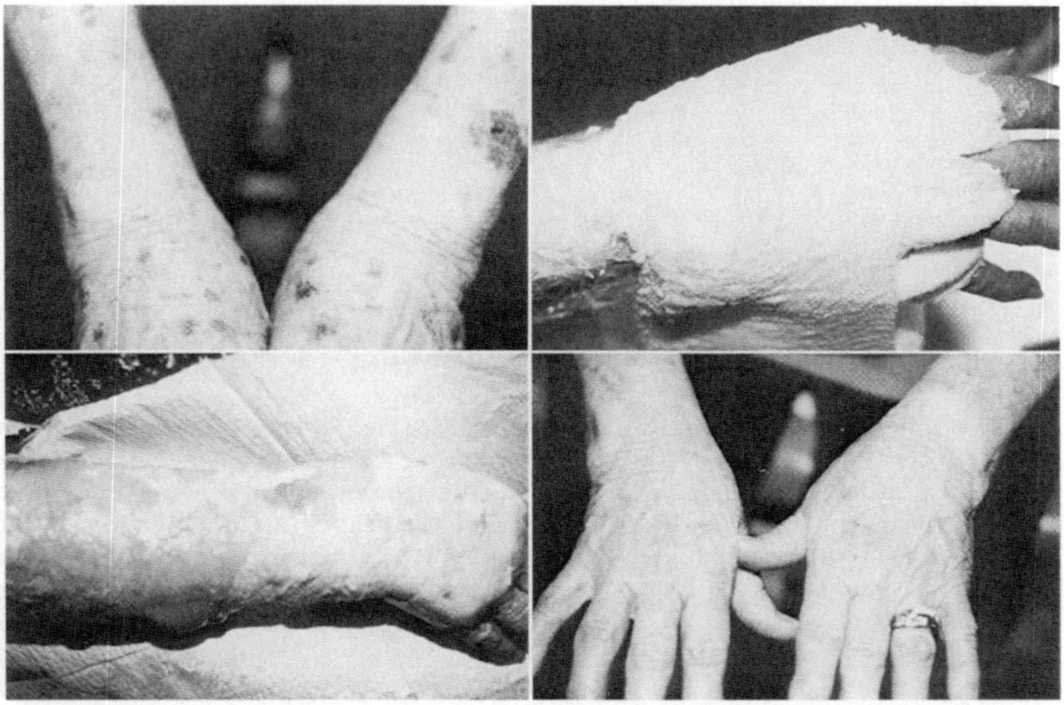

FIG. 5-12. A, Multiple actinic keratoses on the back of the hand and arms before salicylic acid treatment. **B,** Bandage dressing. **C,** Maceration after dressing removal. **D,** Two months later. *(Courtesy of Dr. J.M. Swinehart.)*

Salicylic Acid Ointment

Salicylic acid powder, *USP,* 50%*
Methyl salicylate, 16 drops
Aquaphor, q.s. ad†, 4 oz
Croton oil, 1-2 drops (optional)

*Available from Dermatologic Lab and Supply, Council Bluffs, Iowa.
†*q.s. ad,* Quantity sufficient to add up to.

been noted by Silflo replicas and photography. The solution causes mild stinging for 1 to 3 minutes followed by superficial anesthesia to light touch. After 5 minutes of air drying, the face is washed with water. Peeling is delayed, beginning from day 3 to 5 and continuing for 10 days. Erythema and edema are minimal, and the peel can be repeated every 2 to 4 weeks. Epidermolysis does not occur histologically, and overcoating is remote. Comparisons to other superficial agents have not been evaluated.

Solid Carbon Dioxide

Solid carbon dioxide (dry ice) is a physical modality for peeling and not a true chemical peeling agent. Its properties allow it to be used alone or to amplify chemical peeling agents. The agent has been used in dermatology for the treatment of acne and other cutaneous disorders for over 75 years. Carbon dioxide snow is prepared either by releasing the gas from a cylinder through a

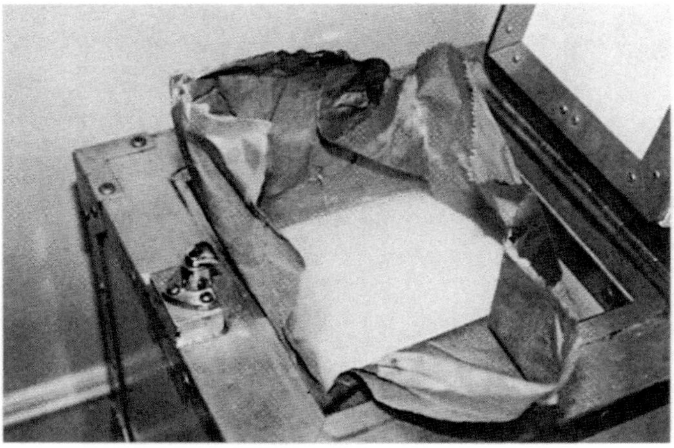

FIG. 5-13. Ten-pound solid CO_2 in an unrefrigerated storage chest.

chamois leather bag and then transferring it to wood or Bakelite-funneled tubes in which the snow is hammered hard or by means of a "Sparkle" machine in which individual cylinders discharge the gas through a small opening into a collecting tube.[35] Dry ice may be purchased from ice plants, but other sources include ice cream manufacturers, dairies, food packing plants, fishing bait supply houses, and pharmaceutical supply companies. Solid blocks at −78.5° C can be delivered to offices twice weekly and stored in standard ice chests or coolers (Fig. 5-13). Five- or ten-pound blocks of ice are broken to hand size for slushing in acetone, ethyl acetate, or sulfur with or without alcohol before application to the skin.[36-38] Acetone serves to dissolve sebum and lowers the temperature of the CO_2 by accelerating the change of CO_2 from a solid to a gas.[39] If the snow is released from a cylinder of gas in the physician's office, hand packing to a hard solid form may be difficult and therefore less effective in performing an adequate medium-depth peel, but in superficial peeling it is efficacious. (See the section on CO_2 plus TCA in Chapter 6.)

We prefer to wrap the dry ice in a small hand towel and dip it in an approximate 3:1 solution of acetone and alcohol, which serves to facilitate application and kill surface bacteria.[40] Either an individual lesion or the entire face may be easily slushed by using slow and even strokes and varying epidermal depth by the pressure of application. Five to eight seconds of moderate pressure per acne area is adequate to freeze comedones (Fig. 5-14). The dry ice is dipped into the solution multiple times during the treatment to allow easy slippage on the skin.[41] The skin reaction ranges from mild erythema to vesiculobullae formation. This treatment speeds removal of comedones and acne resolution. Patients may ask to be "iced" and enjoy the results of this treatment alone. Less destructive than liquid nitrogen, which is over twice as cold at −186° C, the margin of safety of solid CO_2 is wide. It may induce transient hyperpigmentation in dark-skinned individuals, but hard pressure and freezing the skin solid for 12 to 15 seconds has not produced scarring or hypopigmentation in nonpoikilodermatous skin in our experience of over 3000 cases. Care should always be exercised to apply less pressure when peeling over bony prominences. (See the section on cold sensitivity or cold urticaria in Chapter 8.)

Solid CO_2 is used in the BioMedic Micropeel system, a proprietary peel system. Shaving of the skin is followed by the application of 15% to 30% gly-

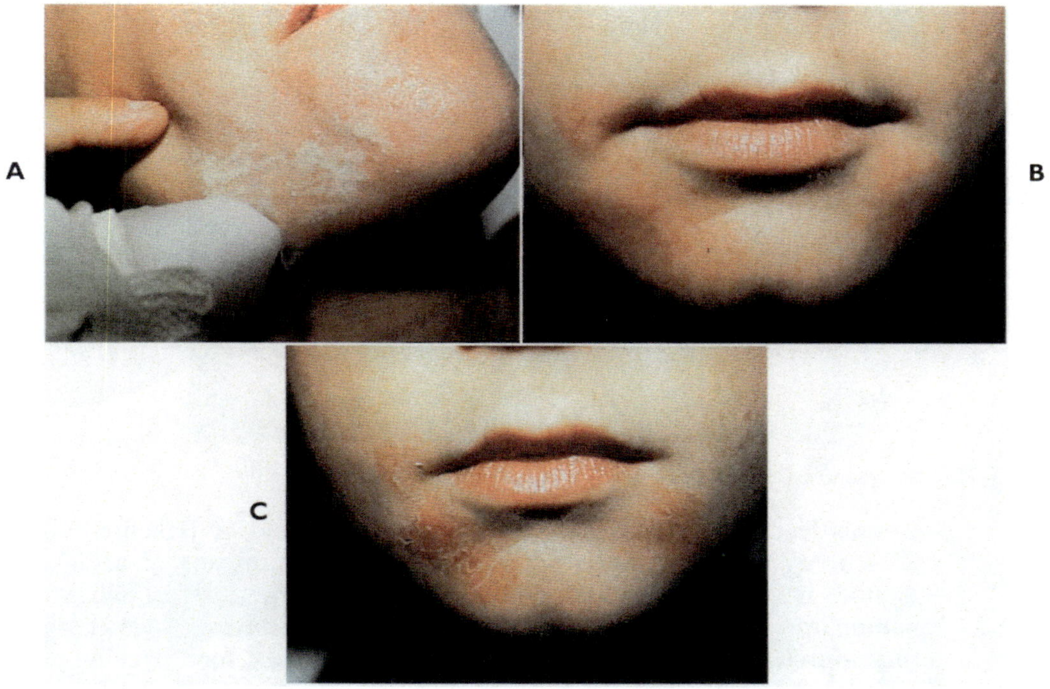

FIG. 5-14. A, Solid CO_2 slushed application, moderate pressure, 8 seconds, for comedones. **B,** Three hours later, microvesiculation. **C,** Two days later, erythema and scaling.

colic acid or a resorcinol combination and by application of selective solid CO_2 slush in a chamois bag. The system is accompanied by and marketed with an extensive product line.[42,43] No clinical or histologic comparisons to other existing superficial peeling agents are available. One case of scarring has occurred allegedly from a Baker's phenol peel performed 3 days after this combination was applied to the face indicating that the patient had sustained substantial epidermal alteration with the initial peel.[44]

Solid CO_2 is a superlative agent for facial and nonfacial neurotic excoriations or acne excoriée. A moderate application to excoriated areas will serve to keep the patient's hands off the lesions long enough to heal and provide inspiration for the patient not to touch the areas for a variable length of time. The result obtained with the application of any superficial or medium-depth chemical agent to excoriated areas is unpredictable in a patient with a tendency to pick at and prematurely remove exfoliating skin.[45,46] Postinflammatory pigmentation as an indication in excoriators may clear with peeling treatments, but it may also worsen if the patient picks at the skin during healing. In our experience the use of a physical agent such as solid CO_2 is less risky in these patients and almost always effective (Fig. 5-15).

α-Hydroxy Acids

α-Hydroxy acids (AHAs)[47-49] are naturally occurring but synthetically mass-produced carboxylic acids that are found in many foods. The AHAs include glycolic, lactic, malic, citric, and tartaric acids. The two shortest carbon chain acids, glycolic (2-hydroxyethanoic) and lactic (2-hydroxypropanoic), are the most commonly used in dermatology (Fig. 5-16). **Glycolic acid** is present in

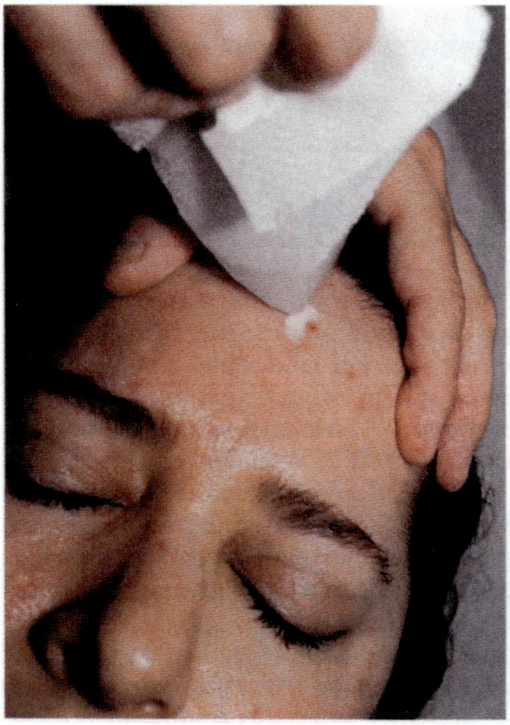

FIG. 5-15. Application of moderate pressure solid CO_2 to excoriations and mildly to surrounding skin of the cosmetic unit promotes healing and discourages patient's tendency to further excoriate during healing.

sugar cane, lactic acid in sour milk, citric acid in fruits, malic acid in apples, and tartaric acid in grapes. (See the box on page 94). Ancient youth remedies such as sour milk baths to smooth the skin or stale wine application to the face for wrinkles may have worked because of their AHA content (lactic and tartaric acid, respectively). Gluconic, mandelic, and benzilic acids are AHAs of larger molecular size. The latter two are derivatives of glycolic acid. Glycolic acid is highly soluble in water, and a saturated solution is approximately 80%. Full-strength 70% glycolic acid, the AHA of smallest molecular size, will cause epidermolysis in 3 to 7 minutes, depending on skin type and thickness of the stratum corneum. **Lactic acid,** 70%, is slower to cause epidermolysis. It is converted physiologically to pyruvic acid, α-keto acid. (See the section on pyruvic acid in Chapter 6.) Five percent to 20% concentrations of lactic acid cause corneocyte detachment and resultant desquamation at the lower, newly forming levels of the stratum corneum.

FIG. 5-16. ALPHA-HYDROXY ACIDS

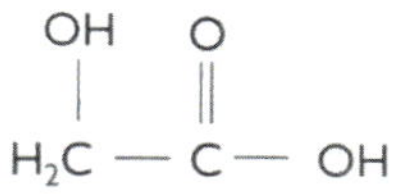

Glycolic acid
(2-Hydroxyethanoic acid)

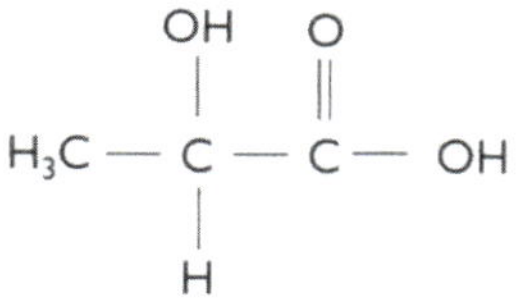

Lactic acid
(2-Hydroxypropanoic acid)

Common α-Hydroxy Acids—Natural Occurrence

Glycolic—sugar cane
Lactic—sour milk
Malic—apples
Citric—fruits
Tartaric—grape wine

Histologic studies of xerotic skin treated daily for 3 weeks with 8% glycolic acid **cream application** in pHs ranging from 3.25 to 4.4 revealed a compacted stratum corneum, a thicker epidermis, and greater deposition of dermal collagen and dermal mucin of an undetermined amount as the acidity of the preparation decreased.[50] Similar results were observed in tests in which the pH was held constant at 3.25 with concentrations ranging from 3.3% to 13%. This suggests that both decreasing acidity and increasing concentration in glycolic acid creams are factors in epidermal reorganization and collagen and mucin deposition. Higher cream concentration suggests faster results if pH is constant. However, application with **glycerin** produced similar changes in the epidermis and dermis.

A comparison of 12% ammonium lactate lotion (pH 4.40) and 8% glycolic acid lotion (pH 4.40) applied to xerotic skin in the same fashion for 3 weeks revealed a similar 19% increase in epidermal thickness and increased papillary dermal mucin deposition by 50%.[51] (See Chapter 2 for detailed light microscopic and ultrastructural effects of AHA cream on skin.)

It has been suggested that more dermal mucin or dermal collagen synthesis may be induced by application of AHA creams with higher pH than lower pH for 3 weeks. The M.D. Forte glycolic acid creams are based on this premise of high concentration and higher pH, but the actual concentration of glycolic acid in some glycolic acid compound mixtures is only 60% to 70% of the listed compound percent.[52] However, acid concentration rather than pH may be the chief factor in achieving more rapid results. The effects of topical treatment longer than 3 weeks are not well documented, but they cannot be assumed to be maintained, especially because it is known that the epidermal effects of continued topical tretinoin rebound or reverse in 1 year. (See the section on tretinoin in Chapter 2.) The amount of "new" dermal collagen synthesis, however, is not a reflection of tensile strength or mature collagen with intermolecular cross-linking.[53] The exact significance and endurance of the increased dermal collagen and mucin seen in response to AHA application is unknown.

Definitions

Chemically the **partial neutralization** of the acid by the addition of a base such as sodium bicarbonate or sodium hydroxide produces a salt plus water with a resulting weaker acid of higher pH. **Buffered solution** is a partially neutralized solution that resists pH changes when an acid or base is added.[54] Partial neutralization of glycolic acid with ammonium hydroxide does not produce a buffered preparation (Table 5-6). There is a greater risk of dermal penetration when unbuffered formulations of glycolic acid with lower pHs of less than 1.0 are used. Increasing the concentration of acid to induce more rapid clinical and histologic results will chemically decrease the pH. The pK_a, the relative strength of the acid to base measured by its proton dissociation, is the more appropriate parameter for evaluating acidity rather than pH, but the pK_a

TABLE 5-6.
pH of Selected Commercially Available 70% Glycolic Acid Peel Products with pH under 2.75.*

PRODUCT	pH†
Glyderm (citrates)	0.5
Delasco	0.5
Neostrata	0.6
Dermatopics	1.2
Humitech	1.3
M.D. Formulations	2.75
Jan Marini	2.75

*Adapted from Rubin M: AHA Symposium, Orlando, Fla, Dec 1994.
†The higher values indicate partial neutralization and less free acid availability (bioavailality). Variation in free acid depends on preparation method from saturated solution versus from crystals.

is not directly associated with potency of the biological action.[55] The pK_a really has little relevancy for chemical peeling but is a measure of the dissimilarities between different acids at different concentrations and pHs. The pH is also a function of the vehicle as well as the acidity of the compound. **Although irritancy of a product is often directly related to lower pH, vehicle irritancy must be considered also and may change the credence of pH as a sole indicator of patient intolerance.** There is not a truly adequate method to ascertain the actual available free acid (bioavailability). Higher pHs reflect less bioavailability of AHA relative to the labeled concentration.

Histologic comparison of 50% and 70% glycolic acid peels using varying pHs in two patients suggests that both a more acidic pH below 2.0 and a higher concentration are two factors to induce more skin necrosis in peeling. With AHA cream application of less acidic pH, increased dermal mucin deposition has been noted. Application of this study of AHA creams to repetitive peeling is uncertain, but it may suggest less dermal benefit to increased direct tissue damage.[56]

The factors that determine whether AHA peels result in desquamation or epidermolysis are the concentration of the acid, the pH, the degree of buffering or neutralization with sodium bicarbonate, the vehicle formulation, the frequency of application, the conditions of delivery, the amount of acid delivered to the skin over a given period, and most important, the duration of time that the acid remains on the skin.(See the box below.)

Factors Affecting Glycolic Acid Penetration

Acid concentration(%)
pH Bioavailability
Amount of buffering or neutralization to salt
Type of formulation—gel, liquid, lotion, or cream
Frequency of application
Skin condition before application
Volume of acid applied to the skin
Duration of time acid remains on the skin

Application Technique of Glycolic acid

Suggested starting application times with 50% and 70% unbuffered glycolic acid are listed in Table 5-7.[57] There is evidence that the 50% concentration will penetrate to half the depth of the 70%, but it takes twice the time and is less efficient. Variation in these application times based on the patient's skin and sebaceousness and also the preparation of acid will be generally harmless and may simply produce a little more erythema and scaling. This peeling is very forgiving, and complications are rare. When partially neutralized products with pH greater than 2.5 are used, much longer exposure times are required.

The skin is first cleaned gently with a defatting agent in the manner described in Chapter 4. However, glycolic acid peels become more unpredictable after overzealous scrubbing. A gentle wipe with acetone or alcohol after makeup has been removed is adequate instead of the extensive defatting that is suggested with TCA peels. This is especially true when treating patients with atopic skin or with sensitive, less sun-damaged but melasma-laden skin in Fitzpatrick type V patients. The agent is applied rapidly, covering the entire face within about 20 seconds with a large cotton applicator to the facial cosmetic units in any order desired. After the desired time for the indication has elapsed as indicated by a timer, or alternatively if severe erythema occurs first, the AHA is wiped off with copious water-soaked gauze. Because all times are approximate the exact moment during the application to set the timer is not crucial. The patient then goes to the sink and splashes water on his or her face to ensure complete removal of the acid. Purified water or neutralizers with sodium bicarbonate marketed to the physician have no advantage over water as long as all acid is removed thoroughly from all rhytides and cosmetic units. Peels may be repeated weekly, biweekly, or monthly.

Specific Application for Indications: Acne, Melasma, and Wrinkles

Seventy percent glycolic acid can be applied to **acne** lesions or the lesions of pseudofolliculitis barbae with a cotton ball by using a gloved hand or with a large cotton-tipped applicator (Fig. 5-17). After 3 to 5 minutes, acne papules begin to blanch, and acne pustules and comedones are "unroofed" (Fig. 5-18). Rinsing with water or 1% sodium bicarbonate prevents further penetration of the glycolic acid. Ensuing erythema fades in several hours followed by inconspicuous desquamation. If exposure time is increased to provoke epidermolysis, erythema may persist, denudation may occur, and the stratum corneum may separate in a sheet.

Glycolic acid can be used to treat **melasma** in all Fitzpatrick skin types. Its mechanism of action may be to allow more effective penetration of bleach and tretinoin with continued repetitive peels. This is supported by Lawrence and

TABLE 5-7.

Suggested Starting Duration of Glycolic Acid Peel Contact for Varying Indications

INDICATION	% GLYCOLIC ACID (pH = 2.5 OR LESS)	TIME (MINUTES)
Acne	50-70	1-3
Melasma	50-70	2-4
Actinic keratoses	70	5-7
Fine wrinkles	70	4-8
Solar lentigines	70	4-6
Back or chest (any indication)	70	5-10

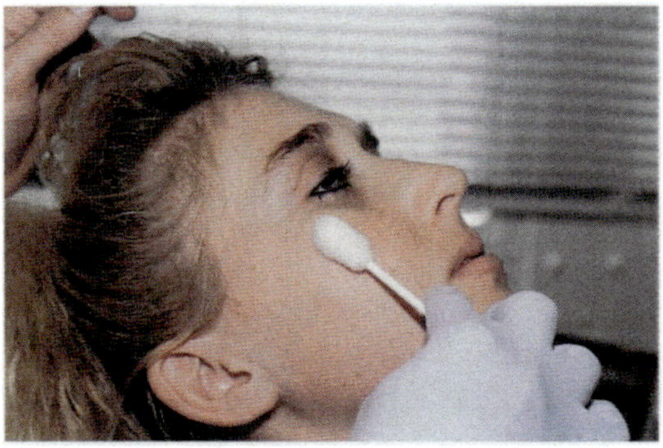

FIG. 5-17. Application of glycolic acid. A large cotton-tipped applicator or a cotton ball in a gloved hand may be used to apply glycolic acid.

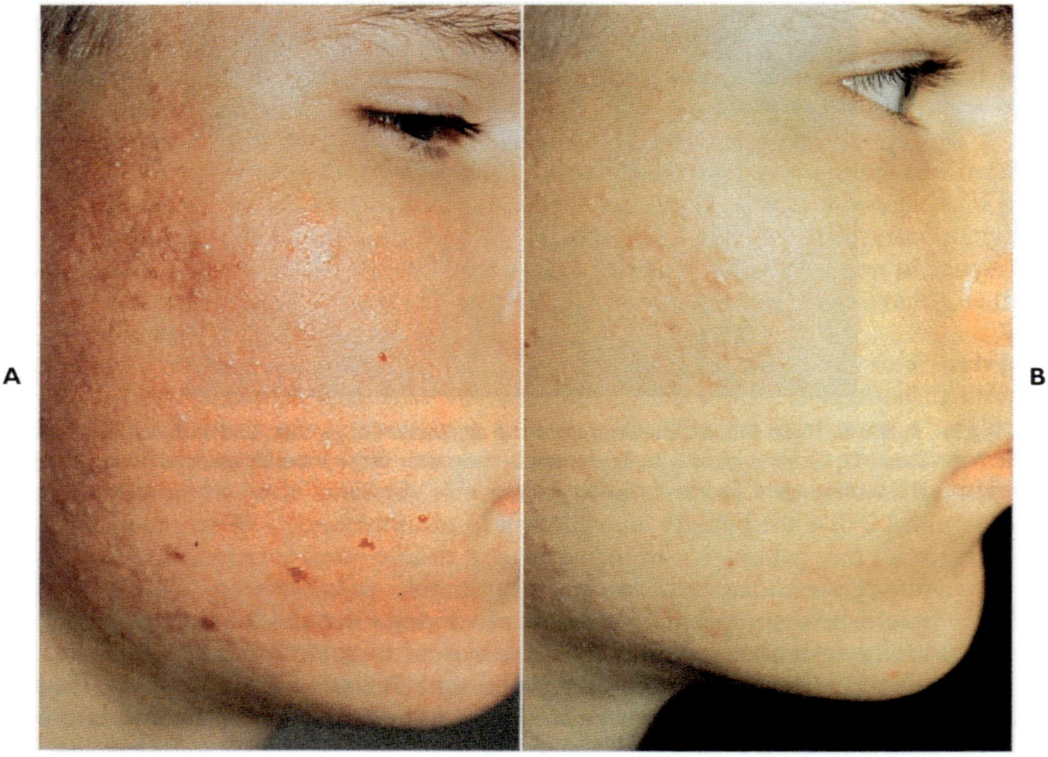

FIG. 5-18. A, Four minutes after application of 70% glycolic acid for comedones and pustules. Note "unroofing" of pustular lesions with pinpoint hemorrhage. **B,** One month later with improvement in the number of comedones and pustules.

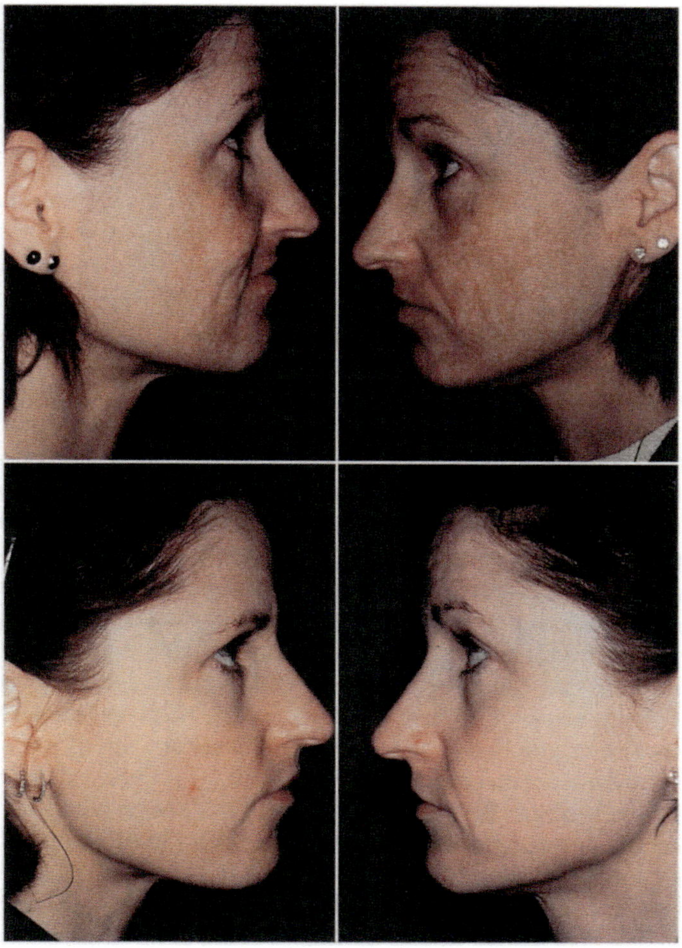

FIG. 5-19. **A** and **B,** Right and left cheeks before the application of glycolic acid and Jessner's solution, respectively. **C** and **D,** Commensurate improvement is seen after three monthly peels, allowing increased penetration of bleaching agent. See text. *(Photos courtesy of Dr. Sue Ellen Cox and Dr. Naomi Lawrence.)*

co-workers' study[58] of 16 patients of varying Fitzpatrick skin types from II to VI, 12 of whom were previously resistent to topical therapy. Melasma was treated with 70% unbuffered glycolic acid (Delasco—Council Bluffs, Iowa) on the right cheek and Jessner's solution on the left cheek in the standard application described in this textbook for three peels spaced 1 month apart. They were treated with tretinoin alone for 2 weeks before peeling and with tretinoin and 4% hydroquinone gel after reepithelialization. Evaluation with colorimetry and by blinded clinical observation using a melasma area and severity index (MASI) demonstrated equivalent substantial statistically significant improvement with both modalities.[59] Ten of the sixteen patients reported more pain with glycolic acid, and only four out of sixteen found the Jessner's peel more painful. The Jessner's peel was better tolerated overall (Fig. 5-19).

Inadvertent overreaction occurred with glycolic acid only and not with Jessner's solution, possibly because of prepeel overscrubbing with acetone. Glycolic acid is inherently more unpredictable than Jessner's solution, and occasionally deeper peeling occurs unexpectedly. Jessner's solution is much less likely than glycolic acid to be influenced by exogenous parameters and is better tolerated by patients. This is supported by the clinical experience of many dermatologists.[60]

Both modalities used in this study worked in the treatment of melasma by decreasing the MASI by 63% and increasing light reflectance by approximately 3 units. When compared with two previous studies[59,61] in which tretinoin alone was used to treat melasma, this study showed that improvement with peels occurred in a much shorter time period (3 vs. 10 months). A paired comparison trial has greater credence than attempting to compare randomized studies done with different modalities at different times and places. The peels alone have improved the penetration of the topical treatment with tretinoin and hydroquinone applied between and after peeling. They have also increased the effectiveness of the bleach in the dermis by stripping away the upper epidermis. Because no topical treatment with glycolic acid was used in the study, the bleach is the critical cream irrespective of adjuvant. Topical glycolic acid can be used between peels but is not critical for good results.

In a related study, 20 patients with melasma and Fitzpatrick skin type III through V were compared clinically and with colorimetry after the daily facial application of 2% hydroquinone/10% glycolic acid partially neutralized gel and tretinoin over 5 months.[62] When three weekly 70% glycolic acid peels were performed on a subgroup using this regimen there was more rapid improvement in the group receiving the peels.

In summary, the studies show that glycolic acid peels alone can improve melasma with the use of hydroquinone/tretinoin creams. Glycolic acid peels improve the efficacy of the combination of hydroquinone/tretinoin/glycolic acid creams alone. Whether glycolic acid peels alone improve melasma any better than glycolic acid peels and glycolic acid creams concurrently, without the use of bleaching agents, is not known.

The same concentration of glycolic acid can be used to treat **wrinkles**. After removing cutaneous oils with acetone, the acid is applied to the skin with a damp gauze sponge or a large cotton-tipped applicator. The glycolic acid is rinsed off at the commencement of erythema. This procedure may be repeated weekly, biweekly, or monthly. One study of 100 patients treated with a 50% to 70% concentration of glycolic acid applied for 3 to 7 minutes every 2 to 3 weeks for three or four total applications concluded that there was moderate improvement in skin texture and mild to moderate improvement in wrinkles and pigmentation, comparable to that seen with tretinoin.[55,57] A 50% to 70% solution of glycolic acid does not vesiculate and causes less epidermal and papillary dermal damage than does 30% TCA. A double-blind study of the application of 50% unbuffered, pH 1.2, glycolic acid gel applied weekly for 4 weeks to the face and hands showed similar clinical results.[64]

Between AHA peels patients incorporate 5% to 15% AHA creams into their skin regimen once or twice daily. Some elegant formulations are available, including Aqua Glycolic facial cream (10%), body lotion (14%), and astringent (11%), all pH 4.4 (Herald Pharmacal, Inc.); NeoStrata 15% nonprescription products (NeoStrata Co., Inc.); M.D. Formulations and M.D. Forte—up to 14% creams for sale in physicians' offices (Herald Pharmacal, Inc.); prescription products such as Viquin Forte (4% hydroquinone and 12% glycolic acid—ICN Pharmaceuticals) or Lac-Hydrin, 12% (Westwood-Bristol Meyers/Squibb).[65] (See Chapter 12). A reduction in fine wrinkles may be apparent with 2 to 12 months of repetitive peels and concomitant daily application of these AHA-containing creams (Fig. 5-20). Some patients report that their skin feels

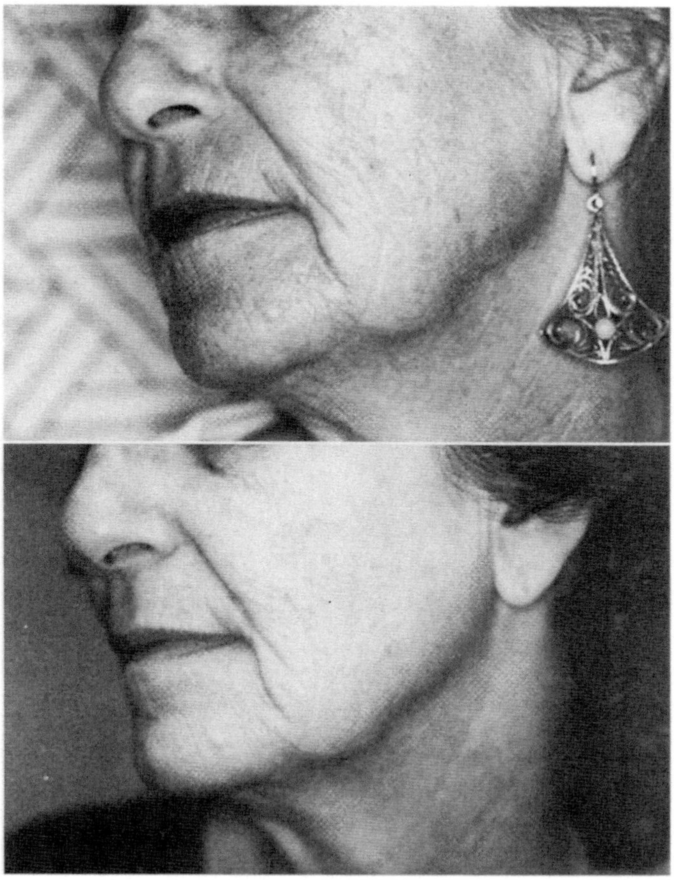

FIG. 5-20. A, Prior treatment with glycolic acid peel. **B,** Improvement in mild wrinkling and solar lentigines after 70% glycolic acid applied for 3 minutes with continuous daily 10% acid lotion. *(Courtesy of Dr. Lawrence S. Moy and Dr. Howard Murad.)*

smoother and softer even though objective changes may not be assessible. There is a prominent placebo effect in trials for cosmetic therapeutic agents based on potential hope for beauty that the trial represents. Piacquadio and co-workers[66,67] could see no definite histologic changes 4 months after monthly 70% unbuffered glycolic acid peels for 3 to 6 minutes with concomitant 10% glycolic acid cream application in 12 patients. Clinical improvement in fine wrinkles and skin roughness occurred in patients who supplemented their peels with 10% glycolic acid lotion concurrently.[66,67] This study underlines the subtle changes in histology that sometimes occur with the AHAs. Monthly peels alone or a concentration of 10% cream application may either not be frequent enough or not strong enough to produce histologic change for wrinkles. Melasma responds, however, to monthly peeling, as noted.

The effectiveness of the peels and creams depends on the many factors discussed herein, and the lack of standardization between the myriad of companies promoting the AHAs makes objective scientific data difficult to attain.

A mixture of glycolic acid and citric acid (a "glycocitrate") has been marketed as less irritating and possibly superior to other glycolic products, but these claims have yet to be substantiated.[54]

Additional Uses of α-Hydroxy Acids

The AHAs can potentiate 5-FU application in the fluorhydroxy pulse peel as discussed earlier in the section on Jessner's solution. Topical 8% glycolic acid also provides a photoprotective effect to pretreated skin yielding an SPF of approximately 2.4. In addition, when 12% glycolic acid is applied to skin after sun irradiation, it acclerates resolution of erythema. Hypothetically glycolic acid may act as an antioxidant because its molecular structure is similar to the antioxidant ascorbic acid. Alternatively, glycolic acid may chelate free iron in the skin and thus reduce free radical production.[68] It may also enhance dermal perfusion similar to other peeling agents.

In the guinea pig model, if 70% glycolic acid remains on the skin for 15 minutes, a dermal wound may be induced.[55] Scarring has been reported in a human subject when 70% glycolic acid was not properly washed off after 3 minutes in the treatment of melasma (personal communication, ASDS Annual Meeting, Orlando, Florida, March 1991.) The length of time that the acid is left on the skin is an important factor in the use of glycolic acid as a peeling agent.

Perspective on AHAs

1. The federal Food and Drug Administration (FDA) monitors the safety and toxicity of AHA creams. The number of reactions reported to FDA concerning AHAs have been small compared with the frequency of their use. The FDA's office of cosmetics and colors relies in part on the Cosmetic Ingredient Review (CIR) expert panel composed of physicians and scientists, including dermatologists. This panel was formed in 1976 by the cosmetics industry. Their initial concern was that the compaction of the stratum corneum noticed after AHA use might lead to increased dermal UVA irradiation or increased penetration by other cosmetic ingredients. However, large amounts of safety data indicate no safety or health hazards associated with the use of these products.[69] Over-the-counter glycolic acid creams are available to consumers and through physician offices in concentrations of up to 14%.
2. Regulation of the use of higher strengths of AHAs is necessary to avoid their misuse by unsupervised nonphysicians. Deeper penetration beyond exfoliation of the stratum corneum increases the risk of complications. The threshold for restriction to physician use for AHA peeling agents will likely fall between 11% and 25%.
3. Comparative studies of AHAs with TCA, JS, and other superficial peeling agents should be performed to substantiate claimed benefits.
4. Standardization of buffered, partially neutralized AHA solutions is needed to control variation in results. Uncontrolled studies with these glycolic acid cream applications and repetitive peels may show no or variable histologic change over the course of a year. There are no convincing studies to confirm that partially neutralized AHAs with higher pH buffered to reduce burning and irritation offer any therapeutic advantage to unbuffered, unneutralized AHAs or vice versa. More rapid results are a function of acid concentration.
5. Both patients and physicians should have realistic expectations regarding the subtle benefits of the AHAs. The results are not overwhelming. Patients need not purchase entire cosmetic lines of AHAs, nor do physicians need to market products extensively to perform AHA peels. Good consumer value should be considered.
6. The FDA recognizes AHAs as cosmetics, not as drugs or "cosmeceuticals." (See Chapter 9.)

(Continued)

7. Results are unpredictable. Some patients experience fading of pigment and softening of wrinkles; others do not. Some patients develop persistent erythema and reactivity; others do not.
8. Peels performed by aestheticians tend to be more highly buffered and possess lower concentration. Therefore they produce little if any reaction until after several peels have been performed. Considering the variablity, cost-effectiveness, and lack of standardization of physician-performed glycolic acid peels, aesthetician-performed glycolic acid peels would be likely to be even more variable, especially with the plethora of cosmetic peel marketing regimes.
9. The exact mechanism of the AHAs in improving wrinkles is unknown. They act to enhance the synthesis of intercellular ground substances and collagen[70,71] but the action is apparently different from and independent of that of tretinoin. Discontinuing glycolic acid cream application will result in return to baseline in 7 to 8 months on the average depending on the degree of improvement obtained. The exact number of peels with unbuffered or buffered glycolic acid or cream applications of varying acidic pHs to achieve desired effects is unknown. It remains to be determined exactly how valuable AHAs will be as another therapy in the cosmetic prophylaxis and treatment of aging and photodamaged skin. It also remains to be demonstrated that the results from the use of the AHAs are equal to or superior to those obtained with other already established superficial peeling agents.[71]

Tretinoin

Topical **tretinoin,** all-*trans*-retinoic acid, is not a true chemical wounding agent. Because of its usage in the treatment of photodamaged skin it may be employed in conjunction with chemical peeling, both before and after. Before its reported usage as a treatment for photoaged skin, topical tretinoin was used in acne therapy since the early 1970s and with chemical peeling and dermabrasion since the early 1980s to mid-1980s, respectively. Its action at the cellular level to stimulate new collagen synthesis is described in Chapter 2. New collagen remains intact histologically for at least 4 months after the last application of the drug.[72] Tretinoin cream (Retin-A, Ortho Pharmaceuticals, Raritan, New Jersey) and tretinoin emollient cream (Renova, Ortho Pharmaceuticals, Raritan, New Jersey), in concentrations from 0.025% to 0.1%, have been demonstrated to reduce rhytides, actinic keratoses, and pigmentary actinic change in the skin when used for greater than 6 months.[73,74] After 48 weeks there was no difference in efficacy between the low and high strengths in reversal of clinical signs of photoaging. Fine and coarse wrinkling, mottled hyperpigmentation and lentigines were equally improved. Histologically the restoration of corneal layer compaction and epidermal thickening were comparable, but the granular layer thickness was significantly thicker in biopsies of skin from patients treated with 0.1% compared with 0.025% cream.[75] However, the presence of a retinoid skin reaction consisting of xerosis and erythema in roughly 70% to 90% of patients is a use-limiting side effect of topical tretinoin in higher strengths and may occur in a few patients regardless of drug concentration. The reaction gradually resolves in 2 to 12 weeks with proper encouragement, guidance, and temporary reduction of the application frequency or concentration.

Perspective on Tretinoin

The lowest strength 0.025% topical tretinoin (Retin-A) is sufficient for clinical and histologic improvement in photoaging. In chemical peeling, the drug is also used to decrease wound healing time after peeling and to potentiate the effects of topical hydroquinone. The minimum dose for the latter two functions is unknown. Tretinoin application before and after TCA does not significantly enhance the efficacy of the peel.[83] Pushing the patient to the maximum dose of tretinoin tolerated is not as important as previously thought, but the physician should not hesitate to raise the dose of tretinoin if the patient is experiencing no irritation. Tretinoin emollient cream 0.05% (Renova), less irritating to the skin in some patients because of the vehicle, accomplishes the same basic functions as Retin-A. Overgreasing with multiple moisturizers and underapplication of the drug may be responsible for less efficacy in some patients.

Catrix cream (Donell DerMedex, New York), a protein bovine mucopolysaccharide complex, may be used as a noncortisone antiinflammatory agent in these reactive patients. If tretinoin is poorly tolerated, using an AHA cream for a week in the morning alone may successfully allow reinstitution of nightly tretinoin. Retinoid concentration may then be increased again to tolerance. A plateau of benefits is reached after 12 to 24 months, at which time the patient may use the drug either daily or two to four times weekly as maintenance. The separation between clinical improvement and irritation suggests that the tretinoin-induced repair of photoaged skin is not dependent on the irritation.

Tretinoin is a supplement to most peel regimens along with daily sunscreen moisturizers or aftershaves. Vehicle-controlled trials of 0.1% tretinoin cream application alone have shown slow lightening of actinic lentigines in Chinese and Japanese patients and lightening of postinflammatory hyperpigmentation and melasma in black patients over a 40-week period.[76-78] Most of the time chemical peeling and hydroquinone supplementation in a regimen are required for total ablation of the pigmentation, and response is quicker than with tretinoin alone. Physicians may encounter patients who have used tretinoin for some time before undergoing chemical peeling. The frequency of application and concentration of tretinoin used in the past should be considered when performing the peel because it will hasten frosting. (See the regimen section in Chapter 4.) Tretinoin may be inactivated by certain aldehydes in creams.[79]

Pretreating with tretinoin before dermabrasion reduces the healing time and seems to prolong the results of the procedure.[80] Daily application of 0.1% tretinoin cream for 2 weeks before a 35% TCA peel significantly enhanced the healing time of the facial, forearm, and hand skin in a double-blind, placebo-controlled study.[81] In this study, however, there was no subjective difference in the visual inspection of the skin 3 months after the peel. No knowledge exists regarding dermal collagen quality changes with enhanced reepithelialization from tretinoin usage. Treatment with the drug should be reinstituted as soon as tolerated after reepithelialization from peeling has occurred, usually within 1 to 4 weeks. If used too soon, tretinoin may retard epithelialization.[82] Prolonged erythema with tretinoin usage before and after peeling is often seen, but its potentiation of hydroquinone in the peel regimen and the subjective sustained peel results seen by many patients make its continued use worthwhile. (See Chapter 3 for histologic discussion of retinoids and reepithelialization.)

Post–Skin Peel Instructions—Superficial

You have been peeled with chemicals that contain superficial agents that may contain alpha-hydroxy acids or other mild acids. Typically the skin turns dark the following day and peels without blistering over the next 3 to 5 days. Flaking may persist longer than this. Stop your skin cream treatment regimen, wash and shampoo normally, and apply only sunscreen moisturizer or bland moisturizer if the sunscreen stings. You may return to your regimen after the skin has peeled and is pink, usually by 5 to 7 days. Do not pick at the peeling skin, or scarring could result. Allow the skin to come off naturally with cream application. Sometimes the first peel produces very little reaction. Successive superfical peels may result in more redness and reactivity, but this can usually be adjusted by you and your doctor. You may apply make up over this peel at any time, but coverage of the peeling skin may not be complete.

Severe swelling or crusting of an area does not usually occur but may happen if you are sensitive to one of the ingredients. Any swelling that occurs is not permanent and will recede in several days. If you develop a fever blister during the recovery period after your peel, you should begin acyclovir (Zovirax), valacyclovir (Valtrex), or your antiviral pills immediately as prescribed. Please contact our office if severe swelling, local crusting, or fever blisters develop.

FIG 5-21. Post–skin peel instructions—superficial.

Aftercare for Superficial Peels

Minimal postoperative care is needed for all superficial peels with glycolic acid, Jessner's solution, or TCA, 15% to 25% (Fig. 5-21). In most cases, patients may return to their normal daily activities immediately and wear cosmetics to conceal erythema. Restriction of water and emollients to the treated skin for 24 to 48 hours after superficial chemical peels to promote epidermal dessication and separation was first advocated by Roberts[4] in 1926 based on his clinical experience. Benefit from this restriction is uncertain. Most patients tolerate normal skin-washing procedures immediately after the peels. Tretinoin should not be applied for the first 3 to 7 days during the healing period because it may impair healing of wounded skin.[81] It is necessary to avoid sun exposure. Sunscreen use may have to be temporarily discontinued for 3 to 7 days after a superficial peel if stinging occurs on application. The patient's daily regimen may then be reinstated. (See the regimen section in Chapter 4.)

Except for occasional persistent erythema, mild burning or stinging, contact photoirritation, acne exacerbation, or hyperpigmentation, complications are rare for all skin types.

THE ROLE OF THE AESTHETICIAN IN SUPERFICIAL CHEMICAL PEELING

The French word "esthétique" is a branch of philosophy relating to art, nature, and various forms of beauty. From Europe, where aesthetics are a major part of the beauty programs of men and women, techniques and formulas have migrated to America and are being integrated into skin care programs in many U.S. cities. In some cases aestheticians work in concert with dermatologists.[84]

Aestheticians are lay operators who specialize in skin care and conditioning. The practice of aesthetics involves massaging, trimming, dyeing, and beautifying the face, neck, arms, or legs "by any method with the aid of the hands or any mechanical or electrical apparatus."[85] Aestheticians are separately licensed by written and practical examinations on a state-by-state basis, usually under the state board of cosmetology rather than medicine. They may or may not be licensed **cosmetologists,** whose chief thrust is usually hairstyling. The occupation of cosmetology includes services involving the care of hair, face, scalp, and nails. Reciprocity of licensure varies from state to state, and a high school diploma is not always required for licensure. Aestheticians usually operate their own salons where they may manufacture, sell, and apply cosmetics; practice massage therapy and body conditioning; and perform skin treatments to manually remove comedones. State skin-care licensure uniformly requires less training hours than licensure for cosmetology. The range of hours required varies from 300 in Delaware, Maryland, and Pennsylvania to 900 in New Mexico, with an average of around 550 hours.[86]

A paramedical esthetician (PME) or a clinical aesthetician as opposed to a facialist in a salon is trained in the effects of and reactions to certain medications on the skin and the causes and treatment of certain skin disorders. These disorders are chiefly acne and photoaging skin with accompanying dryness. The PME works closely with the physician, and each complements the other's expertise. Any liability questions ultimately rest with the physician, although the PME should also carry malpractice insurance. The variation in perspective, education, and expertise is tremendous, and the physician's responsibility

TABLE 5-8.
Types of Masks Used by Aestheticians (Ref. 88)

MOISTURIZING	CLEANING	REVITALIZING
Mineral oil	Bentonite	Glyceryl stearate
Sorbitol	Kaolin	Disodium monooleamide
Animal collagen	Titanium dioxide	Salicylic acid
Glycerin	Magnesium aluminum silicate	Magnesium aluminum silicate
Propylene glycol	Witch hazel	Allantoin

is to train the aesthetician and to define the boundaries between acne treatment or peel instigation and massage or product promotion.[87] An aesthetician's training or salon's perspective may include many scientific misconceptions. An aesthetician may help teach corrective cosmetic application after cosmetic surgery or deep peels and assist with patient chemical peel education and treatment.

A typical facial treatment in a salon consists of makeup removal, moisturizing, comedone extraction, cleansing, and application of a **mask**. The original aesthetic mask is the application of warm melted wax with a brush, which after hardening can be removed in toto to lift the stratum corneum, purge the skin of blackheads, and trap perspiration at the skin surface. Masks for salon or home use are classified as moisturizing/nourishing, cleansing/firming, or revitalizing/stimulating. Examples of their ingredients are listed in Table 5-8.[88] Not all of these products are nonirritating or noncomedogenic.[89] Allergic or irritant dermatitis may accompany their usage.

The performance in salons of other superficial chemical peels, commonly called **fruit acid peels,** utilize stratum corneum sloughing agents or stratum granulosum peeling agents that slough follicular orifices. These are more properly called "washes" or "exfoliations" rather than peels because only the dead cell layer is removed. These may consist of strawberries, avocadoes, egg whites, honey, or oatmeal. Yogurt and buttermilk masks contain lactic acid, an AHA. They do not induce vesiculation, but epidermabrasion may be induced with papaya enzyme, pumice-containing cream, or mechanical brushes. This removal of the desquamative layer allegedly stimulates cell turnover and produces a fresher appearance.[90]

The newest agents used by aestheticians are glycolic acid in concentrations up to 30% or mixtures of AHAs and non-AHAs that are left on the skin for 1

Perspective on Aestheticians

Recognizing that dermatology is the medical specialty dealing with the science, treatment, and prevention of skin disease, and recognizing that aestheticians are lay operators who specialize in care and conditioning of the skin, some dermatologists may find the services of a properly trained and aligned aesthetician to their liking. Alternatively, the physician may find that individualized training of a qualified dermatology nurse may be more or less helpful to the needs and ethics of the practitioner. Skin care professionals should work in concert toward the goal of healthy patient skin. The dermatologist and the aesthetician may work together to achieve this goal if there is agreement on philosophy of skin maintenance, treatment, and ethics. (See Chapter 9 for further discussion of aestheticians and marketing.)

or 2 minutes initially. The depth of chemical peel produced by glycolic acid as administered by aestheticians is related not only to the strength of the solution but also to the duration of time it is left on the skin. Ten weekly treatments constitute a typical series of formal treatments by an aesthetician. Usually the acid is partially neutralized to minimize complications, and many applications are required for results to be apparent. Sometimes a modified Jessner's solution without resorcinol is used, but this also abbreviates its efficacy. Acids are marketed to aestheticians by many companies. (See Chapter 12.) Single agents are safe if prepared properly before commercial distribution, but little research has been published on the safety, depth, and effectiveness of combinations of different acids.

State laws may regulate peeling agents that may be used by aestheticians. Low concentrations of resorcinol, salicylic acid, sulfur, lactic acid, and phenol can be used. In California, it is legal for the nonphysician to apply "not greater than 10% phenol" to the skin. Ten percent solutions of phenol regularly produce corrosion, and occasionally skin necrosis is seen even with more dilute concentrations.[91] Although prepackaged products contain less than 2% phenol, it is not illegal for a beauty professional to mix chemical peel solutions containing phenol in many states.[92] No additional hours of training are required for licensed cosmetology professionals to perform cosmetic face peeling in all states. Cosmetic peeling is considered an integral part of the licensed practice of aesthetics and facial cosmetology. Cosmetic peeling is generally a safe procedure, but the line between the aesthetician's usage of superficial peeling agents in the United States and the dermal invasion of chemosurgery is limited by the fear of litigation that permeates this country regardless of profession. Some state laws concerning what does and does not constitute the practice of medicine are written in a way that would include the performance of all types of skin peels. Indiana state laws, for example, define the practice of medicine as "the performing of any kind of surgical operation upon a human being, including tattooing, or the penetration of the skin or body orifice by any means for the intended palliation, relief, or cure."[93] Other state laws may not be specific on penetration and vague on motivation. State medical board rulings may restrict the concentration of phenol, as in Florida where a concentration of 2% phenol in chemical peeling solution may not be exceeded unless the peel is performed under the direct supervision of a physician.

The National Cosmetology Association supports criteria for chemical face peeling by state legislation that restrict the amount of phenol used by aestheticians to "not greater than 2%." They support prepackaged phenol products and the proscription on phenol mixing by cosmetologists. Encouragement of additional hours of training for cosmetologists and aestheticians who perform cosmetic face peeling is endorsed.[94] Unless these recommended criteria are taken directly to state licensing agencies or state medical boards for action, the existing variation between states will continue.

Although many aesthetician organizations exist, the American Society of Esthetic Medicine in Scottsdale, Arizona (602-368-0108) and the National Center for Competency Testing (913-383-8700) are organizations that support certification for aestheticians.

Acknowledgment

The author is indebted to Lyn Ross-Ingram, Dermess Therapeutic Skin Care Center, Atlanta, Georgia, for her assistance in preparing this chapter.

REFERENCES

1. Murad H, Shamban AT, Premo PS: The use of glycolic acid as a peeling agent, *Dermatol Clin* 13(2):285-307, 1995.
2. Stegman SJ, Tromovitch TA, Glogau RG: *Cosmetic dermatologic surgery,* ed 2, St Louis, 1990, Mosby, p. 50.
3. Matarasso SL, Glogau RG, Markey AC: Wood's lamp for superficial chemical peels, *J Am Acad Dermatol* 30:988-992, 1994.
4. Roberts HL: The chloracetic acids: a biochemical study, *Br J Dermatol* 38:323-391, 1926.
5. Monash S: The uses of diluted trichloroacetic acid in dermatology, *Urol Cutan Rev* 49:119-120, 1945.
6. Resnik SS: Chemical peeling with trichloroacetic acid, *J Dermatol Surg Oncol,* 10:549, 1984.
7. Bridenstine JB, Dolezal JF: Standardizing chemical peel solution formulations to avoid mishaps, *J Dermatol Surg Oncol* 20:813-816, 1994.
8. Spinowitz AL, Rumsfield J: Stability-time profile of trichloroacetic acid at various concentrations and storage conditions, *J Dermatol Surg Oncol,* 15:974-975, 1989.
9. Dolezal JF: Stability study of trichloroacetic acid, *J Dermatol Surg Oncol,* 16:489-490, 1990 (letter).
10. Stagnone JJ: Superficial peeling, *J Dermatol Surg Oncol,* 15:924-930, 1989.
11. Rubin MG: The efficacy of a topical lidocaine/prilocaine anesthetic gel in 35% trichloroacetic acid peels, *Dermatol Surg* 21:223-225, 1995.
12. Taylor MB: EMLA for effective pain relief following chemical peeling, *Dermatol Surg* 21:738-739, 1995.
13. Collins PS, Farber GA, Wilhelmus SM, et al: Superficial repetitive chemosurgery of the hands, *Am J Cosmet Surg,* 1:22-24, 1984.
14. Collins PS: Trichloroacetic acid revisted, *J Dermatol Surg Oncol,* 15:933-940, 1989.
15. Morrison RT, Boyd RN: *Organic chemistry,* ed 2, Boston, 1967, Allyn & Bacon, p. 789.
16. Rook A, Wilkinson DS, Ebling FJG: *Textbook of dermatology,* Oxford, England, 1972, Blackwell Scientific, pp. 2072-2075.
17. Fisher AA: Reactions to selective topical medications. In *Contact dermatitis,* Philadelphia, 1986, Lea & Febiger, pp. 146-147.
18. Goodman LS, Gilman AG: *The pharmacological basis of therapeutics,* New York, 1975, MacMillan, pp. 990-991.
19. Letessier SM: Chemical peel with resorcin. In Roenigk RK, Roenigk HH, editors: *Dermatologic surgery: principles and practice,* ed 2, New York, 1996, Marcel Dekker, pp. 1115-1119.
20. Karam PG: 50% resorcinol peel, *Int J Dermatol* 32:569-574, 1993.
21. Letessier S: Chemical Peeling Seminar, International Society for Dermatologic Surgery, Edinburgh, September 1989.
22. Hernandez Perez E: Different grades of chemical peels, *Am J Cosmet Surg,* 7:67-70, 1990.
23. Hernandez-Perez E, Carpio E: Resorcinol peels: gross and microscopic study, *Am J Cosmet Surg* 12(4):337-340, 1995.
24. Pascher F: Systemic reactions to topically applied drugs, *Bull N Y Acad Med,* 49:613-627, 1973.
25. Fisher A: Resorcinol—a rare sensitizer, *Cutis* 29:331, 1982.
26. Matarasso SL, Glogau RG: The role of chemical peeling in the treatment of photodamaged skin, *J Dermatol Surg Oncol* 17:622-623, 1991 (letter).
27. Monheit GD: The Jessner's + TCA peel: a medium depth chemical peel, *J Dermatol Surg Oncol* 15:945-950, 1989.
28. Horvath PN: The light peel, *Bull Assoc Milit Dermatol* 18:2, 1970.
29. Slagel GA, McMarlin SL: Chemical face peels, *J Assoc Milit Dermatol* 10:38-43, 1984.
30. Katz BE: The fluor-hydroxy pulse peel: a pilot evaluation of a new superficial chemical peel, *Cosmet Dermatol* 8(4):24-30, 1995.
31. Rook A, Wilkinson DS, Ebling FJG: *Textbook of dermatology,* Oxford, England, 1972, Blackwell Scientific, p. 2073.
32. Swinehart JM: Salicylic ointment peeling of the hands and forearms, *J Dermatol Surg Oncol* 18:495-498, 1992.
33. Aronsohn RB: Hand chemosurgery, *Am J Cosmet Surg* 1:24-28, 1984.
34. Kligman D, Pagnoni A, Sadiq I, et al: A new approach to superficial facial chemical peels using salicylic acid. Presented at the American Society for Dermatologic Surgery, Palm Springs, Calif, May 15, 1996.
35. Rook A, Wilkinson DS, Ebling FJG: *Textbook of dermatology,* Oxford, England, 1972, Blackwell Scientific, p. 2099.
36. Dobes WL, Keil H: Treatment of acne vulgaris by cryotherapy (slush method), *Arch Dermatol Syph* 42:547, 1940.

37. Zugerman I: A formula for cryotherapy for acne and postacne scarring, *Arch Dermatol Syph* 54:209, 1946.
38. Dobes WL: A simplified method of cryotherapy for acne vulgaris, *South Med J* 44:546, 1951.
39. Moseley JC, Katz SI: Acne vulgaris: treatment with carbon dioxide slush, *Cutis* 10:429-431, 1972.
40. Wolf R, Landau M, Berger SA, et al: Transfer of bacteria associated with cryotherapy, *Cutis* 51:276-277, 1993.
41. Brody HJ: Medium-depth chemical peeling of the skin: a variation of superficial chemosurgery, *Adv Dermatol* 3:205-220, 1988.
42. W magazine, Fairchild Publications, 22(11):60-62, 1993.
43. BioMedic brochure, 8757 East Via de Commercio, Scottsdale, AZ 85258.
44. Expert Witness, Legal Case, 1995.
45. Wang B, Carey WD: Chemical peeling as adjuvant therapy for facial neurotic excoriations, *J Am Acad Dermatol* 30:669-70, 1994.
46. Rubin MG: Chemical peeling as adjuvant therapy for facial neurotic excoriations, *J Am Acad Dermatol* 32:296-297, 1995 (letter).
47. Van Scott EJ: Alpha hydroxy acids: procedures for use in clinical practice, *Cutis* 43:222-228, 1989.
48. Van Scott EJ, Yu RJ: Hyperkeratinization, corneocyte cohesion and alpha hydroxy acids, *J Am Acad Dermatol* 11:867, 1984.
49. Van Scott EJ: The unfolding therapeutic uses of the alpha hydroxy acids, *Mediguide Dermatol* 3:1-5, 1989.
50. DiNardo JC, Grove GL, Moy LS: Clinical and histological effects of glycolic acid at different concentrations and pH levels, *Dermatol Surg* 22:421-428, 1996.
51. Lavker RM, Kaidbey K, Leyden JJ: Effects of topical ammonium lactate on cutaneous atrophy from a potent topical corticosteroid, *J Am Acad Dermatol* 26:535-544, 1992.
52. Leyden JJ, Lavker RM, Grove G, et al: AHAs are more than moisturizers, *J Geriatr Dermatol* 3(suppl A) (3):33A-37A, 1995.
53. Alvarez OM, Mertz PM, Eaglstein WH: The effect of occlusive dressings on collagen synthesis and reepithelialization in superficial wounds, *J Surg Res* 35:142-148, 1983.
54. Yu RJ and Van Scott EJ: Alpha-hydroxy acids: science and therapeutic use, *Cosmet Dermatol* 7(suppl):12-20, 1994.
55. Rosan AM: The chemistry of alpha-hydroxy acids, *Cosmet Dermatol* 7(suppl):4-6, 1994.
56. Becker FF, Langford FPJ, Rubin MG, et al: A histological comparison of 50% and 70% glycolic acid peels using solutions with various pHs, *Dermatol Surg* 22:463-468, 1996.
57. Moy LS, Murad H, Moy RL: Glycolic acid peels for the treatment of wrinkles and photoaging, *J Dermatol Surg Oncol* 19:243-246, 1993.
58. Lawrence NL, Cox SE, Brody HJ: A comparison of Jessner's solution and glycolic acid in the treatment of melasma in dark skinned patients: a double blind study, *J Am Acad Dermatol* 37:589-593, 1997.
59. Kimborough-Green CK, Griffiths CE, Finkel LJ, et al: Topical retinoic acid (tretinoin) for melasma in Black patients, *Arch Dermatol* 130:727-733, 1994.
60. Clinical discussions, breakfast focus sessions on chemical peeling, Annual meetings of the American Academy of Dermatology and American Society for Dermatologic Surgery, 1993-1996.
61. Griffiths CEM, Finkel LJ, Ditre CM, et al: Topical tretinoin improves melasma. A vehicle-controlled clinical trial, *Br J Dermatol* 129:415-421, 1993.
62. Burns RL, Lawry M, Prevost-Blank P, et al: The use of glycolic acid chemical peels for the treatment of melasma and post-inflammatory hyperpigmentation in patients in diverse ethnicity. Presented at the American Society for Dermatologic Surgery, May 15, 1996, Palm Springs, Calif.
64. Newman N, Newman A, Moy LS, et al: Clinical improvement of photoaged skin with 50% glycolic acid: a double-blind vehicle-controlled study, *Dermatol Surg* 22:455-462, 1996.
65. Ridge JM, Siegle RJ, Zuckerman J: Use of alpha-hydroxy acids in the therapy for "photoaged" skin, *J Am Acad Dermatol* 23:932, 1990.
66. Piacquadio D, Dobry M, Hunt S, et al: Short contact 70% glycolic acid peels as a treatment for photodamaged skin: a pilot study, *Dermatol Surg* 22:449-454, 1996.
67. Piacquadio D, Grove MJ, Dobry M: Efficacy of glycolic acid peels questioned for photodamaged skin, *Dermatol Times* p.52 May 1992.
68. Perricone NV, DiNardo JC: Photoprotective and antiinflammatory effects of topical glycolic acid, *Dermatol Surg* 22:435-438, 1996.
69. Mechcatie E: Review of alpha hydroxy acid safety well under way, *Skin Allergy News* 26(10):1-4, 1995.

70. Ditre CM, Griffin TD, Murphy GF, et al: The effects of alpha hydroxy acids on photoaged skin: a pilot clinical, histological and ultrastructural study, *J Am Acad Dermatol* 34:187-195, 1996.
71. Brody H, Coleman WP, Piacquadio D, et al: Round table discussion of alpha hydroxy acids, *Dermatol Surg* 22:475-477, 1996.
72. Weiss JS, Ellis CN, Goldfarb MT, et al: Tretinoin treatment of photodamaged skin: cosmesis through medical therapy, *Dermatol Clin* 9:123-129, 1991.
73. Kligman AM, Grove GL, Hirose R, et al: Topical tretinoin for photoaged skin, *J Am Acad Dermatol* 15:836-859, 1986.
74. Weiss J, Ellis CN, Headington JT, et al: Topical tretinoin improves photoaged skin: a double-blind vehicle controlled study, *JAMA* 259:527, 1988.
75. Griffiths CEM, Kang S, Ellis CN, et al: Two concentrations of topical tretinoin (retinoic acid) cause similar improvement of photoaging but different degrees of irritation, *Arch Dermatol* 131:1037-1044, 1995.
76. Griffiths CEM, Goldfarb MT, Finkel LJ, et al: Topical tretinoin (retinoic acid) treatment of hyperpigmented lesions associated with photoaging in Chinese and Japanese patients: a vehicle-controlled trial, *J Am Acad Dermatol* 30:76-84, 1994.
77. Bulengo-Ransby SM, Griffiths CEM, Kimbrough-Green CK, et al: Topical tretinoin (retinoic acid) therapy for hyperpigmented lesions caused by inflammation of the skin in black patients, *N Engl J Med* 328:1438-1443, 1993.
78. Kimbrough-Green CK, Griffiths CEM, Finkel LJ, et al: Topical retinoic acid(tretinoin) for melasma in black patients, *Arch Dermatol* 130:727-733, 1994.
79. Leyden JJ: Retin-A for wrinkles: inactivated by aldehydes, *Skin Allergy News* 19:3, 1988.
80. Mandy S: Tretinoin in the preoperative and postoperative management of dermabrasion, *J Am Acad Dermatol* 15(suppl):878-879, 1986.
81. Hevia O, Nemeth AJ, Taylor JR: Tretinoin accelerates healing after trichloroacetic acid chemical peel, *Arch Dermatol* 127:678-682, 1991.
82. Hung VC, Lee JY, Zitelli JA, et al: Topical tretinoin and epithelial wound healing, *Arch Dermatol* 125:65-69, 1989.
83. Humphreys TR, Werth V, Dzubow L, et al: Treatment of photodamaged skin with trichloroacetic acid and topical tretinoin, *J Am Acad Dermatol* 34:638-44, 1996.
84. Ross-Ingram L: Personal communications from Personal Aesthetics Skin and Body Care Institute, Atlanta.
85. State of Georgia Official Code, Annotated (OCGA). Chapters 43-10-1(4) and (5).
86. Warfield SS: Confusion surrounds the esthetician's role in the dermatology practice, *Cosmet Dermatol*, 6(5):42-46, 1993.
87. Bridgeford L, Harris V, Padilla S: The aesthetic alliance: nurses and medical facials, *Dermatol Nurs* 2(4):205-208, 1990.
88. Lupo ML: Knowledge of facial masks important to dermatologists, *Cosmet Dermatol* 5(5):16-22, 1992.
89. Draelos ZD: A dermatologic evaluation of facial treatment salons, *Cosmet Dermatol* 5(1):24-26, 1992.
90. Draelos ZD: Understanding the techniques of the esthetician: part I, *Cosmet Dermatol* 7(4):15-18, 1994.
91. Gleason MD, Gosselen RE, Hodge HC, et al: *Clinical toxicology of commercial products*, Baltimore, 1969, Williams & Wilkins, pp. 189-192.
92. Communication to all State Presidents, *National Cosmetology Association*, November 3, 1989.
93. Indiana Code for Professions and Occupations, Article 22.5, Physicians, 1988.
94. Legislative Policy of the National Cosmetology Association. Adopted by the Delegates to the 70th Annual Convention of the National Cosmetology Association, Washington, DC, July 14-16, 1990.

6 Medium-Depth Peeling

EVOLUTION OF THE MEDIUM-DEPTH PEEL

Medium-depth peeling is defined as the application of a wounding agent or agents to produce an initial dermal wound, usually in the upper reticular dermis. (See Chapter 2.) It is usually performed as a single procedure to achieve a desired result, specifically the removal of actinic keratoses and mild rhytides, the resolution of pigmentary dyschromias, and the flattening of depressed scars. (See the section on indications for peeling in Chapter 4.) Medium-depth peeling may be repeated approximately every 6 to 12 months based on the amount of actinic damage still remaining or recurring after the peel or for continued scar effacement (see the box below).

Traditionally, the classic peel for this depth category is the 50% trichloroacetic acid (TCA) peel, used extensively for three decades as the classic peel for the patient who did not warrant, tolerate, or desire a "phenol peel." Trichloroacetic acid, however, is an agent that is prone to produce increased scarring with higher concentrations.[1] In 1980 this author and his associate became aware of the need for an intermediate procedure that would achieve a similar depth but still not approach the toxicity of the phenol formulas. We reasoned that insulting the epidermis with a refrigerant might allow a less potent concentration of TCA such as 35% to penetrate to the depth of a higher-strength 50% solution.

Of the cryosurgical agents available, we chose solid carbon dioxide (CO_2), or dry ice. Although the temperature of the ice block of CO_2 is $-78.5°$ C, the skin temperature is considerably higher, as demonstrated by clinical experience and rapid thaw time. Liquid nitrogen when used alone to treat scarring is approximately 100° C colder than solid carbon dioxide and can achieve dermal depth destruction and induce melanocyte toxicity, hypopigmentation, and scarring with improper technique.[2] Carbon dioxide alone, however, does not usually induce scarring or hypopigmentation and therefore has a wider margin of safety when combined with TCA.

Medium-Depth Peeling Modalities

- Combination peels
  - Solid carbon dioxide + TCA
  - Jessner's solution + TCA
  - Glycolic acid + TCA
- TCA, 50%
- Full-strength phenol, 88%
- Pyruvic acid (α-keto acids)

Ethyl chloride as a consideration produces a skin temperature of −10° C, about 70 degrees warmer than the carbon dioxide block.[3] It is both inflammable and explosive and does not destroy tissue.[4] The newer preparations of Frigiderm (dichlorotetrafluoroethane) and Fluoroethyl (25% ethyl chloride and 75% dichlorotetrafluoroethane) are more expensive and lack the precise control that carbon dioxide has when used to freeze depressed scarring or specific keratoses. Frigiderm, which is nonflammable and nonexplosive, chills the skin to between 0 and −32° C.

With a long history of safety as a single agent in the last 75 years, solid carbon dioxide is a reliable modality to combine with TCA for **combination medium-depth chemical peeling**. Over 4000 combination peels using CO_2 and TCA confirm the safety. The combination of two superficial agents to reach the depth of one single agent to increase safety is the rationale of medium-depth peeling. (See also Chapters 2 and 4 and the section on CO_2 in Chapter 5.)

A **second combination medium-depth peel** using Jessner's solution (JS) was introduced in 1989. This combination of resorcinol, salicylic acid, and lactic acid acts as an epidermal absorbing agent before TCA application. This has subsequently been shown to achieve a similar peel depth and comparable results to CO_2 plus TCA. The JS plus TCA peel is also satisfactory for pigmentation and actinic damage, but we have found it to be less successful for treating depressed scarring because of the lack of ability to concentrate the peel around the rims of depressed scars, which is more easily performed with solid CO_2. (For detailed discussions on depth measurements and peel application theory, see Chapters 2 and 4, and the section on Jessner's solution in Chapter 5.)

A **third combination medium-depth peel** capitalizing on the use of glycolic acid was introduced in 1994. Depending on the properties of glycolic acid to fractionate the upper epidermis before the sequential application of TCA, this peel is more superficial than the original medium-depth peel but succeeds in reliably penetrating well into the papillary dermis. It can be used in darker skin types. (For detailed discussions see Chapters 2 and 4, and the section on glycolic acid in Chapter 5.)

CHOOSING THE PROPER MEDIUM-DEPTH COMBINATION PEEL

Choices and indications for the combination medium-depth peels appear in Table 6-1. Although all three combination peels are used for photodamage, their pros and cons make knowledge of all peels desirable for maximal correction depending on the patient's needs.

Procedural Differences

Fitzpatrick Skin Type

Jessner's solution plus TCA and glycolic acid plus TCA may be performed on any skin type for pigmentary dyschromias, including darker skin types with the usual caution. Carbon dioxide plus TCA is intended only for skin types I through III and type IV using CO_2 mild only.

Lesion Debridement

First, only the CO_2 plus TCA peel provides inherent debridement of lesions as does cryosurgery. The identification and removal of any exophytic actinic or

TABLE 6-1.
Degree of Effectiveness of Combination Medium-Depth Peels*

PROCEDURAL DIFFERENCES	CO_2+TCA	JS+TCA	GLYCOLIC+TCA
Fitzpatrick skin type	I-III only, IV with caution	All	All
Prepeel lesion debridement	++	0	0
Wound depth and histologic correction	+++	++	++
INDICATIONS:			
Scarring	+++	0	0
Actinic keratosis	++++	+++	+++
Melasma	++	+++	+++
Postinflammatory hyperpigmentation	++	+++	+++
Fine rhytides	+++	++	++
Coarse rhytides	+	+	+
Molluscum contagiosum	+++	+	+

*0, Not effective; +, poor; ++, good; +++, very good.

seborrheic keratosis is required before peeling. This may be done by traditional dermatologic surgery with curettage, cryosurgery, or electrosurgery, and biopsy can be submitted if indicated. Subsequent peeling over these areas is not harmful and will not usually result in hypopigmentation if carefully performed. Cryosurgery with liquid nitrogen, twice as cold as CO_2, can be the exception, and aggressive overfreezing of keratoses will result in depigmented macules with or without peeling with TCA. Extra coating with JS, glycolic acid, or repeated TCA coats on these individual hypertrophic lesions may not result in total ablation. Solid carbon dioxide eliminates this extra step.

Wound Depth and Histologic Correction

Carbon dioxide plus TCA has the greatest wound depth and histologic correction of elastotic changes with the widest papillary dermal Grenz zone. Jessner's solution plus TCA and glycolic acid plus TCA are slightly less deep in penetration but are technique sensitive and can be roughly equivalent in depth. (See Chapter 2 for details.)

Indications

Scarring

Solid carbon dioxide is a physical modality and can be combined with electrosurgery around depressed scars before TCA application. It is the only peel to predictably efface depressed scarring.

Actinic Keratoses

Actinic keratoses are improved by all three peels. However, more progressive keratoses exhibit more mucinous change in the dermis. Depth of peel is important in length of remission.

Melasma and Postinflammatory Hyperpigmentation

All three peels are effective, but CO_2 cannot be used in darker skin types. Risk of rebound pigmentation exists in all peels without use of the regimen as outlined in Chapter 4.

Rhytides

Fine rhytides are improved by all medium-depth peels and are a reflection of changes in papillary and reticular dermal quality. Coarse rhytides may be softened but not removed by any medium-depth combination.

Molluscum Contagiosum

Because cryosurgery alone is effective for this indication in HIV patients, CO_2 + TCA is deepest and most effective as a general peel. See the following discussion.

SEDATION FOR MEDIUM-DEPTH PEELING

Preoperative sedation is optional for all medium-depth peels. Aside from occasional sublingual diazepam, 5 to 10 mg, to allay anxiety before peeling, we almost never use local nerve blocks or intramuscular or intravenous sedation. The discomfort from these peels is not long lasting, and even the most anxious patients can be relaxed by taking the time to give a little "talkasthesia." One exception is the 50% TCA peel described later, which electively may benefit from intramuscular analgesia. Also, if extensive peeling is performed on a bald scalp for actinic keratoses, pain from peel application may be tolerated more easily with intramuscular meperidine (Demerol, Winthrop), 50 mg, or ketorolac tromethamine (Toradol, Syntex), 30 mg.

TECHNIQUES

Solid Carbon Dioxide and Trichloroacetic Acid

The details of each superficial agent[5,6] are described in Chapters 2 and 5. After thorough cleansing of the skin with povidone-iodine followed by an alcohol wipe and acetone scrub for 3 minutes by the patient to remove makeup and debris, the skin is evaluated so that superficial vs. deep defects are noted by the physician. These are mapped on a diagram or facial rubber stamp imprint so that the physician may follow the defects when icing the skin with CO_2 (Fig. 6-1). After verifying that all makeup is removed with an additional acetone scrub for 1 minute, a block of solid CO_2 is broken to hand size and continually dipped in a 3:1 solution of acetone and alcohol so that the dry ice will move freely over the skin (Fig. 6-2). Varying pressure is applied to induce microepidermal vesiculobullous formation where desired. Pressure by the operator determines depth, and this is noted on the diagram of the entire face or of the areas being treated. Mild pressure is 3 to 5 seconds, moderate pressure is 5 to 8 seconds, and hard pressure is 8 to 15 seconds (Table 6-2).

When freezing an individual scar, it is permissible to freeze the rims for 10 to 15 seconds to afford greatest TCA penetration so that the scar edges will be clinically blunted. Immediately after freezing a deep scar, the skin may be wiped dry of flammable acetone, and the rim may be electrodessicated with monopolar current for further effacement. This is painless with attendant

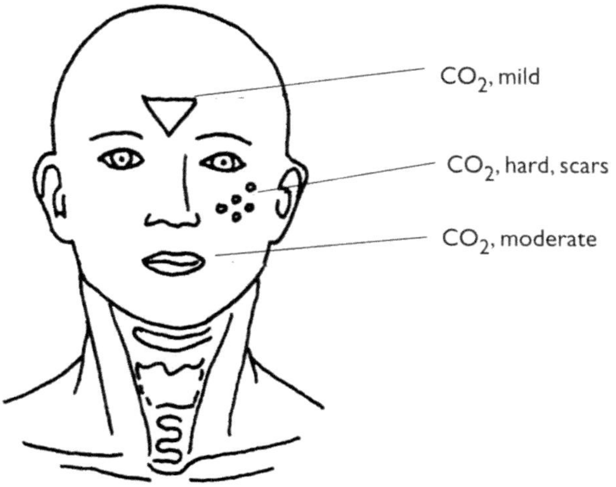

FIG. 6-1. Mapping of CO_2 pressure before TCA application.

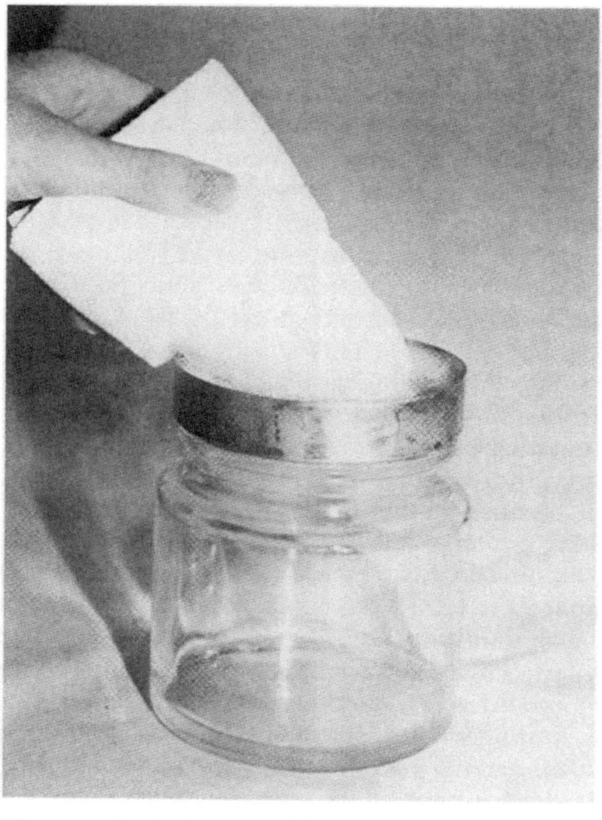

FIG. 6-2. Dipping of CO_2 cut to hand size into a 3:1 solution of acetone:alcohol.

cryoanesthesia. (See Fig. 11-14.) Similarly, individual keratoses may be frozen hard for additional penetration. (See also the section on CO_2 in Chapter 5.)

Patients may not tolerate hard pressure for long periods over certain areas such as the upper portion of the forehead, which is very sensitive. If freezing hard is absolutely necessary here, a nerve block of the forehead may be helpful. The seconds given are general guidelines, and the actual time and pressure will vary slightly with patient tolerance and the surgeon. All areas of the face may

TABLE 6-2.
CO_2 Pressure

PRESSURE	TIME (SEC)
Mild	3-5
Moderate	5-8
Hard	8-15

be iced, with defect size and patient tolerance being the chief limiting factors. The cheeks are less sensitive, and the glabella is more sensitive. Insertion of gauze into the mouth between the lips facilitates hard freezing over the upper lip onto the vermilion. The crow's feet and lower periorbital area may be frozen hard without difficulty before 35% TCA application. Care should always be taken to apply less pressure when freezing over bony prominences where postinflammatory changes may be more likely. Individual scars may be blunted with hard pressure. An electric fan or assistant's manual fanning to blow away the acetone vapors can facilitate patient breathing and reduce discomfort when freezing around the nose, mouth, and glabella (Fig. 6-3).

Next, the skin is lightly rewiped with dry gauze, and 35% TCA is applied with either two cotton applicators or with a 4 × 4–inch gauze pad held with a gloved hand in the standard fashion.[7] The latter achieves heavier application (Fig. 6-4). A cotton-tipped applicator can be used to apply 35% TCA under the eyes, and a 4 × 4–inch gauze pad held with a gloved hand serves as the mode of application on the remainder of the face.

Begin with the most sensitive lower eyelash area first because the patient is unsedated and alert. The cotton-tipped applicator is moist but not dripping wet. The TCA is applied to both lower eyelids in a single sweeping motion while the patient looks up. Then the patient is told to close his or her eyes, and the applicator is switched to a single 4 × 4–inch gauze pad dipped liberally into TCA from a shot glass. Moving in rapid succession from the upper eyelids to the supratarsal plate, nose, cheeks, perioral area, and the least sensitive forehead area affords greatest ease for the physician and the best tolerance for the patient because of inevitable progressive squirming for 1 to 2 minutes while frosting is occurring. Many times the sebaceous nature of the hairline requires continual application and rubbing to achieve whitening. (See the section on application of 35% TCA in Chapter 4 for rationale for the amount of wounding agent and for the order of application.) Fifty percent TCA can be applied to treat individual scar rims, solitary rhytides or keratoses, or areas at the vermilion border. If 50% TCA is applied to wider areas after CO_2 application, there is an increased risk of scarring. Generally, the perioral area is at greater risk of scarring, and CO_2 plus 50% TCA is not recommended for treatment in this area except at the vermilion, where very small vertical rhytides and increased actinic damage may be present.

After 10 minutes when the patient is again comfortable, the skin may be electively retreated with 35% TCA if actinic elastosis and keratoses are considerable.[8] Medium-depth **neck** peeling is unpredictable and may not yield consistently good results. Multiple superficial repetitive 20% to 35% TCA peeling without CO_2 monthly or every several months is a more consistently reliable treatment for mobile areas such as the neck that can easily scar. (See the section on neck peeling on page 127.)

The burning sensation that accompanies the application of the TCA is lessened by the previous CO_2 and can be minimized by the immediate application

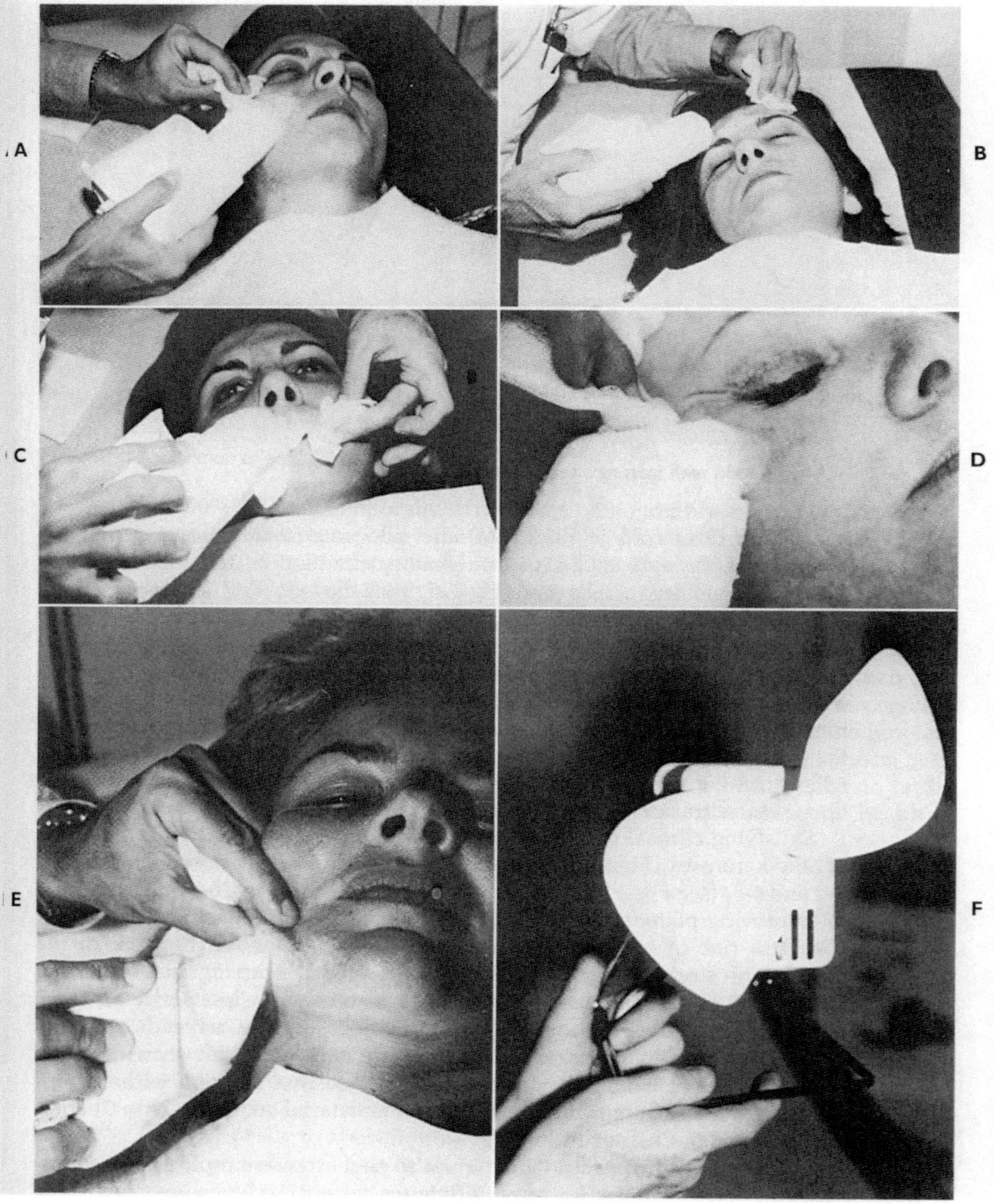

FIG. 6-3. CO_2 application. See the text for details.

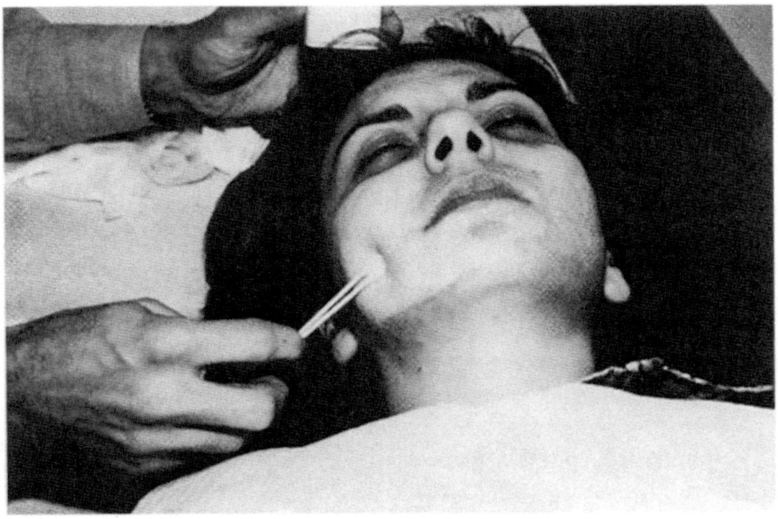

FIG. 6-4. TCA application with frosting after CO_2 application.

of an ice pack or cold gel pack (3M) after adequate frosting has occurred. No aqueous solutions are applied to avoid inadvertent dilution, and after 5 minutes, a soothing emollient can be used (Fig. 6-5). (See the following aftercare section.)

It is especially important with this peel as with any dual-procedure peel to have predetermined exactly which wounding technique and agent are to be applied to each area. This should be mapped immediately before the procedure for ease of decision and rapidity. If this is done, the process can be performed smoothly and quickly, and the patient's discomfort will be minimal. If the peel is prolonged because of last-minute physician indecision, the patient will remember the stinging and heat and be less prepared for a repeat procedure even years later.

Satisfying clinical results can be obtained in correcting mild to moderate actinic keratoses (Fig. 6-6), in flattening the edges of depressed scars (Figs. 6-7 and 6-8) (see Fig. 11-14), in improving fine rhytids (Figs. 6-9 and 6-10), and in improving pigmentation (Fig. 6-11). Scarring on the back can be peeled with less risk of complications than can pigmentation of the back in the absence of scarring, perhaps because the dermal scarring may curb the strength of TCA and because TCA may be metabolically less active on some nonfacial surfaces. (See the section on TCA in Chapter 5.) Carbon dioxide plus 50% TCA can be applied to a back with severe depressed acne scarring, but a nonscarred back would be less likely to tolerate that strength without producing a scar as a complication. (See also the material on back skin in Chapter 2 and Case 4 in Chapter 11.)

We have used this peel in an attempt to peel extensive **molluscum contagiosum** seen in **human immunodeficiency virus (HIV)**-positive patients or patients with the **autoimmune deficiency syndrome (AIDS)**. Because cryosurgery is often used alone to treat molluscum, combined CO_2 plus TCA should be ideal. However, our experience with patients is that the treatment, while moderately effective, is short lived. The molluscum will return usually within 6 to 8 weeks, and repeeling, if tolerated, is necessary. We did not observe delayed healing, Koebner phenomenon, excessive morbidity, or other complications in patients who had CD4 counts of less than 200. The peel is useful to debulk large clumps of virus (Fig. 6-12). Peels of 35% to 50% TCA alone appear to be safe and do not induce lesional spread.[9] Two applications

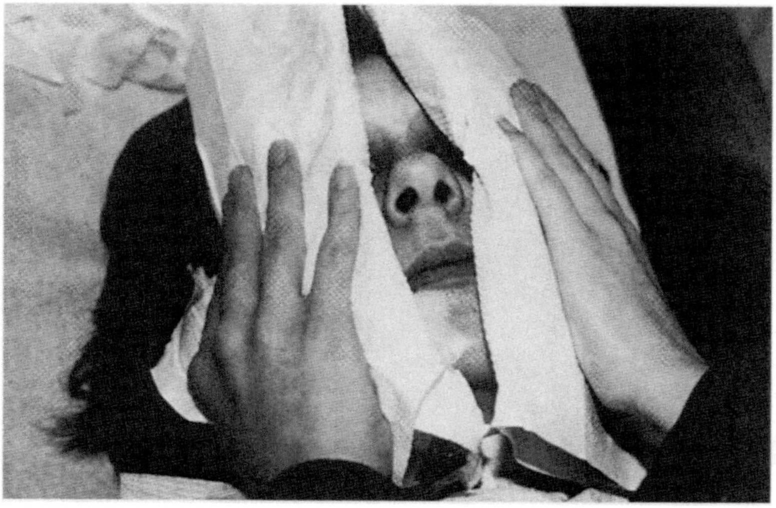

FIG. 6-5. Application of cold gel packs.

of 100% TCA applied locally to mollusca on a monthly interval with a cotton-tipped applicator on the split-face of HIV patients has been shown to be superior to liquid nitrogen cryosurgery with a 20-second thaw time and 3 mm lateral halo thaw.[10] Eight weeks after the initial treatment, the TCA side showed a 90% improvement compared with a 55% reduction on the cryosurgical side. Both agents produced 10% hyperpigmentation, and the TCA produced no hypopigmentation as compared with the cryosurgery, which produced 20% hypopigmentation. All Fitzpatrick skin types were successfully treated. Use of the regimen outlined in Chapter 4 may eliminate the problem with hyperpigmentation in darker skin types. This is not a true chemical peel, but it illustrates the superior destructive potential of TCA, similar to tattoo removal. (See the section on general state of physical and mental health in Chapter 4.)

For a discussion of side effects, see Chapter 8.

Jessner's Solution and Trichloroacetic Acid

The details on the mechanism of each superficial agent[11,12] are described in the corresponding sections in Chapter 5 and Chapter 2. After thorough degreasing of the face with hexachlorophene with alcohol (Septisol) or povidone-iodine followed by an acetone scrub, JS can be applied with two moist cotton-tipped applicators in the manner described in Chapter 4 to the entire face. We prefer to apply it more rapidly with either a 2 × 2–inch or 4 × 4–inch gauze pad or a sable brush and use only one coat to achieve light but even frosting.[13] Overcoating may produce scarring, but the risk is very low. (See the section on scarring in Chapter 8.) The frost achieved with JS is much lighter than that produced with TCA, and the patient is generally not uncomfortable. Extreme hyperkeratotic lesions such as actinic or seborrheic keratoses must be treated with cryosurgery or gently curetted before peeling.

Trichloroacetic acid, 35%, is then applied evenly with one or two cotton-tipped applicators or with a single 4 × 4–inch gauze pad if heavier application is desired in one or all areas. Even application should eliminate the need for reapplication, but if frosting is incomplete or uneven as in an actinic keratosis, for example, the TCA can be reapplied carefully.

(Text continues on p. 125.)

A B C D

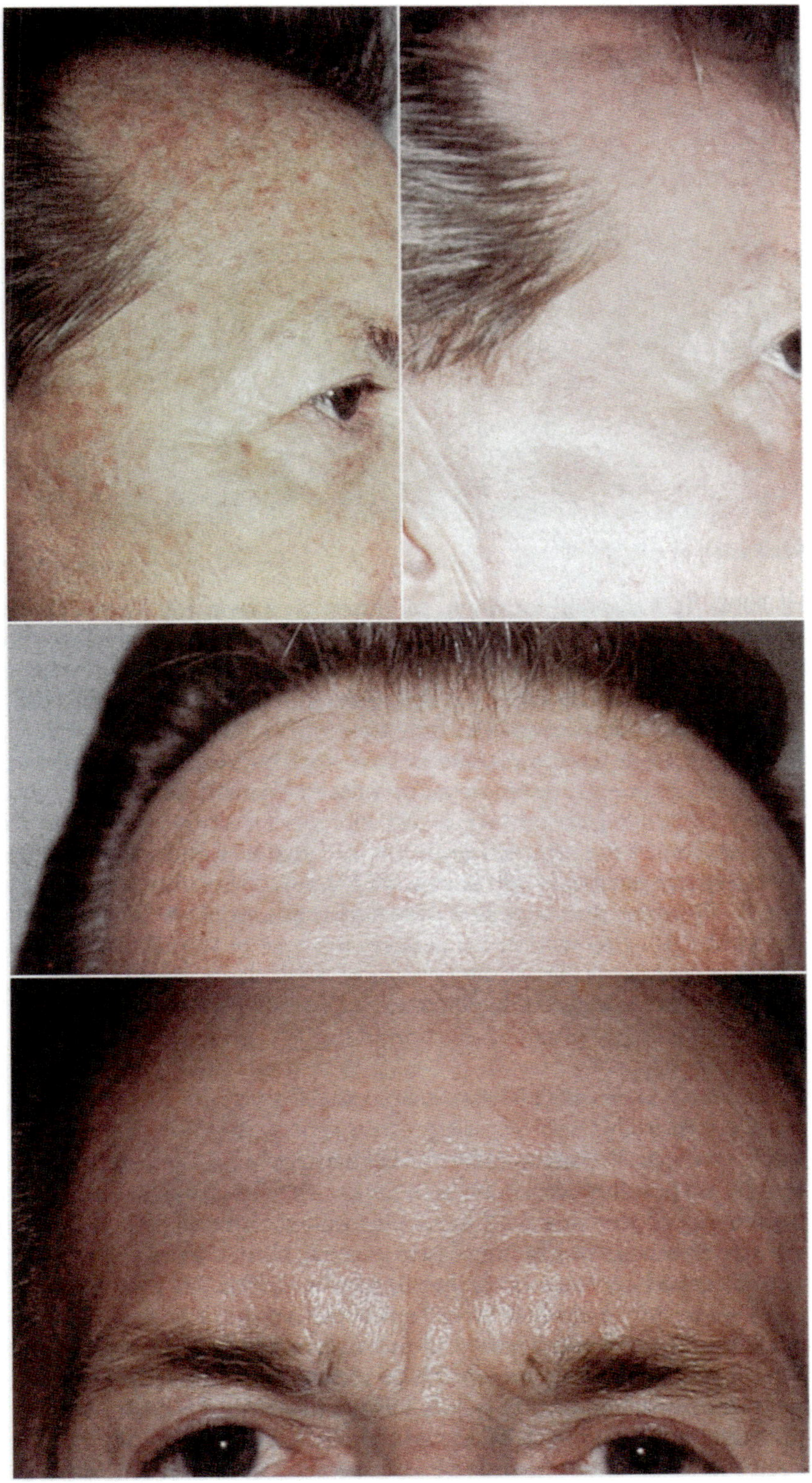

FIG. 6-6. Improvement in actinic keratoses in a Fitzgerald skin type II, Glogau photoaging type IV severely actinically damaged and very sebaceous male. Hard CO_2 was used in all areas followed by TCA, 35%, applied twice with a single gauze sponge and applied three times to the forehead. **A** and **C,** Before peeling. **B** and **D,** Three months after.

(Continued)

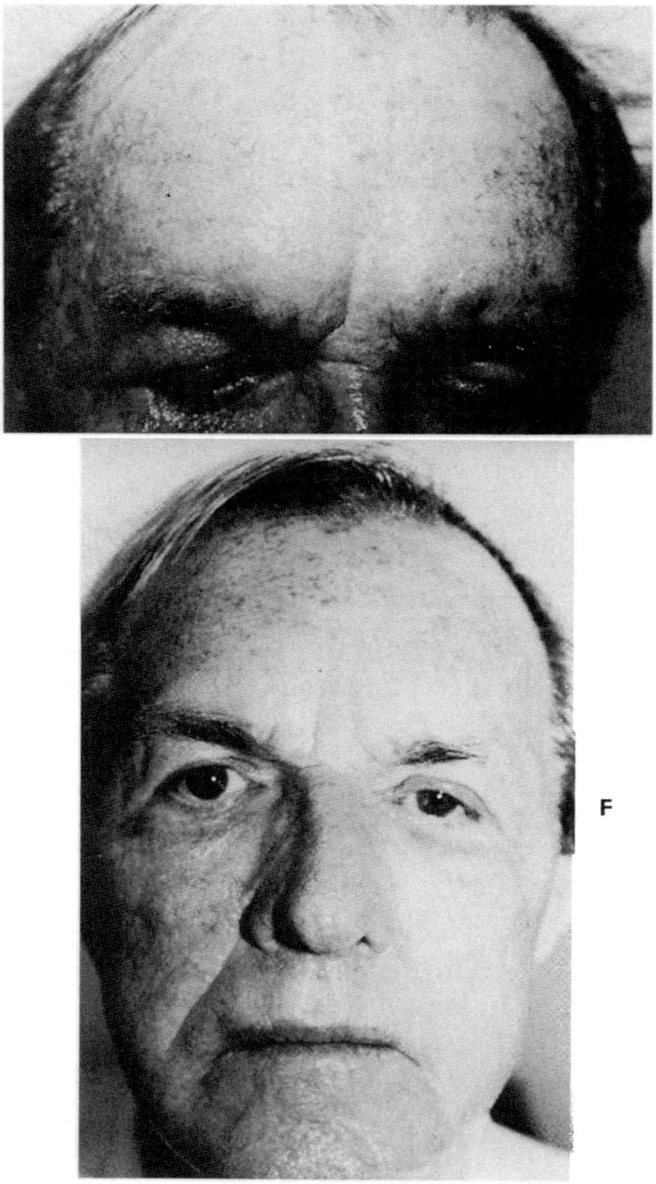

E

F

FIG. 6-6. Cont'd E and **F,** Edema 24 hours after peeling.

A

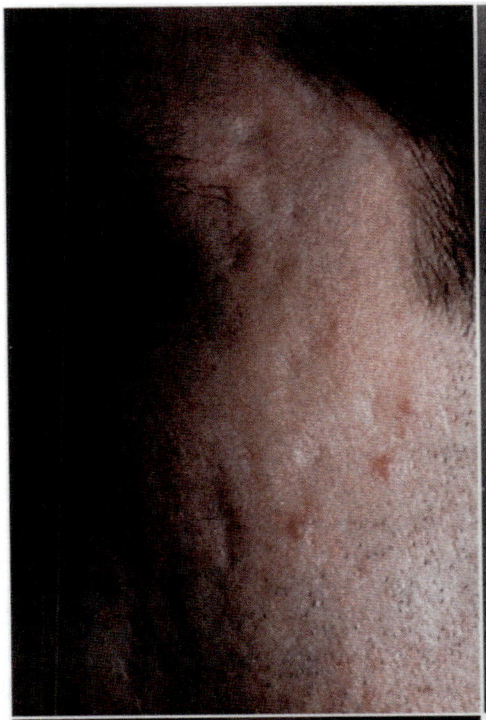

B

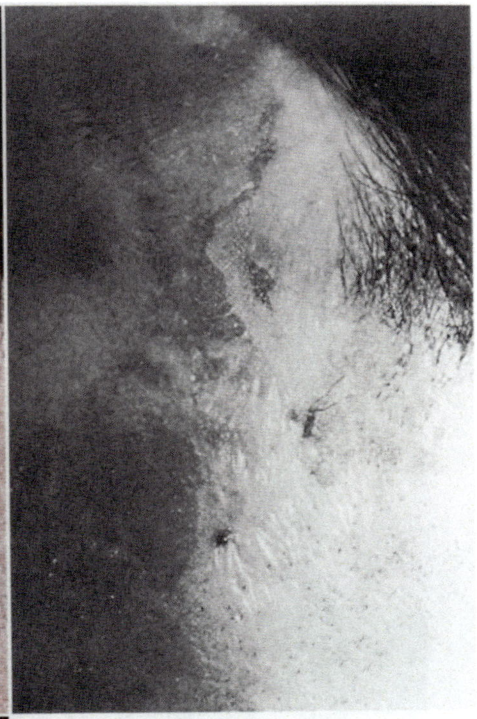

C

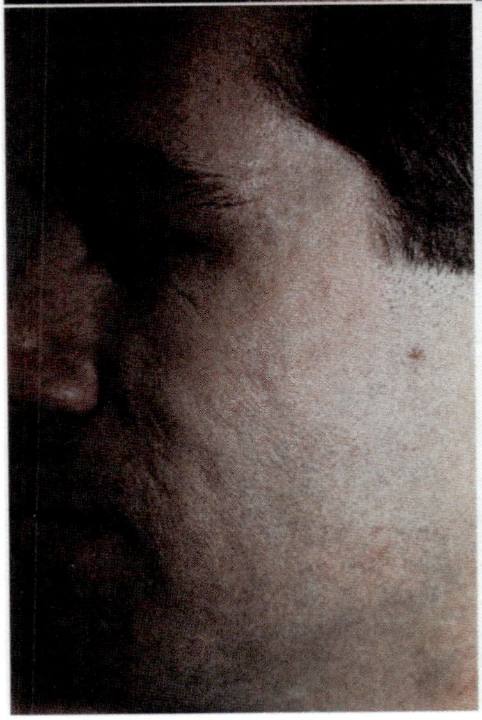

FIG. 6-7. Improvement of depressed scarring with CO_2, hard, to the rims of scars followed by TCA, 50%, to the edges of scars and 35% to the entire remaining area. **A,** Before. **B,** Three days after. **C,** Four months after with effacement of scar rims. *(From Brody HJ, Hailey CW: J Dermatol Surg Oncol 12:1268-1275, 1986. Used by permission.)*

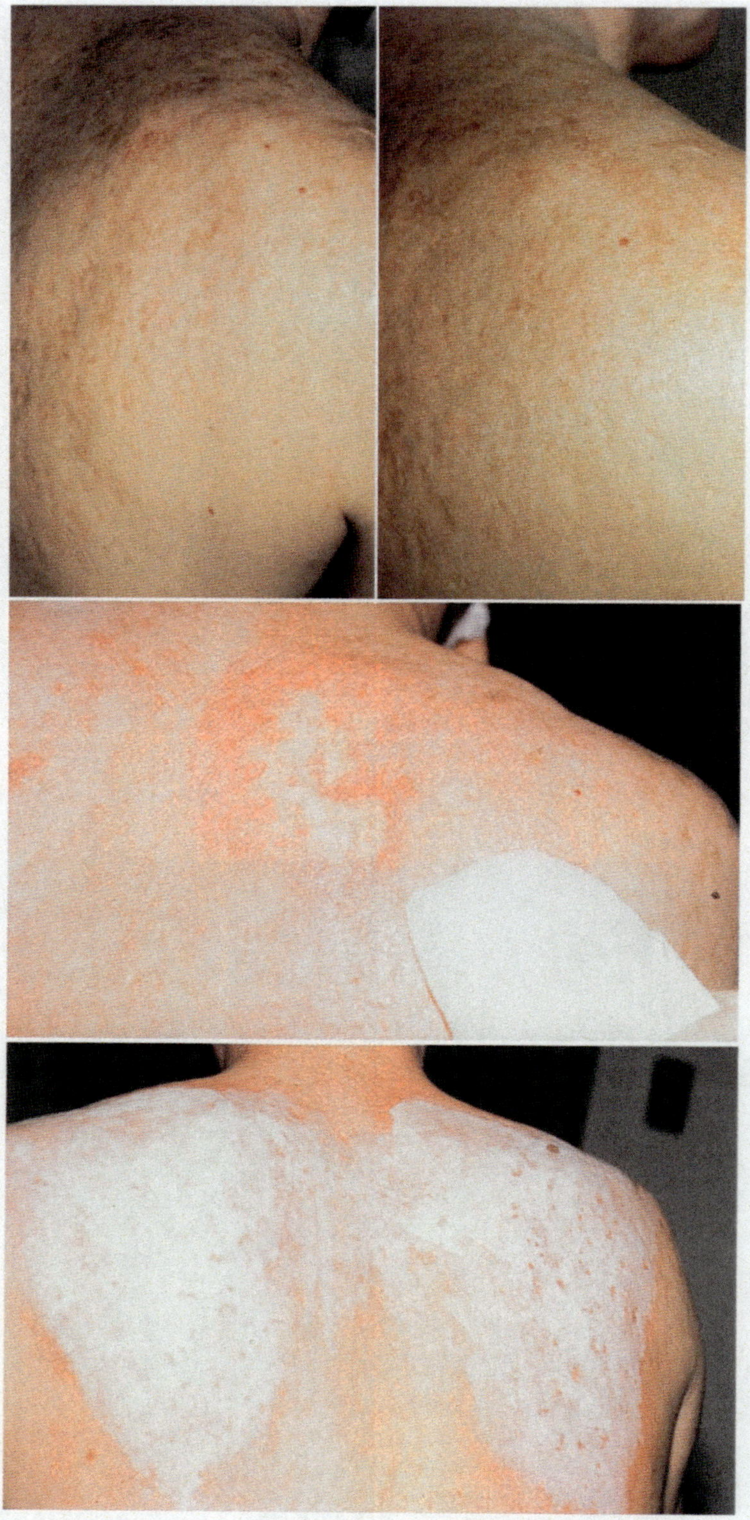

A

B

C

D

FIG. 6-8. A severely acne-scarred back in a Fitzpatrick type I male demonstrates effacement of old acne scarring of greater than 20 years' duration by utilizing three peels of CO_2, hard, plus TCA, 50%, every 6 months. **A,** Before. **B,** Two years after the first peel. **C** and **D,** CO_2 and TCA applications.

A

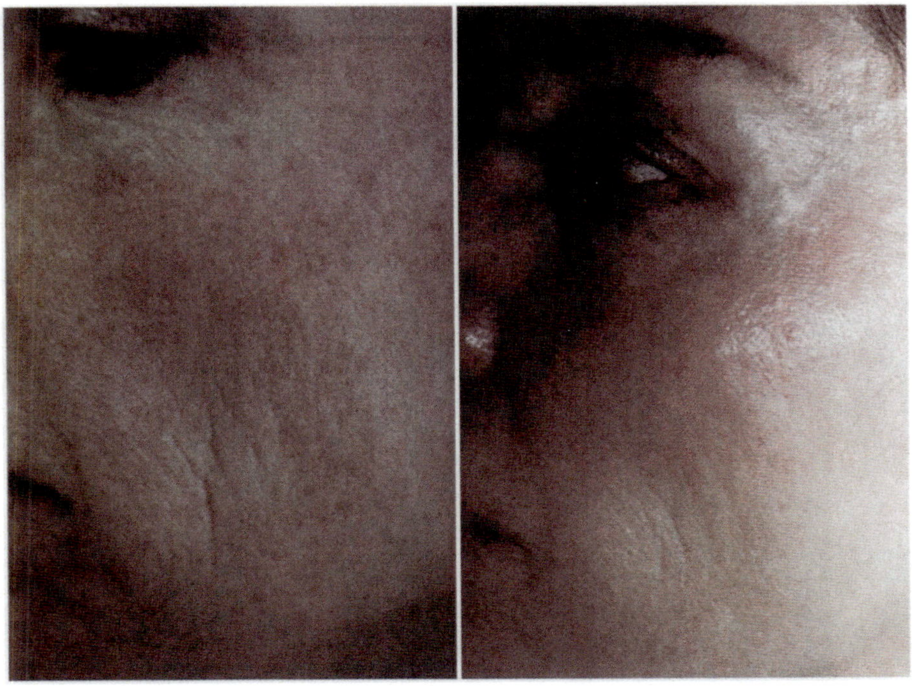

B

FIG. 6-9. A, Before the application of CO_2, hard, plus TCA, 35%, with 50% to cheek rhytides in Fitzpatrick type III, Glogau photoaging group III skin. **B,** Ninety days after peeling there is easing of the rhytides and improvement of mottled pigmentation. *(From Brody HJ, Hailey CW: J Dermatol Surg Oncol 12:1268-1275, 1986. Used by permission.)*

A

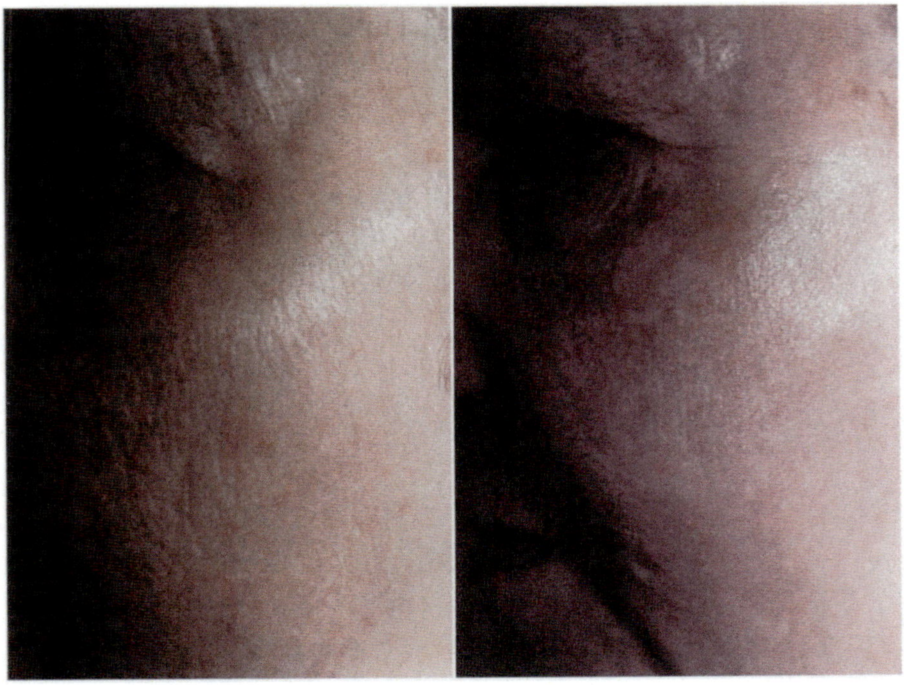

B

FIG. 6-10. A, Moderate rhythides in Fitzpatrick type II, Glogau photoaging group IV skin. **B,** Three months after CO_2 plus TCA, 35%, there is easing of the rhytides at rest and improvement of lentigines and keratoses, but the patient needs rhytidectomy and blepharoplasty for ultimate amelioration of fine wrinkling.

A B C D

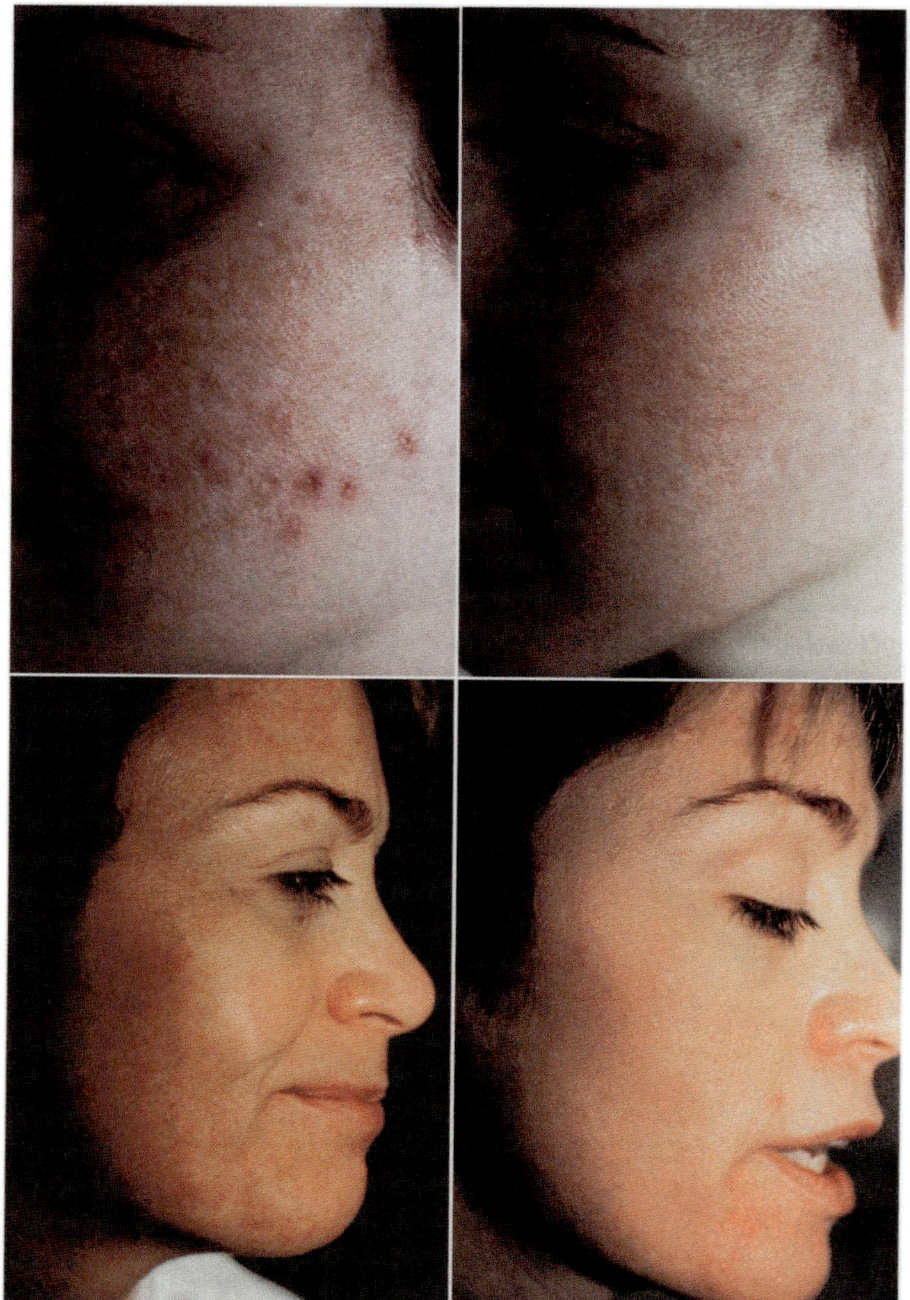

FIG. 6-11. A, Fitzpatrick skin type III, Glogau photoaging group I-melasma, the superficial and deep variety and excoriations with postinflammatory hyperpigmentation. **B,** Ninety days later, there is much resolution after CO_2 moderate plus TCA, 35%. **C,** Fitzpatrick skin type IV, Glogau photoaging group I, melasma. **D,** Four months after CO_2 mild, plus TCA, 35%, resolution is complete with the patient using the peel regimen. *(**A** and **B** from Brody HJ, Hailey CW: J Dermatol Surg Oncol 12:1268-1275, 1986. Used by permission.)*

(Continued)

E

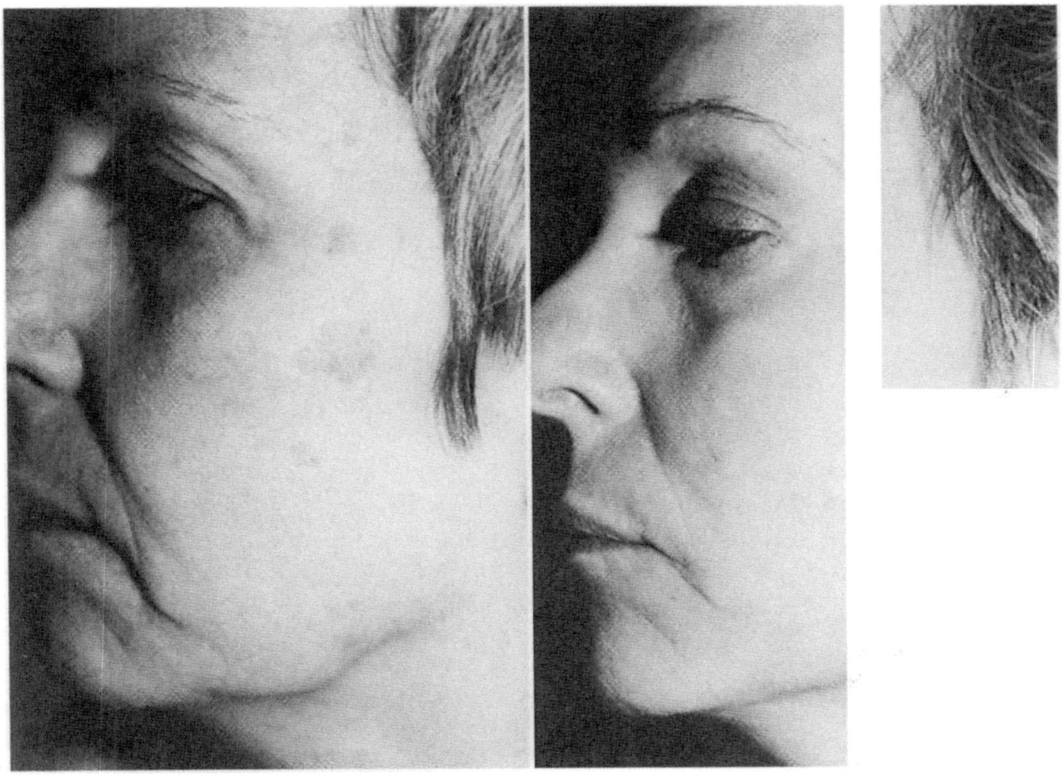

F

FIG 6-11. Cont'd E, Fitzpatrick type II, Glogau photoaging group III, pigmented keratoses. **F,** Three months after CO_2 plus TCA, 35%, with good resolution.

A

B

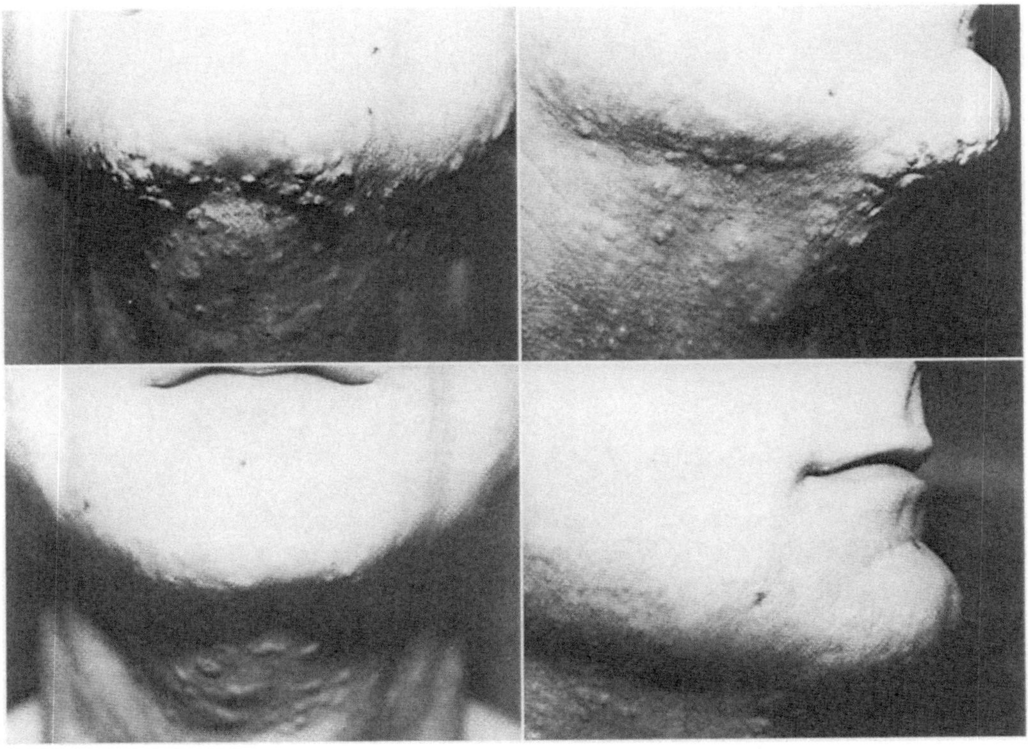

C

D

FIG. 6-12. A and **B,** Immediately after CO_2, hard, plus TCA, 35%, for mollusca. **C** and **D,** Two weeks later there is successful debulking.

Cool compresses of iced saline were originally described for this peel,[11] but we prefer a dry ice pack or cold gel pack, which offers symptomatic relief when applied for about 5 minutes until the patient is comfortable. A soothing emollient may then be applied if desired. (See the section on aftercare later in this chapter.)

This peel produces good results in the treatment of actinic damage, rhytides, and pigmentary dyschromias (Fig. 6-13, *A-D*). (See Chapter 11—case 10 and Fig. 11-10.)

A comparison of the efficacy of JS plus 35% TCA peel on the left side of the face with 5% fluorouracil cream applied twice daily on the right side of the face for 3 weeks to **treat actinic keratoses** was undertaken in 15 subjects. The patients applied tretinoin for 2 weeks before treatment. Equivalency in efficacy with 75% reduction in the number of actinic keratoses was seen, but the peel exhibited superiority in the convenience of a single application with less morbidity and more rapid healing time.[14] The benefits are sustained for at least 1 year and in some patients as long as 3 years. There was loss of the fluorouracil effect after 1 year. Retreatment depends on the original degree of sun damage and aggressiveness of the first peel.

Eleven patients with biopsy-proven actinic keratoses underwent repeat biopsy of the adjacent half of the lesion 2 months after peeling with JS plus 40% TCA and exhibited a 48% cure rate with histologic reconfirmation.[15] Patients resistant to other treatments were selected with significant advanced lesions.

Medium-depth chemical peeling is effective in providing a prophylactic effect against the development of skin malignancies in patients with xeroderma pigmentosum.[16] Although not as effective as dermabrasion, the use of 40% TCA alone in the aforementioned combinations can be repeated at frequent intervals. Dermabrasion may have more sustained results. (See Chapter 10.)

For a discussion of side effects, see Chapter 8. For histologic comparison with other medium-depth peels, see Chapter 2.

Glycolic Acid and Trichloroacetic Acid Peel

The glycolic acid and TCA combination is a predictable method to allow penetration of 35% TCA well into the papillary dermis.[17] The details on each superficial agent are listed in Chapter 5, histology in Chapter 2, and application techniques for TCA in Chapter 4. This peel produces less wounding depth than the first medium-depth combination, but it may be least likely to produce pigmentary dyschromias as a complication.

The chief advantage of this peel is the stratum corneum debridement that the 70% glycolic acid performs, allowing even TCA penetration. No prepeel defatting is necessary. The patients arrive having removed makeup and washed with skin soap. The 70% glycolic acid is applied using a rectal swab over the treated area. After a strict 2-minute contact period, the solution is removed with tap water. Next, 35% TCA is applied to the entire face using 4 × 4–inch gauze pads in the usual fashion up to the lid margins. Spot debridement of hyperkeratotic lesions such as actinic keratoses is necessary before peeling. They may be individually frozen with liquid nitrogen, gently curetted, or retreated with TCA as described in the preceding sections. Cool compresses or packs are used to alleviate burning.

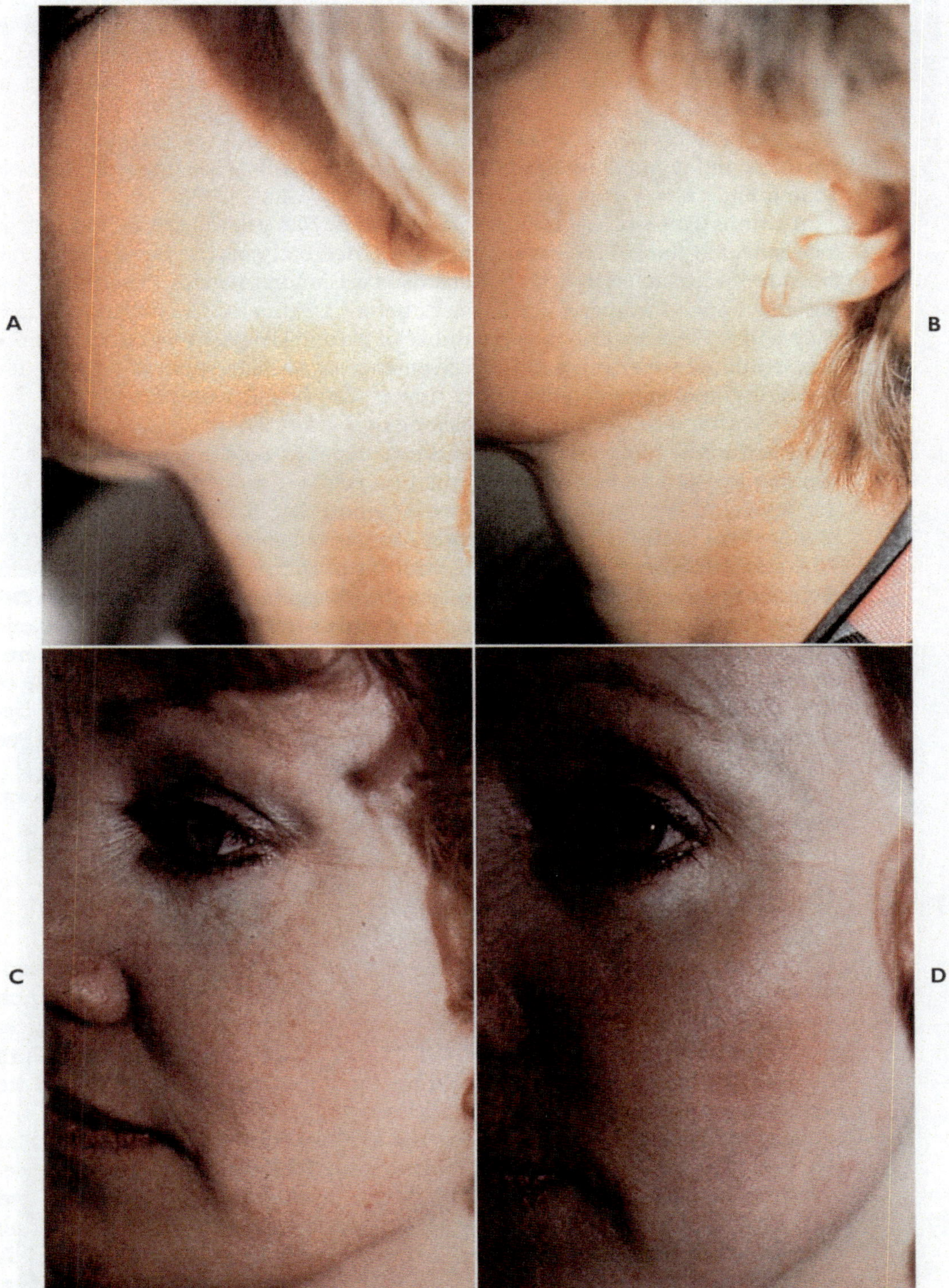

FIG. 6-13. A, Fitzpatrick type II, Glogau photoaging group II, actinic poikiloderma. **B,** After JS applied with two cotton applicators plus TCA, 35%, fading of pigment is apparent. **C,** Fitzpatrick type I, Glogau photoaging group II, mild actinic freckling and rhytides. **D,** Three months after JS applied with two cotton applicators plus TCA, 35%, there is good resolution of pigmentation and small rhytides. Note the retention of a dynamic-related single rhytid in the periorbital area.

The **neck** may be optionally treated with 70% glycolic acid for 2 minutes followed by 20% TCA if photoaging is significant. Petrolatum is applied over the entire area, and the patient is discharged. Nonfacial **body peel** areas such as the **back, upper chest, arms, and legs** are best approached with glycolic acid or alternatively Jessner's solution followed by 20% TCA. Some patients can tolerate 35% TCA after glycolic acid, but this should be done after previously employing the lower concentrations of TCA and observing each patient's individual clinical response. The rejuvenation regimen including tretinoin as outlined in Chapter 4 should be used on nonfacial areas also. Body peels can be repeated every 4 to 12 weeks if needed, but if the skin is too erythematous after healing, inadvertent scarring may result. A light residual erythema from the regimen application is ideal for repeeling.

Applying 70% glycolic acid gel for 2 minutes followed by 40% TCA applied over the gel and washing both off simultaneously when desired frosting has been reached has been suggested as more time efficient for body peels.[18] The glycolic acid gel may slow TCA absorption, but 40% TCA is not safe for all nonfacial areas. There is undefined variation of the acids' time on the skin and uncertainty in washing off both peeling agents at once from the skin. This method is less precise at this time and its safety unestablished.

This peel is excellent for pigmentary dyschromias, actinic damage and mild rhytides (Fig. 6-14). A prepeel acetone scrub will change the depth and safety of this original peel description. As with all peels the original description carries with it the safety record of the author. See the section on aftercare later in

A

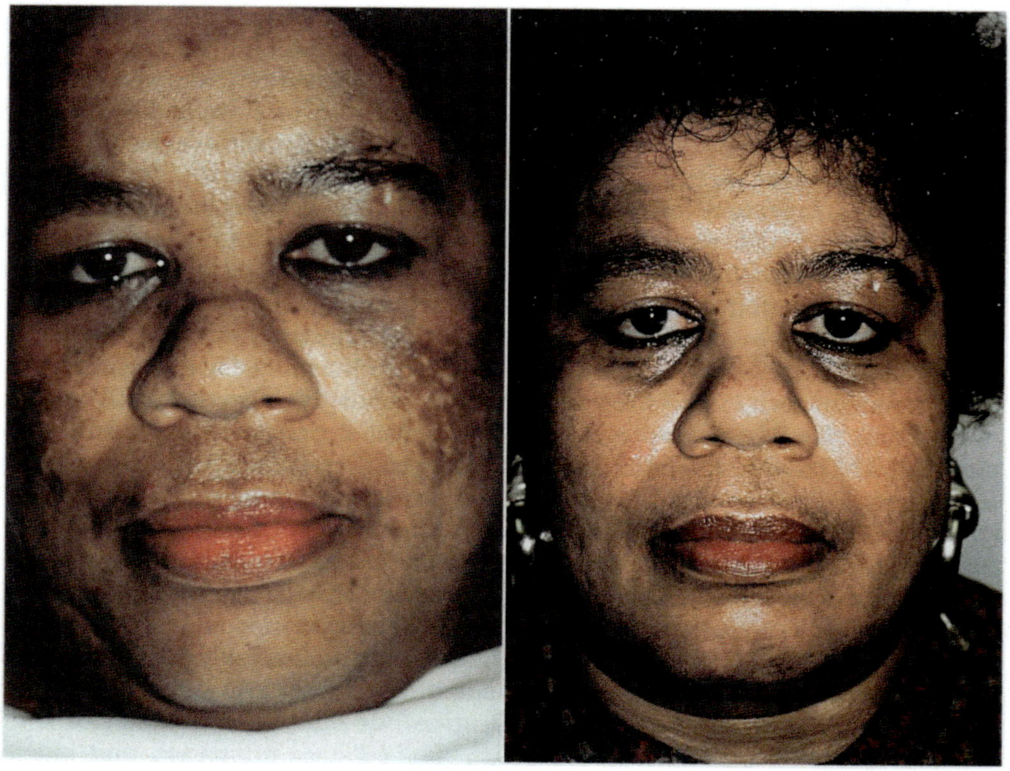

B

FIG. 6-14. A, Fitzpatrick skin type VI patient with melasma peeled with unbuffered glycolic acid, 70%, for 2 minutes followed by TCA, 35%. **B,** Four weeks after. *(Courtesy of Dr. William P. Coleman.)*

this chapter. For a discussion of side effects, see Chapter 8. For histologic comparison to Jessner's solution plus TCA, see Chapter 2.

Fifty Percent Trichloroacetic Acid Peel

The 50% TCA peel does not produce the depth that Baker's phenol solution does, and it is not capable of producing in a single application the same results as a Baker's peel for severe photodamage.[19-27] (See Chapter 2.) However, in properly selected patients with less-than-severe actinic damage, it is an effective chemical peel. The results may be irregular, and individual rhytides may remain at the vermilion. The agent may not be able to penetrate very deep actinic perioral rhytides with uniformity in spite of careful application. (See the section on texture changes in Chapter 8.) These areas may require additional local retreatment. Some feel that TCA in high concentrations is more unpredictable and more likely than phenol to produce scarring.[28] Peeling with **60% to 75% TCA** is much more risky and not recommended as a chemical peel, although spot treatment of localized actinic keratoses with these high strengths can be effective. The destructive effect of 75% TCA and higher to penetrate through the deep dermis to remove amateur **tattoos** can be simple and inexpensive, although hypopigmentation and scarring may result.[29] These improve with time or treatment in 1 or 2 years. (See Chapter 11—Case 8 and Fig. 11-8.)

The 50% TCA peel is more likely than the other three varieties of combination medium-depth peels to result in a texture change or hypopigmentation, which is usually untroublesome to the patient. It is an unpredictable and erratic agent that is more prone to hypertrophic scarring. It has its place, however, in the armamentarium against actinic damage.

For a discussion of the mechanism and preparation of TCA with the exact mode of application as a wounding agent, see Chapter 2; the section on 10% to 35% TCA in Chapter 5; and Chapter 4. For the local use of 50% TCA in the treatment of acne and comedones, see Chapter 4. For the use of additives with 50% TCA, see discussion under frosting in Chapter 4.

This is generally a more painful peel than the previous three medium-depth procedures. There are two methods of application. The first is our preferred method, but either is effective. The application is rapid over the entire face with damp cotton-tipped applicators or a single damp gauze pad, beginning under the eyes and proceeding over the nose, cheeks, chin, and forehead. Dilution is unnecessary, and relief is provided from immediate stinging by compression with ice-cold dry gel packs. Care must be taken not to overcoat any areas that are to be peeled lightly. The eyelids are peeled with 20% to 35% TCA. The concept here is a full-face peel that does not have to be evenly frosted in every aesthetic area in the same fashion. (See the discussion on frosting in the mode of application in Chapter 4.)

The alternative concept is to use TCA in a controlled application with a single cotton-tipped applicator in increments of 1 to 2 cm^2. This achieves slow treatment of each cosmetic unit and prolongs the procedure. Sedation with meperidine, 50 mg, and diazepam, 5 mg, intramuscularly 30 minutes before peeling is helpful to reduce patient discomfort. Applicators are discarded between cosmetic units. "Neutralization," or dilution with water or sodium bicarbonate, has been advocated in the literature after each unit but must occur before complete frosting to be effective and serves only to substitute one sensation for another to ease the stinging. (See the section on dilution in

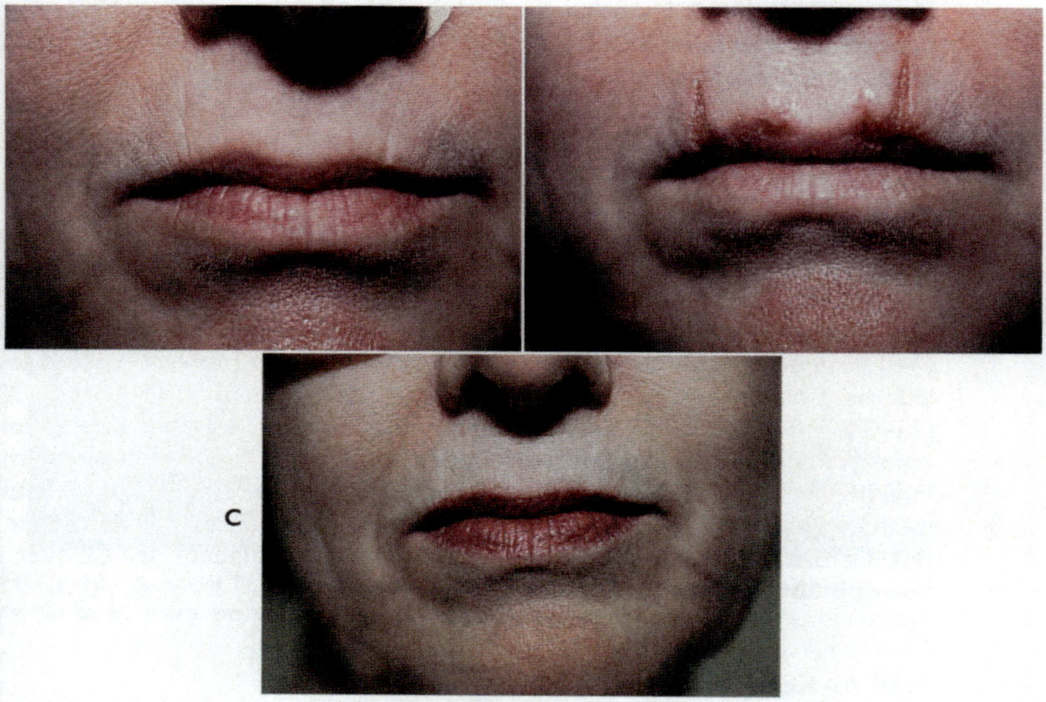

FIG. 6-15. A, Fitzpatrick skin type II patient with Glogau photoaging type III before spot application of TCA, 50%, to isolated actinic rhytides. **B,** One week after application. **C,** One year after two monthly applications showing a hypopigmented linear texture change, preferable to rhytides. (See text.)

Chapter 4.) This peel is unpredictable on the neck area. Blending facial and neck skin with lower concentrations of TCA can minimize the contrast between adjacent unpeeled areas. Repetitive 50% frosting applications may cause scarring and are not recommended on the face or neck.

In patients with isolated rhytides, type III photoaging, and little diffuse yellow clinical actinic damage in the perioral area, 50% TCA may be applied focally to the individual rhytides with the broken wooden end of a cotton-tipped applicator and repeated monthly for 2 or 3 applications (Fig. 6-15). Sometimes these isolated rhytides are amplified by dynamic motion in the cosmetic unit, and these will not be totally ameliorated. A hypopigmented linear texture change may replace the rhytid, which is usually preferable to the wrinkle. This selective application is not indicated for type IV photoaging and is not intended to replace an upper lip peel. The use of selected Baker's phenol in this fashion may produce unacceptable hypopigmented striping.

In the past, occlusion of this peel with tape was thought to increase penetration and create a deeper wound. This is not true. Histologic studies indicate that deeper wound depth does not occur, thus suggesting that taping TCA peels should be discontinued. (See the section on occlusion of TCA in Chapter 2.)

The 50% TCA peel was evaluated and compared in the treatment of actinic cheilitis with topical fluorouracil, lip shave, and the carbon dioxide laser. The latter two procedures showed no dysplasia on biopsy samples after 1 year. Seventy percent of the TCA-treated patients showed a return of actinic cheilitis after 9 months, with all patients showing dysplastic features on biopsy specimens. The peel will succeed in prophylaxis against the eventual development of carcinoma, but it is not as successful as the lip shave or laser. Therefore patients must be reliable in follow-up visits if TCA is used.[30] See the following aftercare section for details.

Full-Strength Unoccluded Phenol Peel

The full strength, unoccluded 88% phenol peel gives a result comparable to any medium-depth chemical peel.[22,31,32] Properly applied doses without excessive amounts of phenol to any one area will give a uniform appearance with barely noticeable hypopigmentation, if any. In a moderately actinically damaged patient, the result may be more predictable and more even with less chance of scarring than with 50% TCA. Its results are commensurate with CO_2 plus TCA and JS plus TCA. However, the disadvantages are that cardiac and renal precautions must be enforced and that the peel is slower to perform. Full-strength phenol is commonly used on the eyelids in conjunction with full-face deep peeling. It can be used for touch-ups in local areas 6 months after a Baker's formula phenol peel. For details on the use of phenol, see Chapter 7. For wounding depth, see Chapter 2.

Pyruvic Acid (α-Keto Acid)

Pyruvic acid is an α-keto acid, a chemical group that has properties of both acids and ketones.[33-36] It converts physiologically to lactic acid, an α-hydroxy acid. Although lactic and pyruvic acids convert to each other, pyruvic acid has additional properties that make it particularly potent as a topical peeling agent. (See the section on pyruvic acid in Chapter 2.) Pyruvic acid is available in pure form as a liquid at 95% to 99% strength. After standing over time, it may decompose to form carbon dioxide and acetaldehyde. The carbon dioxide gas will build up pressure, and the bottle can explode.[37]

The vapors inhaled by patients are pungent and irritating to the upper respiratory tract, and an electric fan is helpful.[38] Epidermolysis occurs in 30 to 60 seconds, and dermal penetration is rapid, occurring within 1 to 2 minutes.

Pyruvic acid is very potent as a chemical peeling agent and has potential for scarring. It should not be used to peel the skin in its full-strength form. Studies in the human model demonstrate that dilutions in ethanol approaching 50% produce increased papillary dermal homogenization and upper reticular dermal penetration.[33] Water decreases the potency of pyruvic acid and is not recommended as a diluent. The agent is painful on application, and scarring on the face has been demonstrated with the use of 80% pyruvic acid utilized as a chemical peel.

Griffin has shown 60% pyruvic acid in ethanol to be effective as a peeling agent. The acid induces more even dermal penetration when 5 cc is combined with 8 drops of an emulsifying agent such as polyethylene laurel ether (Brij 35) and 1 drop of croton oil as an epidermolytic inflammatory agent in a solution similar to Baker's phenol formula. (Griffin TD: Personal communication, 1991.) Phenol penetrates deeper in a 55% than in an 88% concentration, presumably because quick epidermal protein coagulation self-blocks further absorption. The mechanism of action of pyruvic acid is uncertain.

The solution may be applied with cotton-tipped applicators to tretinoin-prepared skin after mild degreasing. No attempt should be made to remove the

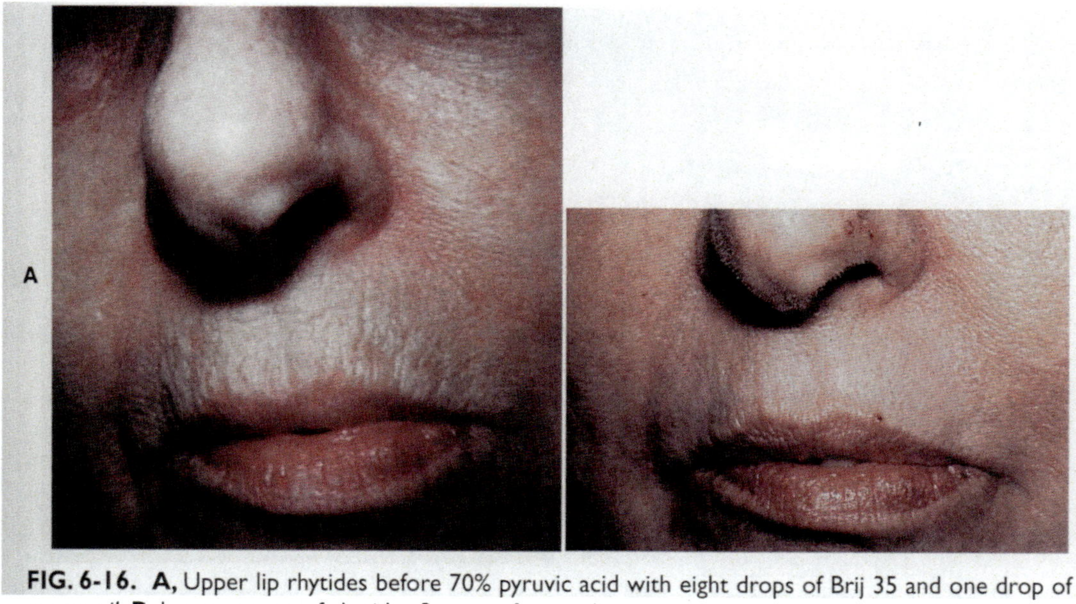

FIG. 6-16. A, Upper lip rhytides before 70% pyruvic acid with eight drops of Brij 35 and one drop of croton oil. **B,** Improvement of rhytides 3 years after peeling. *(Courtesy of Dr. Thomas D. Griffin.)*

stratum corneum by vigorous rubbing because any condition that decreases barrier function may lead to increased penetration. Preexisting dermatitis may be particularly detrimental to this agent. The edges of the peeled area may be feathered with less solution. After 2 to 5 minutes or whenever adequate frosting has occurred, the area is soaked with water, more for patient comfort than neutralization. Reepithelialization occurs between 7 and 14 days. The peeled area is initially erythematous, and this erythema may persist for 2 weeks to 2 months (Fig. 6-16). Focal reapplication may be performed after healing is complete for persistent rhytides. (See the following aftercare section for details.)

Although pyruvic acid does not seem as destructive in wound depth as Baker's phenol, does not seem to have systemic toxicity, and does not cause hypopigmentation as readily as phenol, more research is necessary to further understand its unknown range of penetration with dose and its scarring capability (Fig. 6-17). Scarring is more likely to occur when high concentrations in the range of 80% or above are used on younger, more sensitive, less sun-damaged skin. If used by an experienced operator, pyruvic acid can be an acceptable chemical peeling agent. Because its unpredictable penetration is difficult to standardize, it should be used only with great care and knowledge as a full-face peel.

Spot application of 60% pyruvic acid for 2 to 5 minutes until blanching to treat actinic keratoses has also been described. Five percent 5-fluorouracil (5-FU) cream used for 5 to 7 days before treatment may elicit and highlight the keratoses before application of the pyruvic acid. This is not a true chemical peel but rather a method to reduce the dermatitis that is experienced with 3 to 4 weeks of 5-FU treatment for actinic damage.[39] The resolution of the keratoses, however, is due to the pyruvic acid and not to the 5-FU. The relative effectiveness of pyruvic acid and other spot wounding agents, 50% to 75% TCA, for example, has not been determined.

A

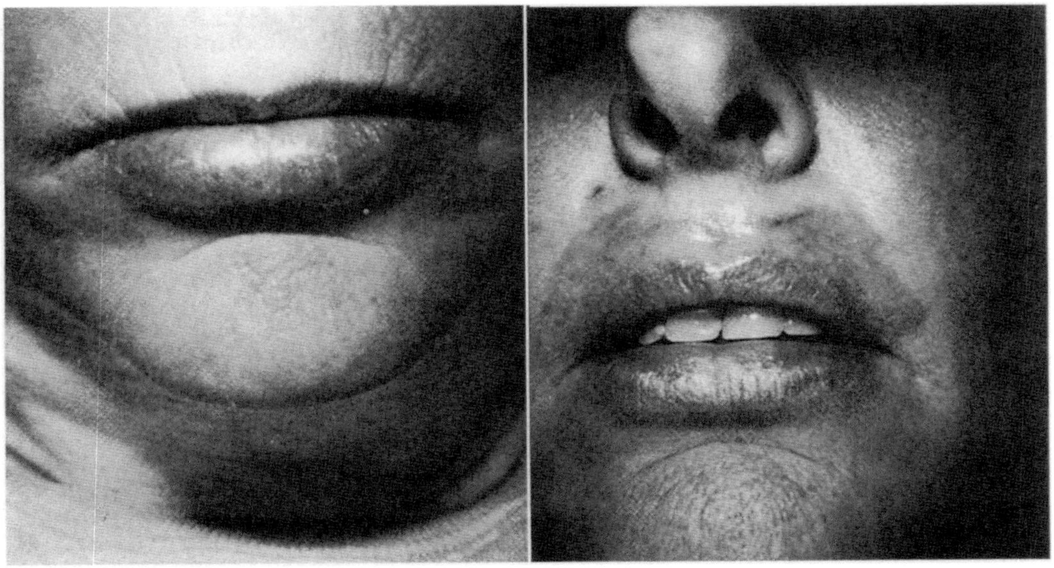

B

FIG. 6-17. **A,** Upper lip rhytides before 80% pyruvic acid peel. **B,** Scarring 6 weeks later with resulting eclabium, which diminished with time. *(Courtesy of Dr. Thomas D. Griffin.)*

A

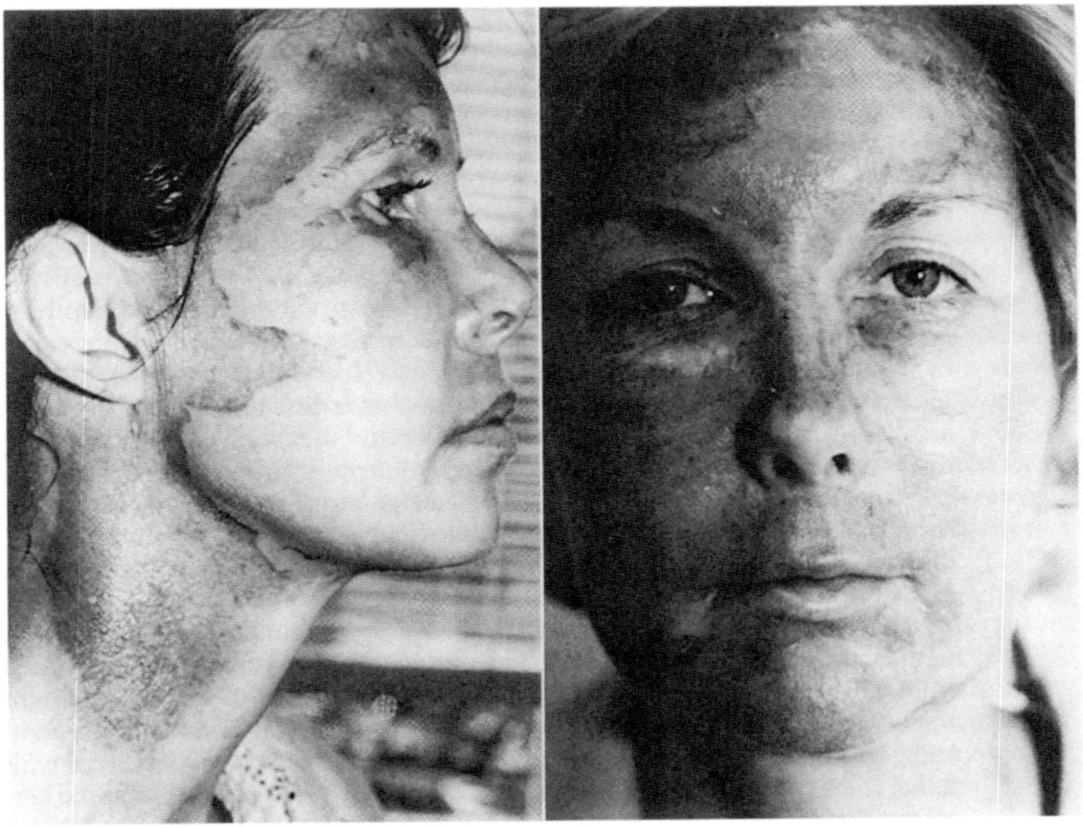

B

FIG. 6-18. Crusting 4 days after medium-depth peeling.

AFTERCARE FOR MEDIUM-DEPTH CHEMICAL PEELS

An hour after the original frost, erythema appears and changes to a brownish hue. Considerable edema is present for the first 48 hours. Discomfort is relatively mild to minimal. After several days when the edema partially resolves, a crust forms. Crust separation generally begins between the fourth and the eighth postoperative day and is completed usually by days 7 to 12, depending on the area and the peel (Fig. 6-18). The patient is encouraged to minimize crusting by washing twice daily with antiseptic compresses and then applying a soothing ointment. We prefer a dilute solution of povidone-iodine lathered in the patient's hands in the shower or basin before facial soaking. Tap water, hydrogen peroxide, or dilute 0.25% acetic acid soaks (1 tbsp of white vinegar in 1 pt of water) are also effective. (See Chapter 3 for details.)

We favor the use of a petrolatum-based shark liver oil and phenylephrine HCl ointment (Preparation H, Whitehall) as the ointment for application in medium-depth peeling. The original formulation increased the oxygen consumption of dermal fibroblasts. Therefore collagen formation was increased, and wound healing rates were increased.[40,41] Sensitizers are present in the new formulation, but in our experience, contact dermatitis is rare, and the ointment's soothing properties outweigh its disadvantages. Bacitracin or Polysporin (Burroughs Wellcome) ointments are also effective and are rarely sensitizing. Petrolatum alone is acceptable. (See the section on pruritis in Chapter 8.) Crisco vegetable shortening, which is sometimes recommended for deep peeling, is too greasy and unnecessary for the thinner crusts of these peels. Overgreasing may produce acne lesions during healing and should dictate a change in ointment. However, healing is more rapid if under an ointment base from the onset. Some physicians use synthetic membrane dressings[42] (e.g., Vigilon, Meshed Omiderm[43]) for the first 2 to 4 days after the peel, but we have found that this is more useful in dermabrasion or laser and offers no advantage in medium-depth peeling. (See Chapter 3 for additional discussion.)

Slight edema and erythema persist for 30 to 60 days, and solar restriction is imperative until the erythema has resolved. Ideally, protection should continue indefinitely. Tretinoin, sunscreens, and optionally hydroquinone in the regimen are reinstituted as soon as the patient can tolerate them. Makeup can be applied at any time to any area that has resurfaced during the healing course. (See the regimen section in Chapter 4.) The makeup applied after this peel does not require special expertise, as opposed to deep peeling. Most water-based foundations will cover the erythema, although a temporary cream-based, blemish-cover makeup (e.g., Clinique Continuous Coverage) may be used for the first 7 days after reepithelialization (Fig. 6-19). (See the section on cosmetic coverage after chemical peeling in Chapter 7.)

Repeat medium-depth peels may be performed in 6 months if there are skip areas or if repeeling in toto or in part would benefit the patient. If all erythema and edema have subsided, the patient can be repeeled sooner, possibly with a lower concentration of wounding agent, but not before 90 days. (See Chapter 2.) If the patient is peeled too soon with another peel of equal depth while erythema is still present, we have seen scarring as a result because the dermal collagen has not completely reorganized. (See Chapter 8 and Chapter 3, Fig. 3-3.) This is not a risk in superficial peeling where it is acceptable to repeel erythematous skin with continual epidermal sloughs incurring little or no risk of scarring.

Post–Skin Peel Instructions

You have been peeled with chemicals that may cause water blisters that may break, crust, turn brown, and peel off over a period of a week.

Washing with a mild soap (Dove) and povidone-iodine skin cleanser twice daily in the shower or over the sink is necessary to prevent any infection. Use your fingertips and not a Buf-Puf, since the skin is very sensitive at this time. A tube of petrolatum-containing ointment (Aquaphor, Vaseline) or Preparation H should be used during this week all over the face after washing; A tube is more sterile than a jar. Do not pick at the peeled skin.

Three (3) aspirin or ibuprofen are to be taken 3 or 4 times daily to reduce swelling. Sleep on several pillows the first night.

Total sunblock and a hat should be used to prevent hyperpigmentation immediately after healing.

Your prescription creams can be applied after the first week, but remember, your skin will be more sensitive than usual.

If *pain* begins, which may signal a fever blister, call us immediately.

FIG. 6-19. Patient instruction sheet after skin peeling.

COMBINING MEDIUM-DEPTH PEELING WITH DEEP PEELING, DERMABRASION, OR LASER RESURFACING

Combinations of various medium-depth peels to effectively blend cosmetic units with deeper methodology are effective and useful. These are described in Chapter 10 and illustrated in Figs. 7-12, 7-13, 10-1, and 10-3.

REFERENCES

1. Ayres S: Dermal changes following application of chemical cauterants to aging skin, *Arch Dermatol* 82:578, 1960.
2. Graham GF: Cryotherapy in the treatment of acne. In Epstein E, Epstein E Jr, editors: *Skin surgery*, ed 4, Springfield, Ill, 1977, Charles C Thomas, pp. 685-697.
3. Bennett RG: *Fundamentals of cutaneous surgery*, St Louis, 1988, Mosby, p. 229.
4. Sutton RL: *Diseases of the skin*, St Louis, 1916, Mosby, p. 83.
5. Brody HJ, Hailey CW: Medium depth chemical peeling of the skin: a variation of superficial chemosurgery, *J Dermatol Surg Oncol* 12:1268-1275, 1986.
6. Brody HJ: Medium depth chemical peeling of the skin: a variation of superficial chemosurgery, *Adv Dermatol* 3:205-220, 1988.
7. Brody HJ: Trichloroacetic acid application in chemical peeling, *Operative Techniques Plast Reconstr Surg* 2(2):127-128, 1995.
8. Brody HJ: Variations and comparisons in medium depth chemical peeling, *J Dermatol Surg Oncol* 15:953-963, 1989.
9. Garrett SJ, Robinson JK, Roenigk HH: Trichloroacetic acid peel of molluscum contagiosum in immunocompromised patients, *J Dermatol Surg Oncol* 18:855-858, 1992.
10. Sadick NS: A comparative study of 100% TCA and cryosurgery in the treatment of disseminated HIV facial molluscum contagiosum. Presented at the American Society for Dermatologic Surgery, Palm Springs, Calif, May 17, 1996.
11. Monheit GD: The Jessner's + TCA peel: a medium depth chemical peel, *J Dermatol Surg Oncol* 15:945-950, 1989.
12. Bloom RF: Combined peels tackle actinic keratoses, *Dermatol Times* 19:25, 1991.
13. Monheit GD: The Jessner's–trichloroacetic acid peel, *Dermatol Clin* 13(2):277-283, 1995.
14. Lawrence N, Cox SE, Cockerell CJ, et al: A comparison of the efficacy and safety of Jessner's solution and 35% trichloroacetic acid vs 5% fluorouracil in the treatment of widespread facial actinic keratoses, *Arch Dermatol* 131:176-181, 1995.
15. Clark RE, Weingold DH, Hirsh E, et al: TCA chemical peel effective for extensive actinic keratoses, *Skin Allergy News* 22:34, 1991.
16. Nelson BR, Fader DJ, Gillard M, et al: The role of dermabrasion and chemical peels in the treatment of patients with xeroderma pigmentosum, *J Am Acad Dermatol* 32:623-636, 1995.
17. Coleman WP, Futrell JM: The glycolic acid + trichloroacetic acid peel, *J Dermatol Surg Oncol* 20:76-80, 1994.
18. Cook K: Chemical peel used on the neck, chest and extremities, *Skin Allergy News* 27(3):5, 1996.
19. Ayres S: Superficial chemosurgery in treating aging skin, *Arch Dermatol* 85:125, 1962.
20. Monash S: The uses of diluted trichloroacetic acid in dermatology, *Urol Cutan Rev* 49:119, 1949.
21. Collins PS: The chemical peel, *Clin Dermatol* 5:57-74, 1987.
22. Stegman SJ, Tromovitch TA, Glogau RG: *Cosmetic dermatologic surgery*, ed 2, St Louis, 1990, Mosby, pp. 35-58.
23. Roberts HL: The chloroacetic acids: a biochemical study, *Br J Dermatol* 38:323-391, 1926.
24. Resnik SS: Chemical peeling with trichloroacetic acid, *J Dermatol Surg Oncol* 10:549-550, 1984.
25. Resnik SS: Chemical peeling with trichloroacetic acid. In Roenigk H, Roenigk R, editors: *Dermatologic surgery: principles and practice*, New York, 1989, Marcel Dekker, pp. 979-995.
26. Brodland DG, Roenigk RK: Trichloroacetic acid chemexfoliation (chemical peel) for extensive premalignant actinic damage of the face and scalp, *Mayo Clin Proc* 63:887-896, 1988.
27. Collins PS: Trichloroacetic acid peels revisited, *J Dermatol Surg Oncol* 15:933-940, 1989.
28. Ayres S: Dermal changes following application of chemical cauterants to aging skin, *Arch Dermatol* 82:578, 1960.
29. Piggot TA, Norris RW: The treatment of tattoos with trichloracetic acid: experience with 670 patients, *Br J Plast Surg* 41:112-117, 1988.
30. Robinson JK: Actinic cheilitis, *Arch Otolaryngol Head Neck Surg* 115:848-852, 1989.
31. Stegman SJ, Tromovitch TA: *Cosmetic dermatologic surgery*, St Louis, 1984, Mosby, pp. 27-46.

32. Mackee GM, Karp FL: The treatment of post-acne scars with phenol, *Br J Dermatol* 64:456-459, 1952.
33. Griffin TD, Van Scott EJ, Maddin S: The use of pyruvic acid as a chemical peeling agent, *J Dermatol Surg Oncol* 15:1316, 1989 (abstract).
34. Van Scott EJ: The unfolding therapeutic uses of the alpha hydroxy acids, *Mediguide Dermatol* 3:1-5, 1989.
35. Van Scott EJ: Alpha hydroxy acids: procedures for use in clinical practice, *Cutis* 43:222, 1989.
36. Brody HJ: Update on chemical peels, *Adv Dermatol* 7:232-245, 1992.
37. Milstein E: Is pyruvic acid potentially explosive? *Schoch Lett* 40:41, 1990.
38. Van Scott EJ, Yu RJ: Alpha hydroxy acids: therapeutic potentials, *Can J Dermatol* 1:108-112, 1989.
39. Griffin TD, Van Scott EJ: Use of pyruvic acid in the treatment of actinic keratoses: a clinical and histopathologic study, *Cutis* 47:325-329, 1991.
40. Goodson W, Hohn D, Hunt T, et al: Augmentation of some aspects of wound healing by a "skin respiratory factor," *J Surg Res* 21:125-129, 1976.
41. Kaplan JZ: Acceleration of wound healing by a live yeast cell derivative, *Arch Surg* 119:1005-1008, 1984.
42. Falanga V: Occlusive wound dressings, *Arch Dermatol* 124:872-877, 1988.
43. Raab B: A new hydrophilic copolymer membrane for dermabrasion, *J Dermatol Surg Oncol* 17:323-328, 1991.

7 *Deep Peeling*

BAKER-GORDON FORMULA PHENOL PEEL

Perspective on Deep Peeling

The deep peel with phenol has received an unwarranted bad reputation from some practitioners who have marketed and advertised TCA peeling to non-dermatologists while overemphasizing phenol's "toxicity" and understressing its excellent 30-year safety record. Emphasizing the "poisonous" effects of the chemical phenol when no one has died from a properly performed peel is deceptive. Emphasizing an alablaster skin after peeling when it does not appear in most patients is unfair. Emphasizing scarring from phenol and ignoring the catastrophic scarring from TCA is also dishonest.

The truth about phenol is that it is increasingly unnecessary to perform a full-face phenol peel if each cosmetic unit has been properly evaluated. When indicated the reliability and predictablity of the deep peel reflects evidence of its 30-year safety record. Laser peeling or resurfacing is being heavily promoted. Laser recovery does not uniformly have less pain, less erythema, less swelling, or quicker recovery, and time and expense are required for the machine, the anesthetic nerve blocks, tumescent anesthesia, or sedation with the laser. The location and severity of photodamage or scarring of a given cosmetic unit may be factors that make one modality preferred over the other, as discussed in this text. The same complications of pigmentation and hypertrophic scarring occur with laser surgery, as well as deep peeling. Candidiasis and contact dermatitis are more common with laser resurfacing. As new technologies are embraced, unbiased and peer-reviewed scientific data that are objectively evaluated and felt to be advantageous will be examined over long-term follow-up. A tried-and-true technique such as phenol peeling will have a position alongside the laser as another complementary resurfacing modality.

Preliminary clinical comparison between the laser and Baker's solution reveals that the laser improves severe photodamage by approximately 50%. In the treatment of Glogau photoaging type III perioral area skin, for example, the laser may eliminate these mild defects in one treatment with little risk of pigmentary change. The peel does the same but may be more likely to slightly hypopigment the skin. In contrast, photoaging type IV skin with severe rhytides may require multiple touch-ups by the laser for adequate treatment.[1] The Baker's peel, however, can eliminate the vast majority of rhytides in one treatment. Neither procedure for this indication leaves bothersome residual hypopigmention, but mild pigment loss is not unexpected. More comparative studies and long-term follow-up will eventually be forthcoming. Further contrast between peels and the laser car. be found in Chapters 2, 8, and 10.

FIG. 7-1. PHENOL

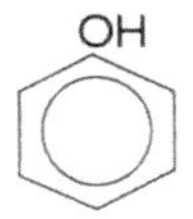

The chemical peel that penetrates the deepest into the reticular dermis to correct most severe actinic damage utilizes a formula containing phenol, or carbolic acid (Fig. 7-1). Lister reported the germicidal effects of phenol in 1867. It is clinically bacteriostatic up to a strength of 1% and bactericidal above this concentration. The compound is a local anesthetic to cutaneous nerve endings. Liquified phenol consists of an 88% solution of phenol in water. As a chemical agent it is soluble in oil and fats and may be rapidly removed from the skin with glycerin, vegetable oils, or 50% alcohol. The addition of salt increases its activity by reducing its solubility in water. Alcohol has the opposite effect, thus the practice of wiping off additional phenol from the skin with alcohol after evulsing a nail, for example. The alcohol has no value in chemical peeling because controlled wounding is desired.[2,3]

Phenol is quickly absorbed percutaneously. For information on its metabolism, inherent cardiac, hepatic, and renal toxicities, and accidental spillage of solution, see the sections on cardiac arrythmias and inherent errors in Chapter 8.

The traditional chemical peel with phenol as described in 1961 by Baker and Gordon is still used today.[4-6] This measured formula (Table 7-1) is the modification made by lay peelers in Los Angeles and Miami that evolved from the use of phenol to treat gunpowder burns in World War I. (See Chapter 1 for details.) This specific formula has been studied histologically and clinically. It remains the chief formula for deep peeling. (See Chapter 2 for histopathologic details, classification, and the duration of results.) Full-strength 88% phenol allegedly causes immediate coagulation of epidermal keratin proteins and self-blocks further penetration of phenol. The specific formula dilutes the concentration to approximately 50% to 55%, and keratolysis resulting from sulfide bond disruption promotes further penetration into the dermis.[7]

This theoretical explanation given by Rothman[8] in 1945 has never been proved. Below about 30%, lesser concentrations are progressively more dilute and weak. Liquid hexachlorophene soap in alcohol (Septisol—Calgon Vestal Laboratories, St. Louis, Missouri) as a surfactant reduces surface tension to promote a more even peel. Croton oil, the fixed oil from the seed of the plant *Croton tiglium,* is an epidermolytic vesicant that may enhance absorption of phenol and increase inflammation. (See the section on croton oil addition in Chapter 2.) The freshly prepared emulsion is not miscible and must be stirred constantly in a clear glass cup immediately before patient application. The

TABLE 7-1.
Baker-Gordon Formula

INGREDIENT	AMOUNT
Phenol, *USP*, 88%	3 ml
Tap or distilled water	2 ml
Septisol liquid soap	8 drops
Croton oil	3 drops

Deep Peeling Modalities

Baker's formula phenol, unoccluded
Baker's formula phenol, occluded

mixture can be stored in an amber glass bottle for short periods, but this is unnecessary because it is easily combined before use.

Weaker variations of the Baker-Gordon formula using phenol solutions between 25% and 50% and less than 2 drops of croton oil may produce good clinical results for lesser degrees of photoaging in certain skin types. However, TCA may produce the same results without the need for systemic precautions of phenol peeling. The role of the amount of croton oil in producing hypopigmentation after various concentrations of phenol application is undetermined.[9]

Litton's formula,[10,11] which substitutes glycerin for liquid soap in the formula (see Chapter 1 for specifics), cannot be quickly formulated because heat is required for dissolution. It may be stored in amber glass bottles, but the emulsion also requires shaking before application.

Baker and Gordon originally described the application of waterproof tape after the peel to increase penetration, presumably through a mechanism of maceration. The modification of this peel by Beeson and McCollough[12] promotes more aggressive defatting of the skin and aggressive removal of the epidermal barrier with acetone before a heavier application of the formula. This elimination of the taping and tape removal discomfort with optional sedation or anesthesia is advantageous.[13,14] However, in spite of claims of similar results and possibly less risk of scarring, histologic evidence supports the increased wound depth of phenol from taping.[15] (See Chapter 2.) Both techniques have merit, and unoccluded Baker's formula produces an excellent peel as long as the wound depth is deep enough to efface defects. It is easier to selectively tape severe, thick, actinically damaged skin and rest assured that the deepest peel possible is produced over these areas. (See the box above.)

Many patients today that are peeled with phenol have been using combinations of tretinoin and α-hydroxy acids before the procedure. They may have had superficial peels before phenol application. These factors should be considered additional risks for increased penetration of the deep peel. Exact time interval precautions to avoid exfoliation before phenol peeling are uncertain because the extent of epidermal insult is highly variable with the many skin care programs and superficial peels in use.

For information on actinic changes persisting after peeling, see also the section on dermal injury in Chapter 2; the sections on Jessner's solution and TCA and on 50% TCA in Chapter 6; Chapter 10; and later in this chapter.

TECHNIQUE FOR FULL-FACE APPLICATION

Immediately before the administration of intravenous fluids and sedation, the patient is placed in a sitting position, and a line of small dots is placed slightly inferior to the mandible* (Fig. 7-2). The peel is extended to this point to minimize possible permanent color change, which would fall into the shadow cast by the mandible.[18] (See the section on pigmentary changes in Chapter 8.)

*References 5,6,13,14,16,17.

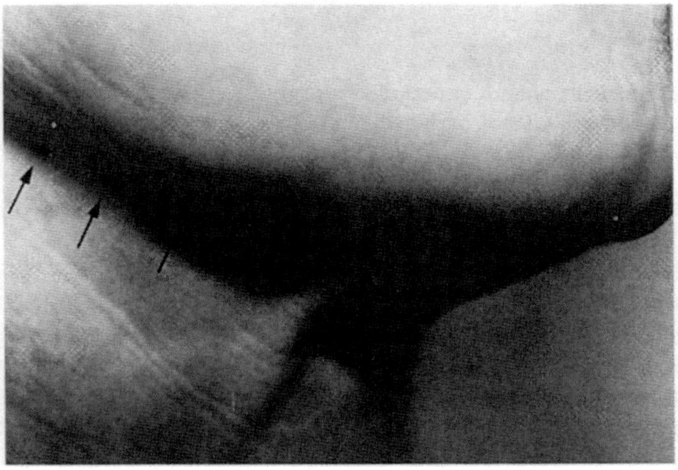

FIG. 7-2. Marking of the peel border under the mandibular ramus.

Intravenous Fluids

Because phenol is partially detoxified in the liver and excreted by the kidney and because phenol may induce cardiac arrhythmias (see Chapter 8), the good health of these organs should be established before peeling. A preoperative history and physical examination to rule out cardiac and hepatorenal disease is performed, and a recent electrocardiogram, complete blood count, hepatorenal profile, and electrolyte values are obtained. Hydration with 500 cc of lactated Ringer's solution before the procedure and 1000 cc during and after the peel will prevent phenol toxicity to these organ systems and ensure an increased output of alkaline urine.[19] Occasionally 250 to 500 cc of dextrose in water may prevent hypoglycemia and nausea.[20]

Sedation and Analgesia

Numerous preoperative sedatives and analgesics have been employed in deep peeling. Intramuscular or intravenous meperidine (Demerol, Winthrop), 50 to 100 mg, and diazepam (Valium, Roche), 2 to 5 mg, have been used extensively for many years. The intravenous combination of fentanyl citrate (Sublimaze, Elkins-Sinn), an analgesic, and midazolam (Versed, Roche), a sedative, can be titrated to the needs of the patient and administered by an anesthetist or anesthesiologist. Oral fentanyl citrate is available but produces nausea and vomiting and may be impractical.[21] The patient is instructed not to eat on the day of surgery. Regional supraorbital, infraorbital, mental, superior alveolar, and preauricular block anesthesia can electively be employed by using the long-acting local anesthetics bupivacaine (Marcaine, Winthrop) or etidocaine (Duranest, Astra). Epinephrine-containing local anesthetics might exacerbate cardiac arrhythmias. (See the section on dermal healing after local skin flaps and chemical peeling in Chapter 2 for theoretical information regarding lidocaine injection in concert with peeling.)

Cardiac monitoring equipment, a pulse oximeter, and blood pressure monitoring are state of the art for intravenous sedation and for monitoring vital signs as phenol is excreted. The cardiac monitoring equipment is available with and without printers in compact, portable, battery-operated form from

Propaq, Protocol Systems, Inc., Beaverton, Oregon, toll free 800-289-2500. After an intravenous infusion of lactated Ringer's solution is begun, Versed can be administered and titrated to avoid respiratory depression at 1 mg per dose to a maximum of 5 mg. Sublimaze is given in 50 µg increments to a maximum dose of 250 µg over a period of 90 to 120 minutes (Fig. 7-3).

Cleansing the Skin

The face should be washed thoroughly with soap and water the night before and the morning of the procedure. No makeup should be employed on the morning of the peel. The fine facial hair is shaved first to avoid the discomfort of depilating these hairs during tape removal after surgery.[18] A thorough 3-minute acetone scrub or a combination of acetone followed by alcohol to degrease the skin is utilized immediately before the application of wounding agent. Ether, which is flammable and less accessible, was used in the past. McCollough and Langsdon believe that hexachlorophene sudsing solutions (PhisoHex and Phisoderm, Winthrop) may deposit an oily residue on the skin that may retard phenol absorption and tape sticking. Hexachlorophene with alcohol (Septisol) can be used instead because of its possible keratolytic action

A B C D

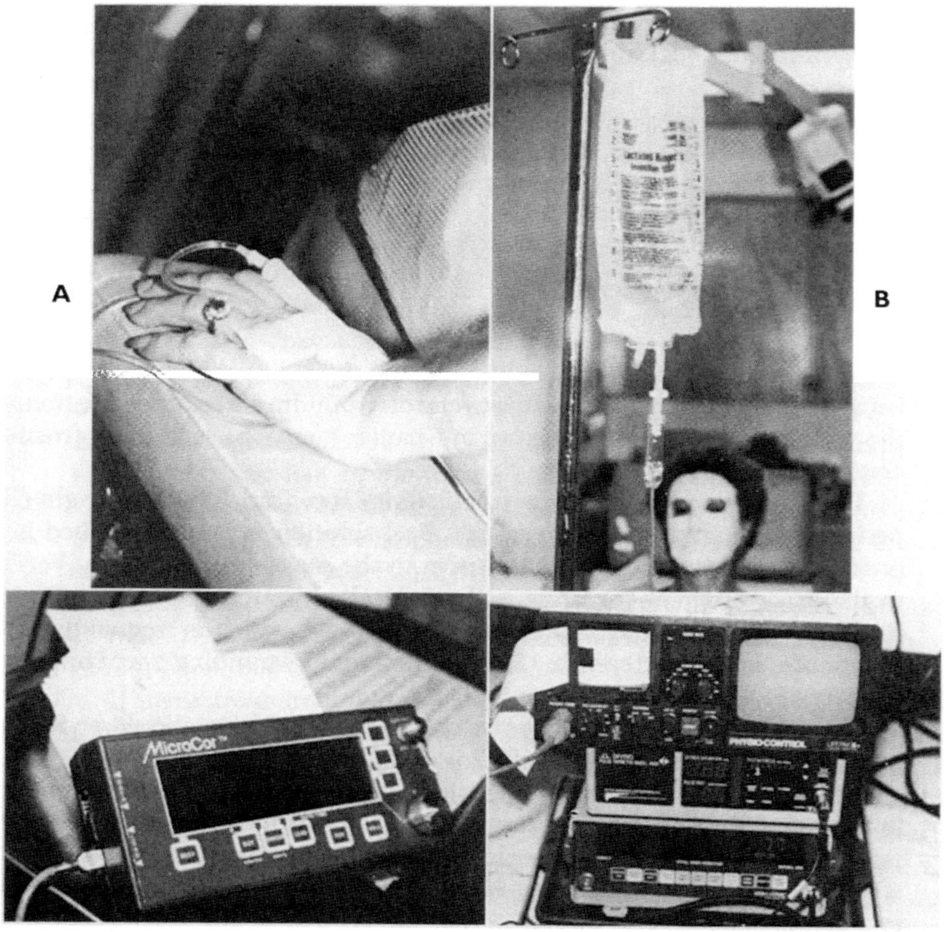

FIG. 7-3. A and **B,** Intravenous solutions in place. **C** and **D,** Compact electrocardiograph (ECG) monitor and combined monitor and pulse oximeter.

and promotion of phenol penetration. The gentle abrasion of the skin with acetone on gauze until a sandpaper-like sound is heard when the sponge is rubbed across the skin may result in more phenol absorption but less need for a taped mask, assuming that more Baker's solution is applied.[13,14] We do not abrade to this aggressive end point because it may result in irregular penetration of phenol. We prefer to occlude only what we judge clinically needs to be taped. Adequate degreasing of each cosmetic unit is imperative for good results and an even peel. (See the section on wounding agent quantitation in Chapter 4.)

Application of Wounding Agent

The application of phenol should be accomplished with moist but not very wet cotton-tipped applicators. Whether continued application and rubbing produces increased penetration has been discussed and argued between different cosmetic surgical specialties. There is no question that phenol penetrates immediately through the papillary dermis to the reticular dermis. The continued penetration for approximately an extra tenth of a millimeter is the item of contention. One study in non–sun-damaged juvenile minipigs suggests that there is no difference in histologic penetration between moist and very wet applications of phenol.[22] However, clinically in actinically damaged human skin one cannot obtain removal of the thickest rhytides of photoaging IV, in the perioral area for example, without continued rubbing and the subsequent application of a greater quantity of phenol with a very moist cotton-tipped applicator past a white color until a gray-white color is seen. A single application with one cotton-tipped applicator to the individual deepest rhytids may be used before the application to the rest of the cosmetic unit. If the rhytides are not very deep and only a photoaging III variety, in the periorbital area for example, a single application with one cotton-tipped applicator that has been "wrung out" against the lip of the peel container with no continued rubbing is adequate. This might be termed a "light" versus a "heavy" application of phenol because the gray-white end point is not achieved here. In relatively non–sun-damaged skin the light application is less likely to be a reality because it is the sun damage that retards wounding agent penetration. (See the section on occlusion of phenol in Chapter 2 and the section on frosting in Chapter 4.)

The face is divided into six cosmetic units: forehead, left cheek, right cheek, perioral, nose, and periorbital areas. Peel solution is usually applied in this order—moving from the least sensitive to the most sensitive areas. Variation in the exact order of the units is the individual preference of the physician. Peeling the most damaged area early in the peel, which is frequently around the mouth, is our preference. (See the section on wounding agent application concepts in Chapter 4.)

Phenol does not affect the growth of hair. The solution should be feathered into all hair-bearing areas, including the scalp and eyebrows (Fig. 7-4). An electric fan to vent the phenol fumes accompanied by good central ventilation in a room with outdoor air access is important for the comfort of the staff. To minimize renal and cardiac toxicity, 10 to 15 minutes are allowed between cosmetic units, so it takes 60 to 90 minutes for the entire procedure. (See the section on cardiac arrhythmias in Chapter 8.) One or two fresh single cotton-tipped applicators are used for each application of solution. These many applicators are discarded during the procedure and are soaked with substantial

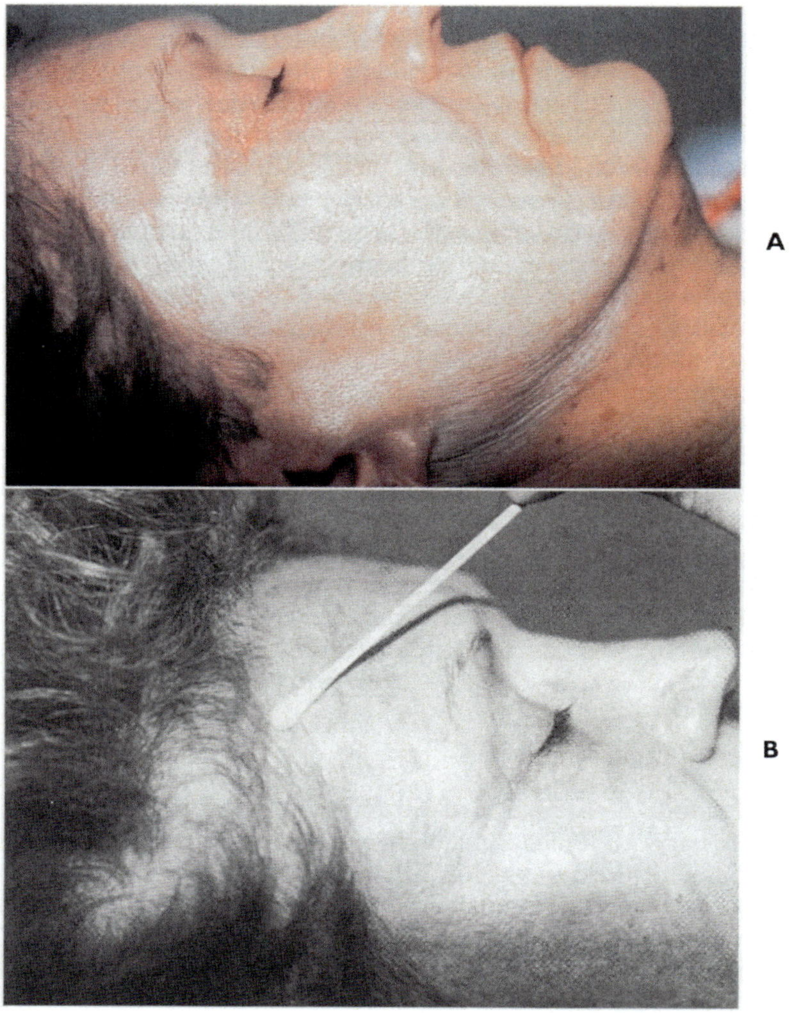

FIG. 7-4. A, Application of phenol to a cheek cosmetic unit. **B,** Feathering into the hairline.

amounts of wasted phenol. In reality the amount of phenol in contact with the skin is less than half of the total 3 cc in the formula. (Gordon HL: Personal communication, cosmetic surgery seminar, October 31, 1991.) This small total amount, along with slow application and hydration, accounts for the excellent safety record of this procedure over the last 35 years. If only one cosmetic unit or less is peeled, no precautions are necessary with regard to cardiac monitoring.[14] Oral hydration with several tumblers of water may be given for such miniapplications but are not essential.

If there are many folds and rhytides indicating more surface area, the cosmetic units may be subdivided, and application may be slower. The extent of cutaneous absorption of phenol depends more on the total area of skin exposed than on the concentration of solution employed. A flow sheet or face peel chart on the operative report that indicates times at which areas are treated is necessary (Fig. 7-5). The peel solution is carefully applied with the cotton-tipped applicators, and care is taken to avoid any spillage. An ivory white frosting occurs on application, but the formula should be applied until a gray cast is perceived in areas that are severely sun damaged. The application should be worked into thick rhytides with moderate pressure.

BAKER'S PHENOL OPERATIVE REPORT

NAME Mary Sundamage AGE 58 DATE 9-10-91

Diagnosis Actinic Keratoses, Rhytides
Skin Type Fitzpatrick Type I, Glogau IV
Actinic Degree Actinic Keratoses Present
Sebaceous Degree 1+

Preoperative Skin Preparation & Degreasing:
3 min. Acetone Scrub, Alcohol Wipe
Hx BCE
Photos Yes

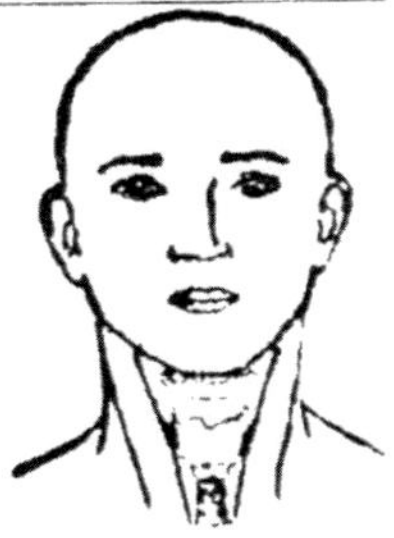

	Type/Amount	Time
Anesthesia:	Versed 1.0 mg	9:45
	Sublimaze, 50 mcg	9:45
	V+S	10:45
	V+S	11:15

Total Amount Used: Versed 3mg; Sublimaze 150mcg; 1500cc, Lactated Ringers
Keloid Former? No
Mixture Used: Baker's phenol, Full face

Area	Time Applied
(1) Forehead	(1) 10:00 a.m.
(2) Left Cheek	(2) 10:20
(3) Right Cheek	(3) 10:40
(4) Perioral	(4) 11:00
(5) Chin	(5) 11:20
(6) Nose	(6) 11:40
(7) Periorbital	(7) 12:00 p.m.

=(Phenol U.S.P. ✓ TCA ___) (to lash cilia not peeled)

Tape Variety: Curity; except microfoam, perioral
Time Left Office: 1:00 p.m.

Return In: 48hrs; call 24hrs.
Condition Upon Discharge: Responsive, sleepy

Post-Op Pain Medications: I.M. Demerol 50mg now; Percodan P.O.

Physician: Brody
Assistant: Whitmire

Comments: Many wrinkles, used 7 cosmetic units. No previous cosmetic surgery or medical problems. CBC, SMA, EKG - normal

FIG. 7-5. Baker's phenol operative report.

An immediate burning sensation is present for 15 to 20 seconds and quickly subsides. Pain returns in 20 minutes and persists for 6 to 10 hours. The use of EMLA once immediately after application on the frost to reduce this pain in untaped peels may have some measure of success in pain relief.[23] Throbbing and burning still persists but may be more tolerable. Rebound stinging may occur if the patient overuses the topical anesthetic at home multiple times.

The applicators are never passed over the eyes of the patient. Baker's solution is usually needed for the crow's feet area, but we switch to full-strength phenol for the upper or lower eyelid unit as determined by actinic damage or a history of previous peels. Some patients have more folds when their eyes are open, and this creates an occlusive phenomenon. There is variation in quality of the infrabrow area, and the physician must choose the appropriate wounding agent.[24] From the superior border of the tarsal plate to the upper eyelash ciliary margin we choose to use 35% TCA.[25] Both Baker and Litton relate that Baker's solution has been applied down to the upper ciliary margin in thousands of cases without complication. (Personal communications, Dr. Thomas Baker, American Society of Plastic and Reconstructive Surgery, September, 1991, and Dr. Clyde Litton, American Academy of Facial Plastic and Reconstructive Surgery meeting, March, 1993.) This is in contrast to the lower eyelid margin where scarring or ectropion has been produced. (See the section on periorbital peeling techniques in Chapter 4.)

Taping the Mask

Tape is applied to each segment as the peel progresses, although one can wait until the entire face is covered with Baker's solution. Waterproof zinc oxide nonporous tape is the most occlusive. Curity tape, ½ inch, can be more adhesive and pliable than the Johnson & Johnson brand. Short strips from 1.5 to 4 cm are cut by an assistant in advance. Shorter-length tapes act as a hinge when overlapped allowing a slight amount of motion and better adherence. At least two layers of tape should cover all treated areas, but this may vary with physician preference (Fig. 7-6, *A* and *C*). Tape must adhere properly, or **skip areas** may result. These areas can be spot peeled when the tape is removed. Taping is stopped immediately adjacent to the hair-bearing areas to avoid a traction alopecia at the time of the removal. The eyebrows, eyelids, and earlobes should be peeled but not taped (Fig. 7-6, *D*). Microfoam tape (3M)[26] can be used to occlude the perioral area because the tape is elastic and will both stretch and contract with lip movement. We apply tape in short vertical overlapping strips and then optionally cover with several long horizontal strips to anchor the area. If deemed appropriate, the skin just superior to the vermilion border can be covered with a thin strip of tape, and the rest of the lip can be unoccluded.[27]

Tape can be placed to a line 1 to 2 cm parallel to the inferior border of the mandible, which corresponds to the line of cosmetic application in most women.[17] We prefer the sawtooth taping method along the mandibular region; this produces an irregular line that may be less noticeable[3,24] (Fig. 7-6, *B*). Alternatively, the last several centimeters of peeled skin under the mandible can be untaped. Most surgeons do not perform deep peeling on the neck because of the risk of scarring. (See Chapters 8 and 10.)

A variation in mask application has been described that uses measured surgical adhesive drape cut to facial size and covered with tape to provide bulk to the mask.[28] Intensely adhesive and watertight, it is thin, easily contoured, and

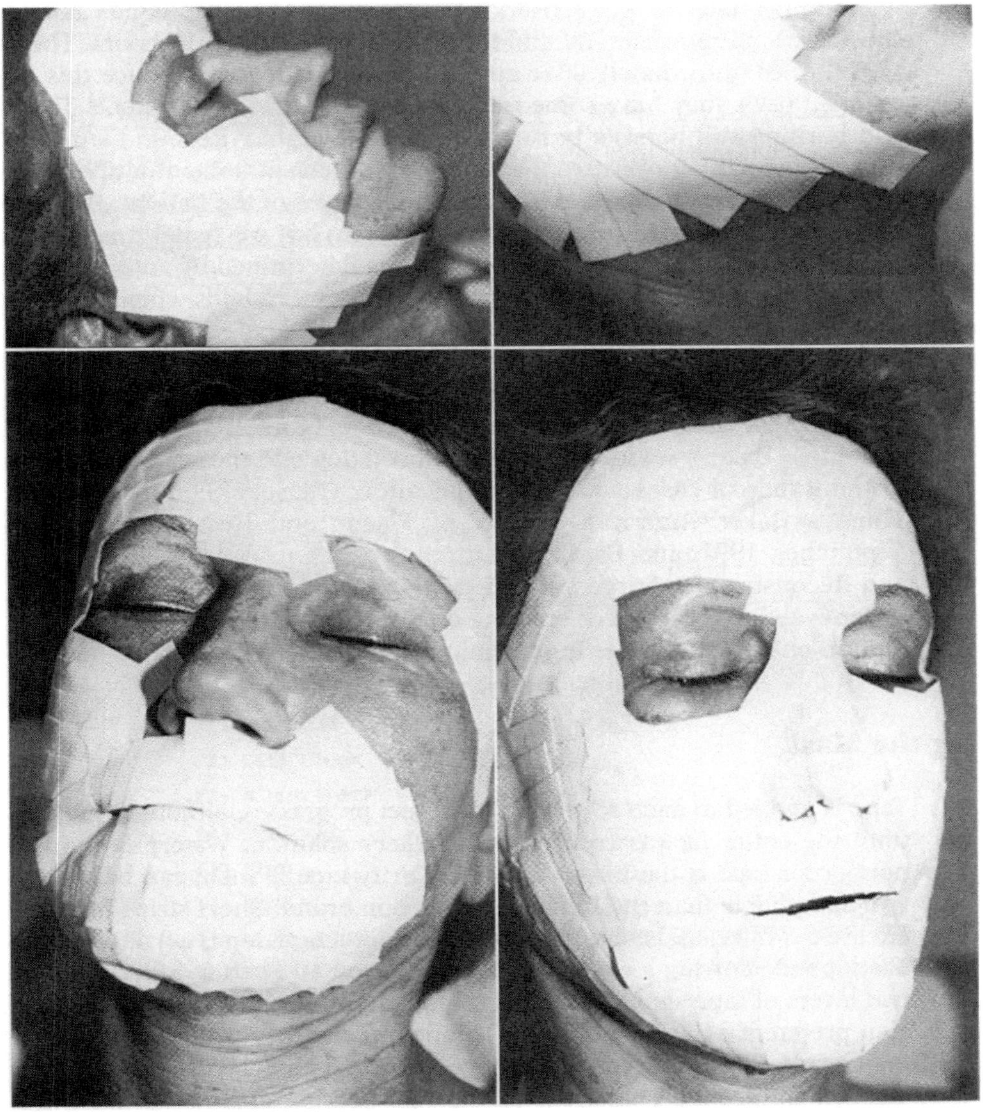

FIG. 7-6. A, Short strips of overlapped tape applied to act as a hinge. **B,** Feathering under the mandible. **C,** Near completion with vertical perioral application. **D,** Tape mask sparing the eyebrows, periorbital area, and earlobes.

rapidly applied. Because the sticky and smooth inner surface of prepackaged unsterilized surgical adhesive tape has been demonstrated to be sterile,[29] the use of this method is acceptable but unnecessarily expensive because of the sterile drape. Salicylic acid–impregnated tape may increase maceration.[30]

Stuzin and co-workers[31] have found that immediate application of petrolatum (Vaseline petroleum jelly) applied only once immediately after the peel may obviate the need for the mask and serve as a vapor barrier to prevent phenol evaporation and increase maceration and penetration. However, they concede that deeply lined faces that appear weather-beaten still require use of the tape. The sun damage of these less actinically damaged patients simply does not require the additional tape artillery for penetration below their wrinkles. The goal, of course, is to choose the technique that penetrates the sun damage but does not unnecessarily overpenetrate.

Corticosteroid Administration during Peeling

Many physicians administer 6 mg of bethamethasone (Celestone, Schering, Kenilworth, New Jersey) in conjunction with a deep peel. We choose to do this to reduce edema, but controlled studies have never been performed. For details and explanation, see the section on corticosteroids in Chapter 3.

Tape Mask Removal

Patients may return in 24 hours for psychologic support, but a phone call may be all that is necessary. Ice packs applied over the tape relieve the burning. A liquid or soft diet is generally encouraged to minimize mastication until tape removal. Although the pain subsides within 6 to 8 hours, the edema is severe, and the eyelids are frequently swollen shut. The patient should sleep with the aid of oral hypnotics and analgesics if necessary in a sitting or semireclining position to reduce this edema. The mask is removed in 48 hours when the exudate has lifted the tape and drainage is beginning under the chin. Analgesia is generally not required by most patients to remove the mask if the face was shaved first. Optionally, some physicians remove the mask at 24 hours, although this is more painful and may delay healing.[32] A gray and deeply edematous face with pinpoint bleeding is cleansed with sterile saline or hydrogen peroxide (Fig. 7-7).

Aftercare

Wet to dry soaking gently three to five times daily with tap water while standing in the shower or dilute antiseptic skin cleansers (Betadine, Hibiclens) can be used to dry the exudative edema, followed by an occlusive moisturizer of Crisco vegetable shortening to reduce the healing time. We prefer to use Bacitracin or Polysporin ointment in spite of a low risk of contact allergy with more rapid reepithelialization. Petrolatum or petrolatum-containing ointments (A & D ointment) may not be as effective. (See the section on medications affecting reepithelialization in Chapter 3.) There is less chance of infection if the wound is kept crust free with a modified wet or semiocclusive technique. Therefore the original thymol iodide powder forming an overlying dry crust, or second "mask," that was used by lay peelers and in Baker's original description should seldom be used today (Figs. 7-8 and 7-9). Its use may be associated with an increased healing time or increased degree of hypopigmentation or depigmentation (See the section on pigmentary changes in Chapter 8.)

Biosynthetic occlusive dressings have been successfully implemented to prevent dessication and speed epithelialization in dermabrasion. (See the section on reepithelialization in Chapter 3 for further details.) Vigilon (Hermal Labs, Oak Hill, New York) may be employed if changed daily for the first 2 days after the unoccluded procedure. The use of a newer synthetic wound dressing, Meshed Omiderm (Doak Dermatologics, Fairfield, New Jersey) after dermabrasion has been heralded as a revolutionary type of dressing that is not removed for the entire healing period.[33] Fully permeable to fluids, ointment is applied to the surface of the dressing, and it is held in place at the edges by Mastisol (Ferndale Labs, Ferndale, Michigan). The dressing is removed after reepithelialization has occurred. The use of Omiderm merits further evaluation after deep

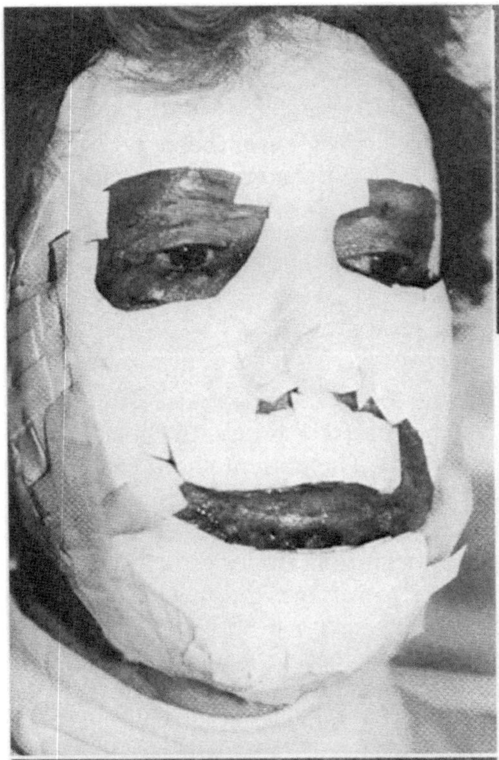

A

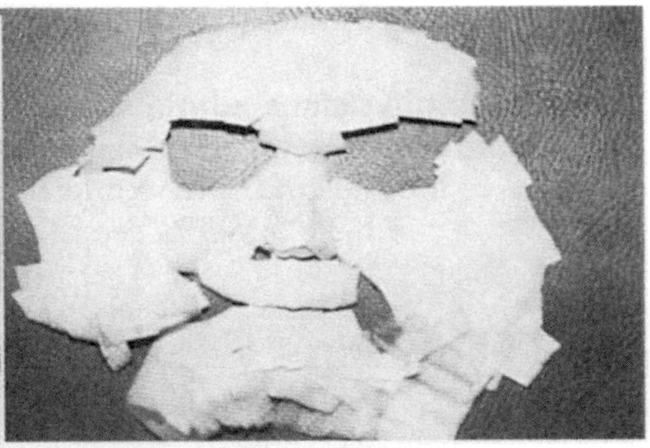

B

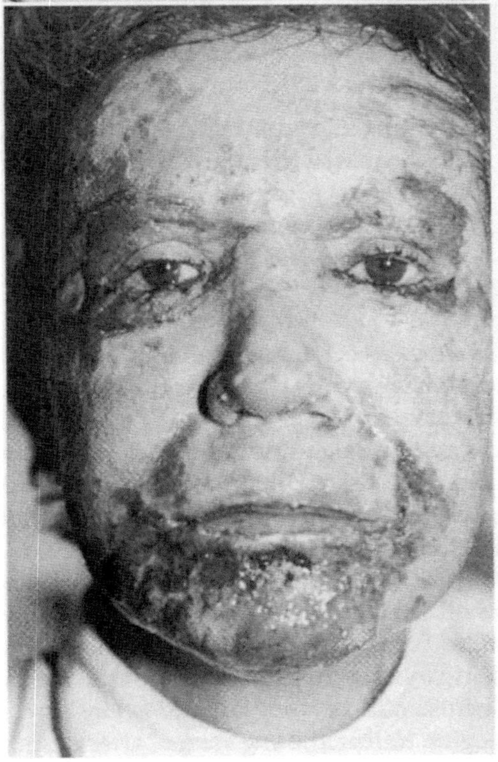

C

FIG. 7-7. **A,** Immediately before mask removal at 48 hours, there is much exudate. **B,** Mask on removal. **C,** Immediately after mask removal.

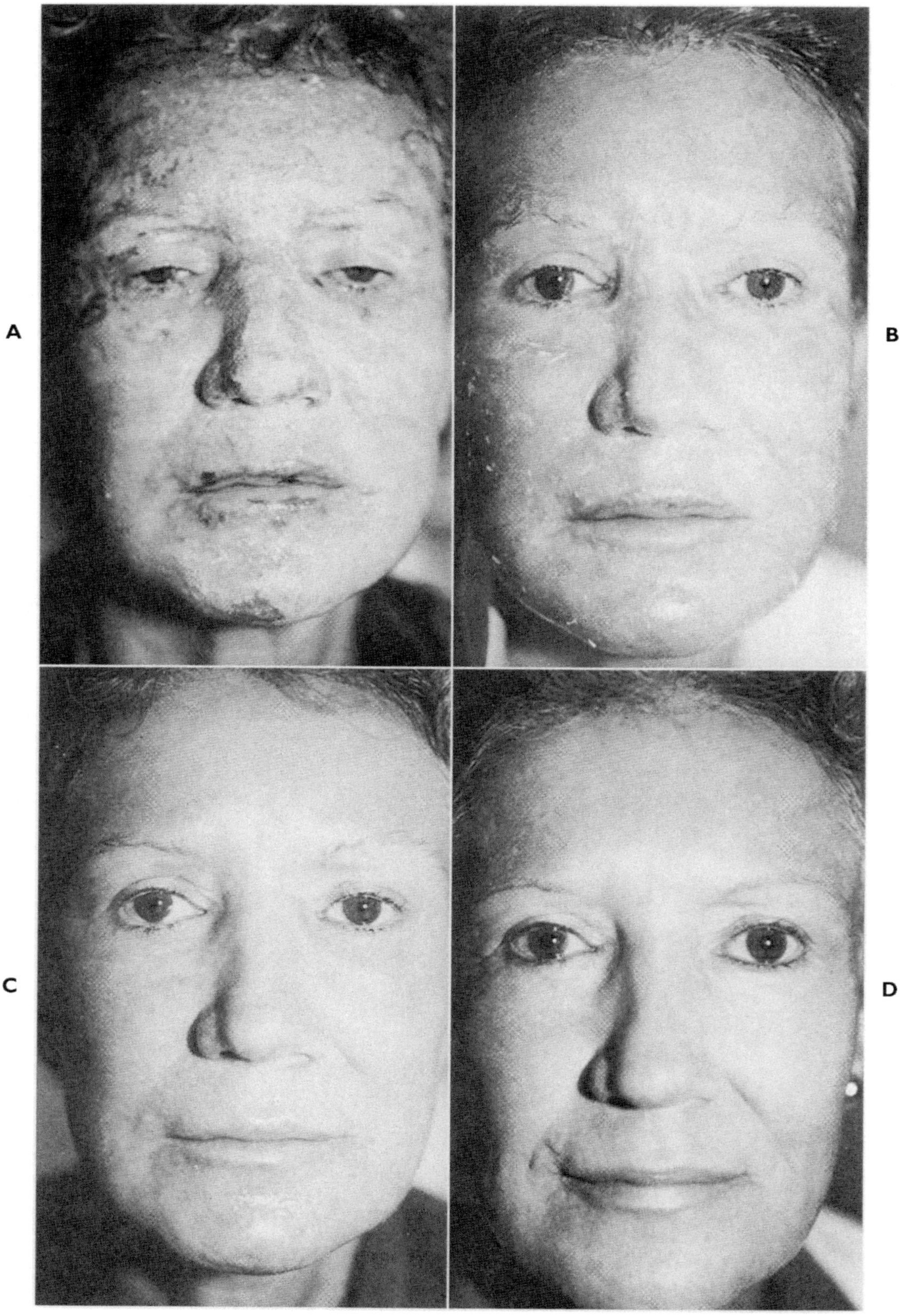

FIG. 7-8. Healing process using povidone-iodine shower soaks mixed with white unscented Dove soap, followed by Polysporin ointment. **A,** Four days. **B,** Seven days. **C,** Ten days. **D,** Twenty-one days.

A B

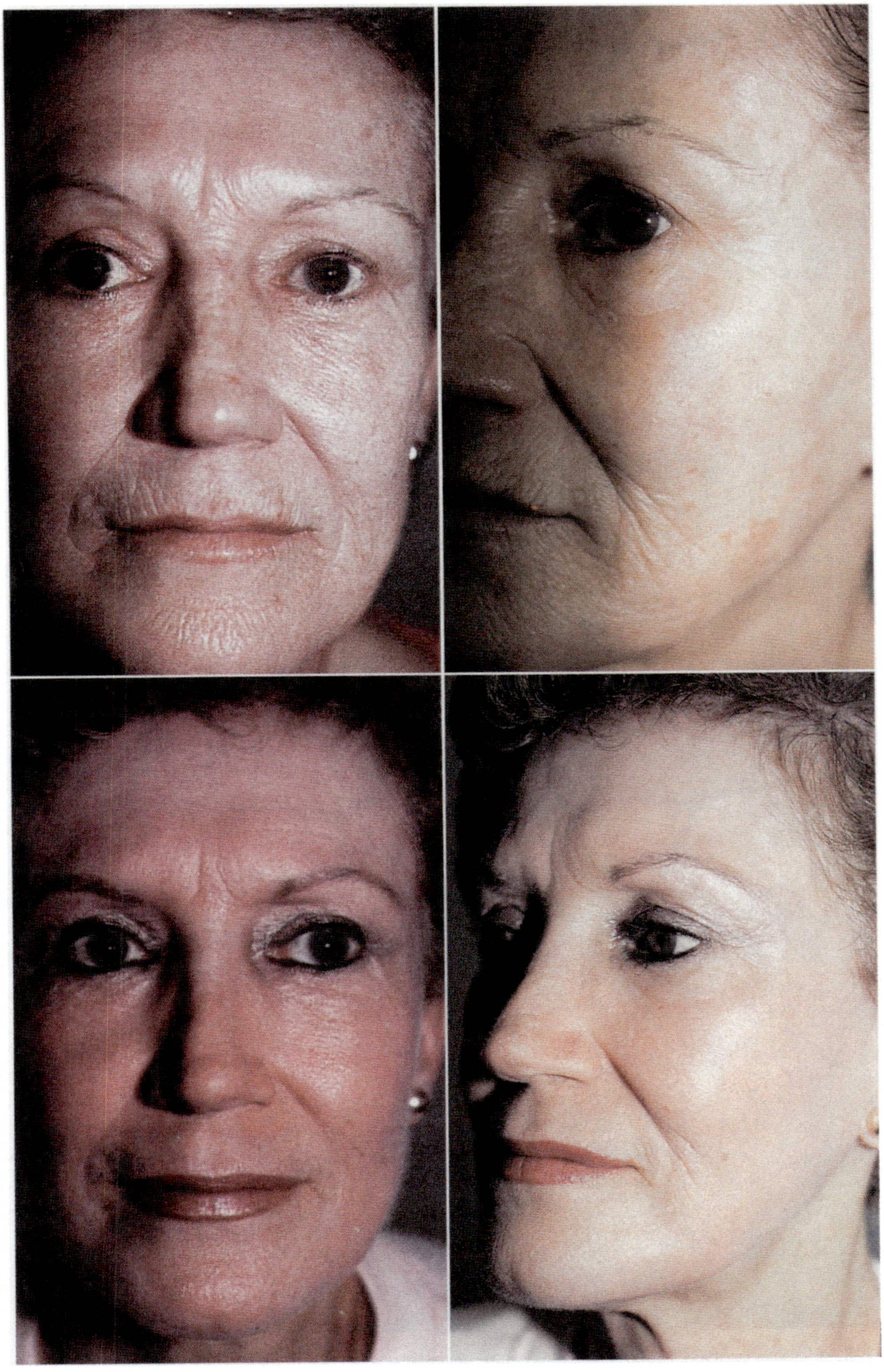

C D

FIG. 7-9. **A** and **B,** Before peeling. Fitzpatrick type II, Glogau photoaging type III. **C** and **D,** Ninety days after peeling.

A

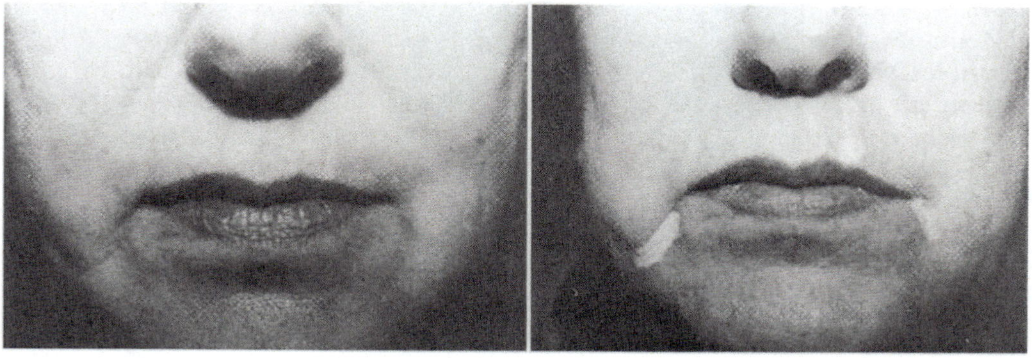

FIG. 7-10. A, One year after unoccluded Baker's peel with three significant residual rhytides. **B,** Loc retouch with unoccluded Baker's solution.

chemical peeling, although by its very nature the peel causes instant vascu coagulation with no bleeding, and therefore less need for the use of permea membrane dressings exists immediately after a peel. Attachment may be d cult without pulling the edges of the hairline that has been peeled. This dress may prove to be useful immediately after tape removal. Whether dermal qua is enhanced or lessened with more rapid reepithelialization is unknown.[17]

The patient should resist the uniform temptation to pick at the face. F ritis is common and is relieved by noncomedogenic moisturizers, hydroco sone ointments, ice packs, and aspirin. (See the section on prolonged e thema or pruritis in Chapter 8.) Daily cream-based sunscreens and tretin

A

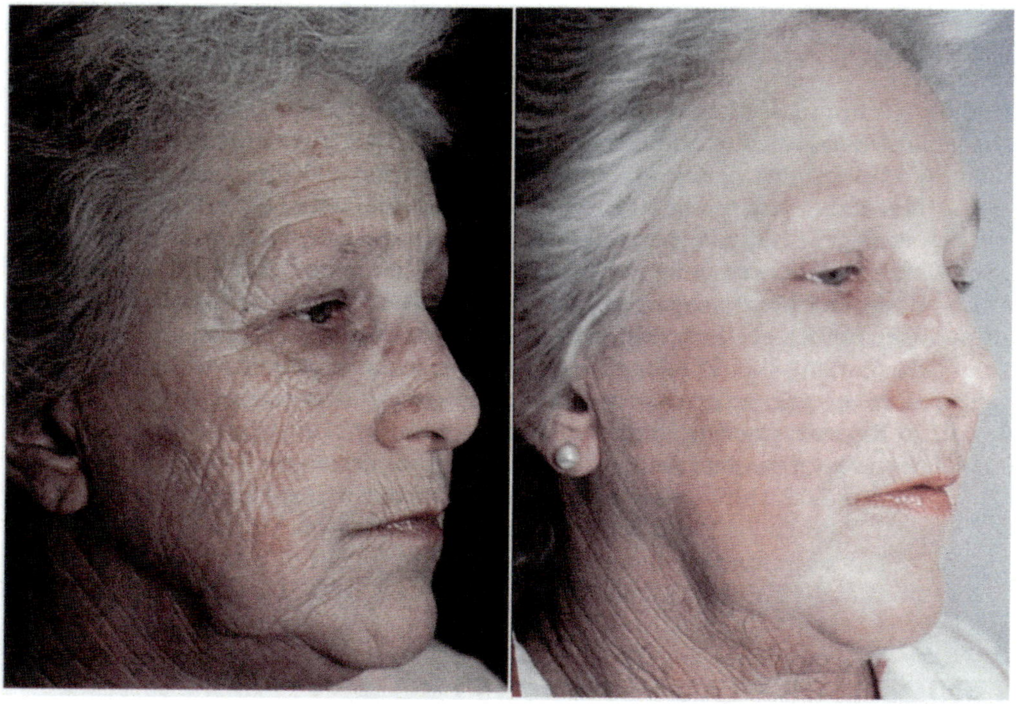

FIG. 7-11. A, Fitzpatrick type II, Glogau photoaging type IV, severe actinic rhytides and keratoses before a full-face occluded Baker's peel. **B,** One year after peeling with substantial improvement. *(Cou tesy of Dr. Robert A. Clark.)*

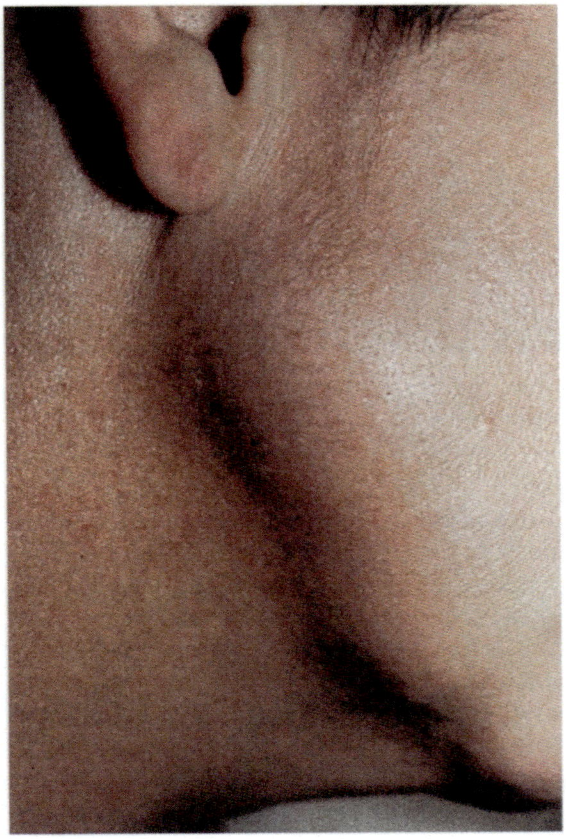

FIG. 7-12. Thirteen years after an occluded Baker's peel new actinic freckling is occurring on the face, through the color line of demarcation, and onto the neck. The peel will retard the appearance of keratoses and freckling but not prevent them completely, especially if the patient returns to the sun.

are reinstituted as soon as tolerated within 1 or 2 weeks of reepithelialization. Complete avoidance of sunlight is imperative during the healing period. Petechiae may result from strenuous physical exercise within a month after peeling.[18] Milia are a common occurrence and may be extracted with a no. 11 scalpel blade or may resolve spontaneously. (See the section on milia in Chapter 8.) It is suspected but unproved that fewer milia result if tretinoin is used before peeling. Tretinoin will prolong erythema if used after peeling, but the patient should return to the maintenance regimen within 21 to 30 days after the peel or as soon as tolerated. (See the regimen section in Chapter 4.)

Repeat peeling may be performed in 12 to 18 months.[34] Individual rhytides or spot areas can be retouched at 6 months (Figs. 7-10 and 7-11). Figure 7-12 shows new actinic freckling occurring 13 years after a Baker's peel. Figures 7-13 and 7-14 are patient information forms.

For an informed consent form see Fig. 4-15. For additional case correlations, see Chapter 11.

TECHNIQUE FOR PARTIAL-FACE APPLICATION

As indicated in the preceding discussion on application of wounding agent, at least half the volume of phenol in the formula is discarded with multiple cotton-tipped applicators. The actual amount of phenol applied to the skin is probably a little more than 1 ml. The amount applied to one cosmetic unit is equivalent to that applied to a nail bed for a phenol nail matrixectomy. No cardiac or renal precautions are needed for this small application. Oral hydration may be given in the form of 8 to 16 ounces of water before the peel if the patient has not been drinking much fluid on the day of the procedure. EMLA applied once after peel application may be helpful for topical anesthesia. (See Figs. 7-16 and 11-13.)

The section on wounding agent application details the method of application. After phenol has been applied to the perioral area, for example, medium-depth peeling or other resurfacing modalities may be used on other cosmetic units. (Figs. 7-15 and 7-16 and Chapter 10.) If necessary, placing small dots of gentian violet at the margins of the applied phenol may assist the physician in changing wounding agents. (See Fig. 11-11 for local periorbital phenol application.)

Cosmetic Coverage After Chemical Peeling

After superficial and medium-depth peeling there is usually no problem in concealing the pink erythema from these peels with ordinary makeup.[14,24] Opaque-coverage concealer cream (e.g., Clinique Continuous Coverage) may be required temporarily instead of a water-based foundation. This will not be irritating if a mineral oil–based dissolver (e.g., Abolene, Menley & James Labs, Horsham, Penn.) is gently applied to the erythematous skin for removal. This technique may also cover temporary hyperpigmentation.

However, after deep peeling the erythema is so intense and the skin so tender that special attention should be paid to assist the patient with cosmetics. Cosmetics with a green foundation that are cream based (e.g., Dermage or Clinique) will mask the intense red erythema for the immediate weeks after peeling and may be applied as soon as the crusts have disappeared. The green foundation is applied first and is followed by a liquid or cream base gently applied with a synthetic sponge. Applications are repeated until the area is covered. The line of demarcation may require repeated thin retouching. Optional setting of the makeup with powder keeps it in place and is permissible. The patient's attempts to hide everything may be difficult in the first 10 days after reepithelialization, but reassurance by a member of the office staff is helpful. Men do not handle erythema even from medium-depth peels very well, and they should be encouraged to use a foundation for self-comfort if only for a short time after deep peeling (Fig. 7-17).

For a discussion of hypopigmentation occurring after phenol peels and comparison with laser, see the section on pigmentary changes in Chapter 8 and the section on combining chemical resurfacing with laser resurfacing in Chapter 10.

CONCURRENT DEEP PEELING AND COSMETIC SURGERY

A suggested interval of at least 1 to 3 months is recommended between any procedure that involves undermining or a flap closure. This includes rhytidectomy, brow lift, and blepharoplasty. This time interval is supported by histologic study because collagen remodeling is not complete in medium-depth or deep peeling until 60 to 90 days later. (See the section on dermal healing after local skin flaps and chemical peeling in Chapter 2; the section on classifica-

(Text continues on p. 159.)

Before Deep Peel

1. Do not wear makeup on the day of surgery; wash the face with Betadine skin cleanser and water the morning of the surgery.
2. Bring someone with you who can take you home.
3. Wear a blouse that you do not have to pull over your head for removal.
4. You might eat a light meal up to 3 hours before the surgery. After that time, only liquids should be taken.
5. You will feel pain for 8 hours after the procedure. You will take your pain medicine for this and sleep so that you will be comfortable.
6. Purchase: 2 tubs of Polysporin ointment
   1 small can of Crisco vegetable shortening
   Betadine skin cleanser
   1 bar of white, unscented Dove soap
7. Let us know if you have a history of keloids, scarring, or fever blisters.

FIG. 7-13. Patient information sheet: before a deep peel.

After Deep Peel

When you return home, you will have some bandages in place and will probably sleep through the initial 8-hour pain period. Pain medication can be taken without difficulty. Clear liquids sipped through a straw or soft foods should be taken for the first 48 hours until the bandages are removed. Cool ice packs may be applied to the outside of the bandages.

If no bandages are in place, those areas should be kept moist consistently with ointment. Swelling will be considerable, and drainage may appear underneath the tape after the first 12 hours until the tape is removed. Sleep by keeping the head elevated on several pillows. When the tape is removed, you should wash in the shower with a mixture of Betadine Skin Cleanser and white, unscented Dove soap by using a splashing action and your fingers only. Do not use a Buf-Puf or washcloth. After each washing, the ointment should be applied in a thick coat. The swelling begins to subside after the fifth day, and the peel is usually healed by the fourteenth day. DO NOT PICK AT THE CRUST.

Prolonged constrictive use of caps, shower caps, eyeglasses, or visors in peeled areas should be avoided until the skin has healed over.

If any pain occurs during the entire peel process, call us immediately so that we may be sure that you do not have a fever blister or herpes attack.

Itching between 7 and 14 days after healing occurs is not uncommon. However, excessive redness and itching may be due to allergy to the ointment. If so, switching to Crisco is appropriate, and call us to come in to receive additional treatment.

We will instruct you regarding special makeup so that you may return to work as promptly as possible, usually after 14 days. Makeup and sunscreen can be applied on any area that has healed.

Working out and jogging should be avoided for 30 days because increased blood flow may cause broken blood vessels in the new skin.

A retouch of specific areas or repeeling 6 months after peeling may be required for selected deep wrinkles. This peel is quite effective, but like any surgical procedure, it may not be 100% effective.

Complete avoidance of the sun is mandatory. Exposure to sunlight, getting pregnant, or administration of birth control pills before the redness has disappeared may cause blotchiness. The redness from deep peeling is not usually gone until 90 to 180 days after peeling. Occasionally, localized areas may persist as long as 18 months.

Minimize talking or biting/chewing after peeling; sipping liquids through a straw is helpful.

FIG. 7-14. Patient information sheet: aftercare for the patient.

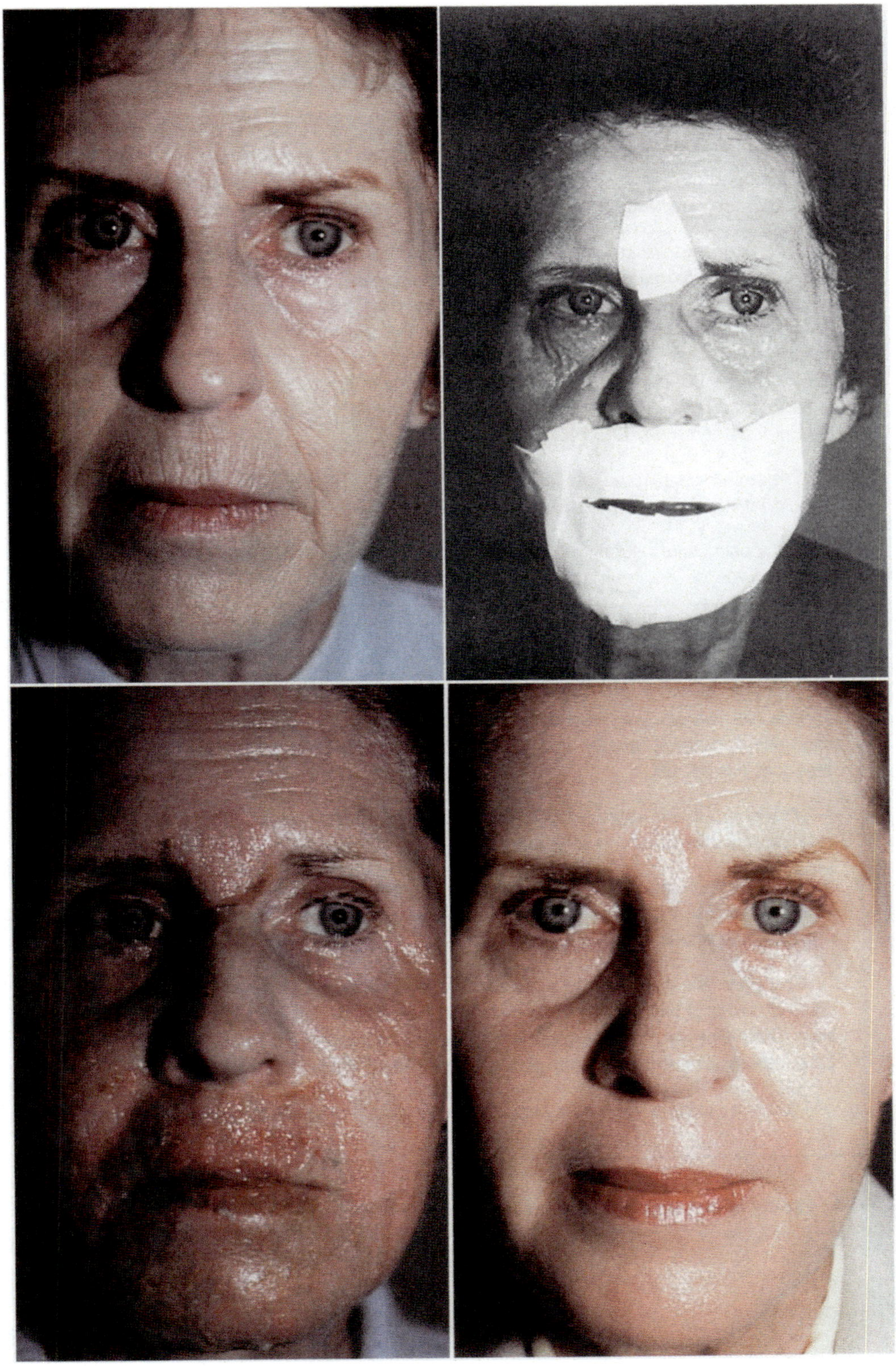

A B C D

FIG. 7-15. Fitzpatrick type II and Glogau photoaging group IV with the most severe defects in the perioral area. The patient was peeled with occluded Baker's solution in the perioral and glabellar areas and CO_2 plus TCA, 35%, on the remaining areas. **A,** Before peeling. **B,** Immediately after peeling. **C,** Immediately after tape removal at 48 hours. **D,** Ninety days after.

(Continued)

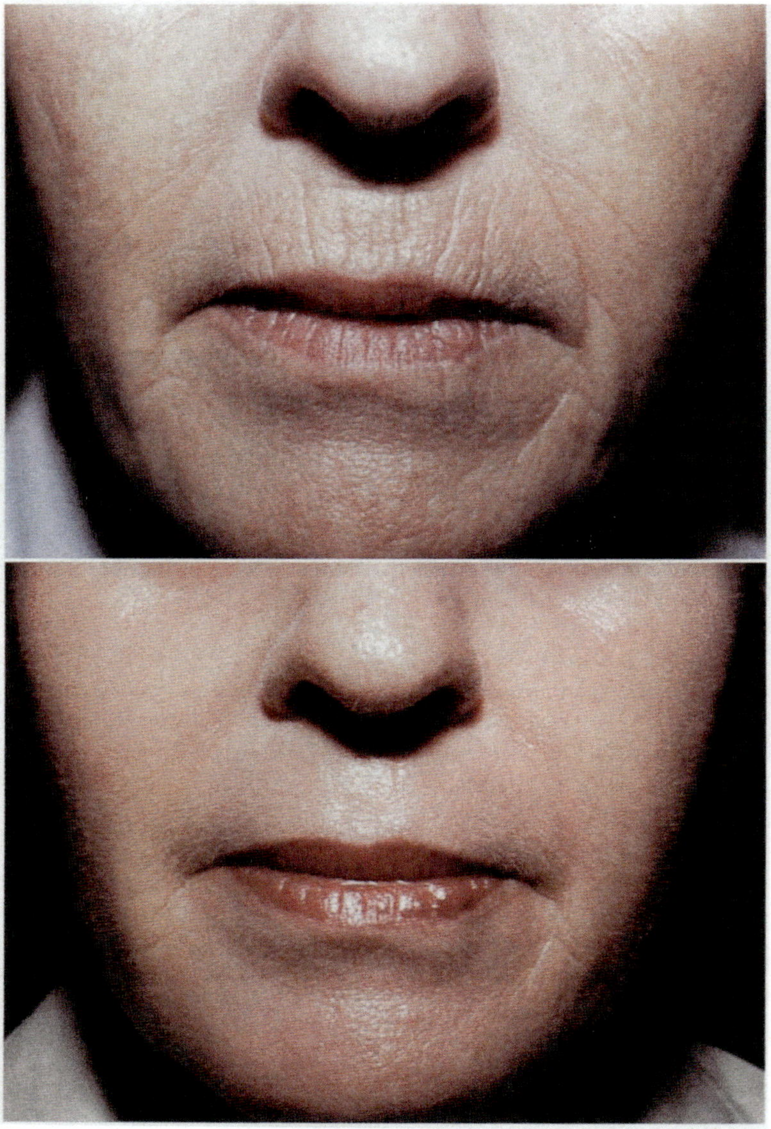

E

F

FIG. 7-15—Cont'd E, Perioral area before. **F,** Ninety days after.

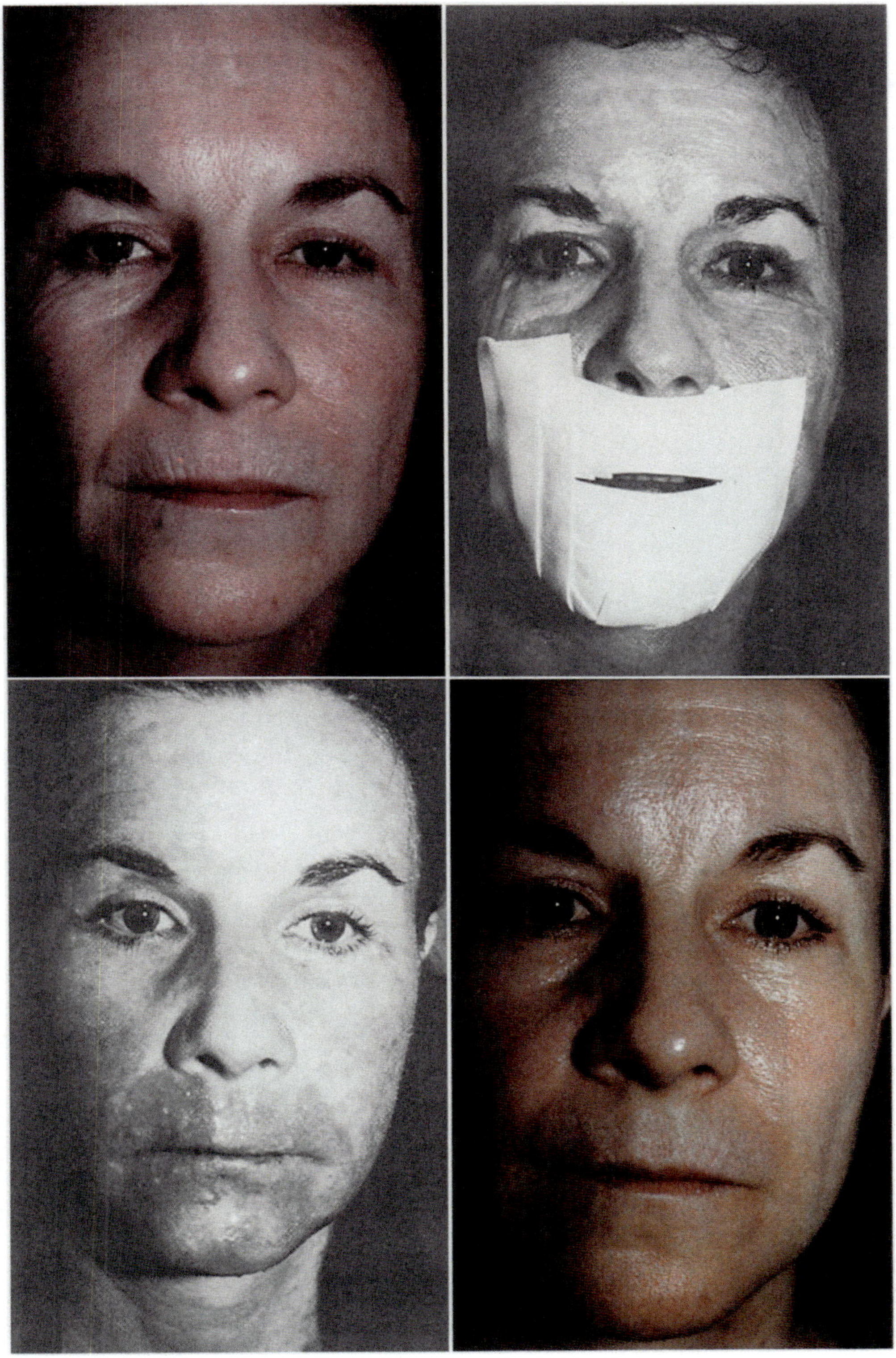

A B C D

FIG. 7-16. Fitzpatrick type III and Glogau photoaging type III intensified only in the perioral area. An occluded Baker's peel was performed periorally, and CO_2 plus TCA, 35%, was used on the remainder of the face. **A,** Before. **B,** Immediately after. **C,** Four days after. **D,** Six months after.

A B

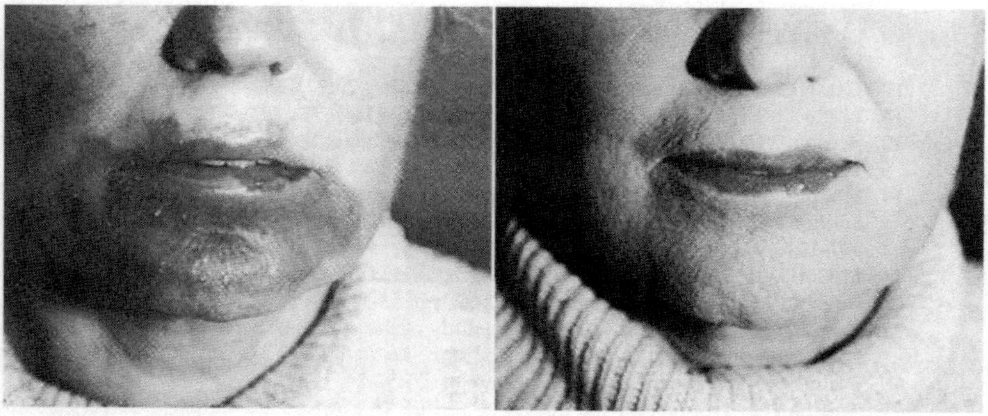

FIG. 7-17. A, Initial deep peel 12 years earlier, now 10 days after a repeat deep touch-up peel before makeup application. **B,** Immediately after makeup application using a green foundation base followed by flesh tone.

tion of wounding agents and techniques in Chapter 2; and the section on collagen remodeling in Chapter 3.) Postrhytidectomy slough may occur, and lower eyelid ectropion has been reported if the peel is performed within 6 months of blepharoplasty.[34-38] (See the section on scarring in Chapter 8.) Regional perioral and periorbital peels can be done at the completion of a face-lift if a blepharoplasty or perioral surgery is not performed.

A transconjunctival blepharoplasty performed by laser or by scalpel does not involve undermining or closure of the skin. Therefore chemical peeling of any variety may be performed concurrently with less risk. The degree of edema that occurs from this blepharoplasty, however, may be considerable, might produce vascular and lymphatic compromise, and might be a theoretical factor in scar formation.

In a review of 100 facial plastic surgeons who had performed a cumulative 5000 blepharoplasties yearly, 66% of the physicians surveyed used Baker's solution after blepharoplasty. Of that 66%, 87% used the peel in fewer than 25% of their patients. Sixty-two percent of the facial plastic surgeons in the survey waited 3 months after blepharoplasty before periorbital peeling.[39]

In a series of 383 primary transconjunctival blepharoplasties during which 70% underwent simultaneous peel with either TCA up to 35% or a phenol formula, no cases of ectropion or scleral show were observed.[40] There was a risk of scarring in using simultaneous phenol peel and repeat secondary transconjunctival blepharoplasty, however.

REFERENCES

1. Fitzpatrick RE, Goldman MP, Sauter NM, et al: Pulsed carbon dioxide laser resurfacing of photoaged facial skin, *Arch Dermatol* 132:395-402, 1996.
2. Rook A, Wilkinson DS, Ebling FJG: *Textbook of dermatology*, Oxford, England, 1972, Blackwell Scientific, p. 2075.
3. Matarasso SL, Glogau RG: Chemical face peels, *Dermatol Clin* 9:131-150, 1991.
4. Baker TJ, Gordon HL: The ablation of rhytids by chemical means in a preliminary report, *J Fla Med Assoc* 48:451, 1961.
5. Baker TJ, Gordon HL: Chemical face peeling. In *Surgical rejuvenation of the face*, St Louis, 1986, Mosby, pp. 37-100.
6. Baker TJ, Gordon HL: Chemical peel with phenol. In Epstein E, Epstein E Jr, editors: *Skin surgery*, ed 6, Philadelphia, 1987, Saunders, pp. 423-438.
7. Brown AM, Kaplan LM, Brown ME: Phenol induced histological skin changes: hazards, techniques, and uses, *Br J Plast Surg* 13:158-169, 1960.

8. Rothman S: The principles of percutaneous absorption, *J Lab Clin Med* 28:1305-1321, 1945.
9. Hetter GP: Facial peeling with different strengths of phenol and croton oil. Abstracts, *Am Soc Aesthetic Plastic Surgery,* May, 1996.
10. Litton C: Chemical face lifting, *Plast Reconstr Surg* 29:371-380, 1962.
11. Litton C: Observations after chemosurgery of the face, *Plast Reconstr Surg* 32:554-556, 1963.
12. Beeson WH, McCollough EG: Chemical face peeling without taping, *J Dermatol Surg Oncol* 11:985-990, 1985.
13. McCollough EG, Langsdon PR: Chemical peeling with phenol. In Roenigk H, Roenigk R, editors: *Dermatologic surgery: principles and practice,* New York, 1989, Marcel Dekker, pp. 997-1016.
14. McCollough EG, Langsdon PR: *Dermabrasion and chemical peel. A guide for facial plastic surgery,* New York, 1988, Thieme Medical, pp. 53-112.
15. Stegman SJ: A comparative histologic study of the effects of three peeling agents and dermabrasion on normal and sundamaged skin, *Aesthetic Plast Surg* 6:123-135, 1982.
16. Collins PS: The chemical peel, *Clin Dermatol* 5:57-74, 1987.
17. Stegman SJ, Tromovitch TA: Chemical peeling. In *Cosmetic dermatologic surgery,* St Louis, 1984, Mosby, pp. 27-46.
18. Alt TH: Occluded Baker/Gordon chemical peel: review and update, *J Dermatol Surg Oncol* 15:980-993, 1989.
19. Hemels HG: Percutaneous absorption and distribution of 2-naphthol in man, *Br J Dermatol* 87:614-622, 1972.
20. Asken S: Unoccluded Baker/Gordon phenol peels: review and update, *J Dermatol Surg Oncol* 15:998-1008, 1989.
21. Gerwels JW, Bezzant JJ, LeMaire L, et al: Oral transmucosal fentanyl citrate premedication in patients undergoing outpatient dermatologic procedures, *J Dermatol Surg Oncol* 20:823-826, 1994.
22. Zukowski ML, Mossie RD, Roth SI,et al: Pilot study analysis of the histologic and bacteriologic effects of occlusive dressings in chemosurgical peel using a minipig model, *Aesthetic Plast Surg* 17:53-59, 1993.
23. Taylor MB: EMLA for effective pain relief following chemical peeling, *Dermatol Surg* 21:738-739, 1995 (letter).
24. Stegman SJ, Tromovitch TA, Glogau RG: Chemical peeling. In *Cosmetic dermatologic surgery,* ed 2, St Louis, 1990, Mosby, pp. 35-58.
25. Goldman PM, Freed MI: Aesthetic problems in chemical peeling, *J Dermatol Surg Oncol* 15:1020-1024, 1989.
26. DiGeronimo EM: Simple taping after chemical peels, *Plast Reconstr Surg* 68:953-954, 1981.
27. Mosienko P, Baker TJ: Chemical peel, *Clin Plast Surg* 5:79-96, 1978.
28. Epstein LI: Taping technique in chemical face peels, *Plast Reconstr Surg* 71:147, 1983 .
29. Bundy AT: Sterility in unsterilized surgical adhesive tape, *Plast Reconstr Surg* 83:880, 1989 .
30. Kotler R: Facial peeling: phenol. In Parish L, Lask G, editors: *Aesthetic dermatology,* New York, 1991, McGraw-Hill, pp. 128-139.
31. Stuzin JM, Baker TJ, Gordon HL: Chemical peel: a change in the routine, *Ann Plast Surg* 23:166-169, 1989.
32. Szachowiez EH, Wright WK: Delayed healing after full-face chemical peels, *Facial Plasti Surg* 6:8-13, 1989.
33. Raab B: A new hydrophilic copolymer membrane for dermabrasion, *J Dermatol Surg Oncol* 17:323-328, 1991.
34. Wood-Smith D, Rees TD: Chemabrasion and dermabrasion. In *Cosmetic facial surgery,* Philadelphia, 1973, Saunders, pp. 213-231.
35. Spira M, Gerow FJ, Hardy SB: Complications of chemical face peeling, *Plast Reconstr Surg* 54:397-403, 1974.
36. Litton C, Fournier P, Capinpin A: A survey of chemical peeling of the face, *Plast Reconstr Surg* 51:645, 1973.
37. Litton C, Trinidad G: Chemosurgery of the eyelids. In Aston SJ, et al, editors: *Third International Symposium of Plastic and Reconstructive Surgery,* Baltimore, 1982, Williams & Wilkins, pp. 341-345.
38. Wojno T, Tenzel R: Lower eyelid ectropion following chemical face peeling, *Ophthalmic Surg* 15:596-597, 1984.
39. Beeson WH: Chemical peel symposium at the Midwestern Section of the American Academy of Facial Plastic and Reconstructive Surgery Annual meeting, Indianapolis, 1989.
40. Newman J, Brandow K, Petmecky F: Transconjunctival blepharoplasty with simultaneous lower lid skin peel, *Int J Aesth Restor Surg* 3:43-52, 1995.

8 Complications of Chemical Peels

The application of wounding agents to the skin to produce a controlled wound is the principal concept in chemical peeling. A thorough knowledge of the histology of the wounding techniques and agents and their behavior on actinic damage and skin types will enable the physician to better control the wound. Despite attempts to standardize the peeling discipline to understand defect depth in addition to specific wounding agent depth, side effects may still occur.

The controlled wounding that is produced by chemical peeling is not a burn, and to refer to it as such is inappropriate and confusing. First- and second-degree burns define neither epidermal erythema nor distinguish between suprabasilar or subepidermal vesiculation. The clinical reclassification of burn injuries to encompass thermal injury is more logical because its application to chemical wounding does not correlate with the histopathology.[1]

The total number of different types of complications that may occur increases with wound depth. (See the box below, and on page 162.) Superficial peels usually produce transient pigmentary reactions only, but scarring can occur if dermal invasion occurs inadvertently. Medium-depth peels can cause pigmentary changes and scarring. Deep peels are associated with the preceding and other, more serious reactions.[2]

Proper informed consent is suggested before all dermal peels. Postpeel instruction sheets leave little room for misunderstanding. (See examples of the consent form in Chapter 4 and instruction sheets at the end of Chapters 5, 6, and 7.)

Good-quality photographs of the patient before and after peeling are good deterrents to patient dissatisfaction or litigation. The patient may not be aware of previous skin defects or may forget the previous appearance of the skin. In addition, more subtle improvements that sometimes follow peeling can be demonstrated photographically. (See the material on photodocumentation in Chapter 4.)

Complications of All Types of Chemical Peeling

- Pigmentary change
- Scarring
- Infection
- Prolonged erythema or pruritis
- Contact dermatitis
- Textural changes
- Milia
- Acne
- Cold sensitivity
- Poor physician-patient relationship

Complications Arising Exclusively from Deep Phenol Peeling

- Atrophy
- Cardiac arryhthmias
- Laryngeal edema
- Exacerbation of concurrent disease
- Toxic shock syndrome infection

A favorable test spot result in patients at higher risk for pigmentation or scarring may allay the fears of the patient and the physician, but it does not guarantee the response of the rest of the facial skin to the procedure[3] (Fig. 8-1). However, an unfavorable test result may help inform the high-risk patient or eliminate him or her from further consideration. We do not perform test spots on every chemical peel patient but usually do in Fitzpatrick type V and VI individuals.

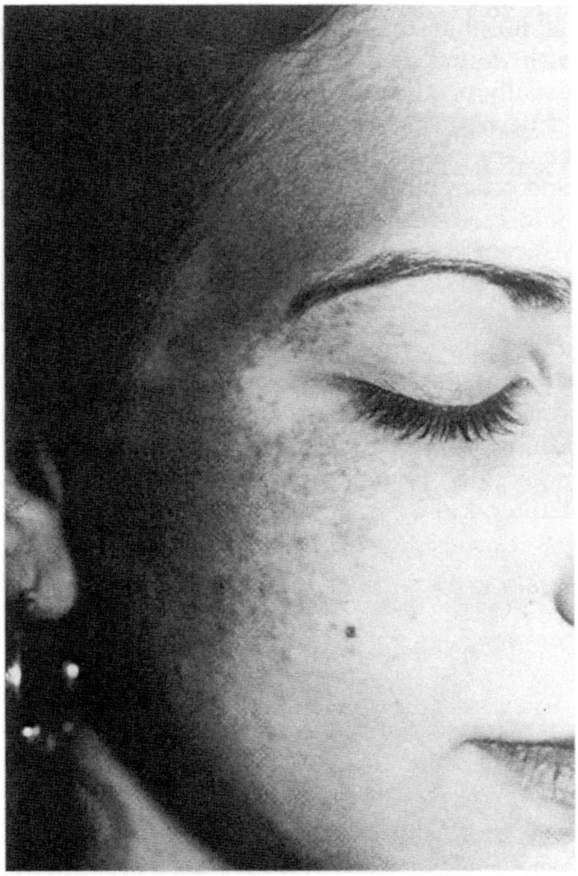

FIG. 8-1. Two months after two test spots at the hairline, deep and medium-depth modalities are compared. This pigmentation anomaly naturally spares the lateral canthal area.

COMPLICATIONS ARISING FROM ALL TYPES OF CHEMICAL PEELS

Pigmentary Changes

A noticeable transition between peeled and nonpeeled skin is a great aggravation to some patients. It may be difficult to cover the line with makeup, which some men especially may not wish to use. Therefore deciding where to stop a peel is an important consideration. Multiple sequential superficial peels may be performed to reduce the color differential on the nonfacial areas. If a single cosmetic unit is to be peeled, applying solutions approximately 5 mm beyond the natural boundaries will make **demarcation lines** less noticeable. For example, when peeling around the eyes, peel to the orbital rims, and periorally, peel beyond the nasolabial fold. Applying a superficial agent on the remainder of the face may be helpful. Similarly, the contrast between phenol-peeled and unpeeled areas may be noticeable in very sun-damaged Fitzpatrick type I skin. Feathering the edge of a peel with a superficial agent such as 25% TCA onto the neck under the angle of the jaw is helpful, especially with diligent electrosurgical or laser ablation of telangiectasia before and after peeling (Fig. 8-2). (See the box on the following page.)

Although **hyperpigmentation** can occur after any depth of chemical peel, lighter complexions (Fitzpatrick skin types I to III) have lower risk. (See the section on Fitzpatrick skin types in Chapter 4 for a detailed discussion.) Type IV skin can be peeled, but the patient must realize that the contrast between peeled and unpeeled skin may be obvious. Type VI skin can also be peeled, but the skin may be hyperpigmented after any nonphenolic wounding agent and may require as long as 18 to 24 months to return to normal. Phenolic peeling

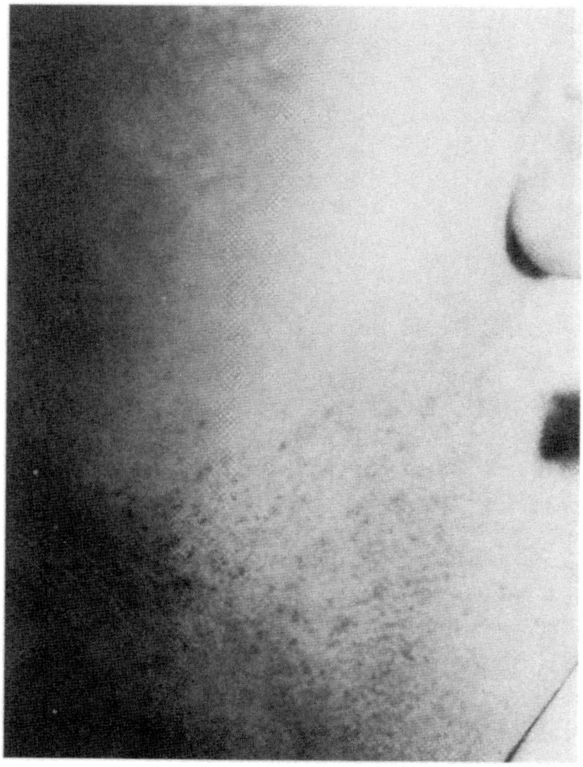

FIG. 8-2. Improper placement of a peel margin above the mandibular line with failure to feather the procedure or wounding agents.

Clinical Pigmentary Dyschromias

Hyperpigmentation
Hypopigmentation
Depigmentation (porcelain)
Mixed combination pigmentation
Lines of demarcation
Nevi accentuation

of type VI skin has resulted in a 10% to 20% lighter skin complexion.[4] In our experience, type V skin is the most unpredictable. It may develop more diffuse pigmentary changes after peeling with any wounding agent than any other skin type (Figs. 8-3, 8-4, and 11-9). (See Chapter 11.)

Although hyperpigmentation is more likely to occur after superficial or medium-depth peels and hypopigmentation after peels involving phenol, this is not always true. Nor can one generalize that freezing agents such as solid carbon dioxide are more likely than nonfreezing agents to cause hyperpigmentation. We have not found this to be true. Most cases of **hyperpigmentation** after peeling, regardless of the wounding agent, are due to minimal sun exposure during the erythematous phase in the months after peeling, but we have also seen it occur spontaneously. In our experience, if a patient is peeled when very suntanned for any indication, the incidence of postinflammatory hyperpigmentation may be greater.

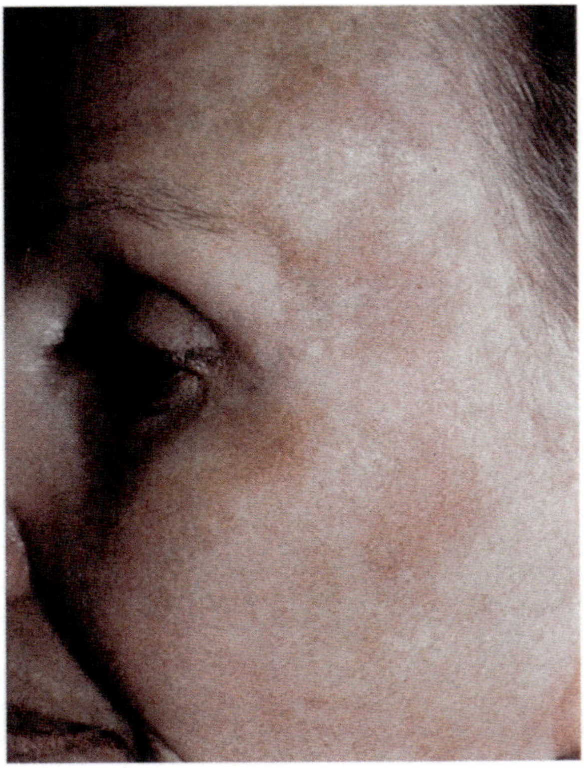

FIG. 8-3. Hyperpigmentation from probable sun exposure 6 weeks after medium-depth peeling in a Fitzpatrick type III skin type.

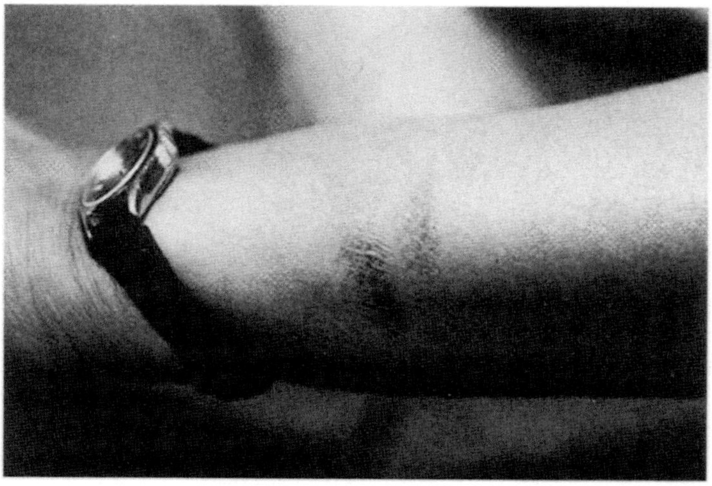

FIG. 8-4. Telltale signs of hyperpigmentation may include previous postinflammatory pigment.

If patients use birth control pills, exogenous estrogens, or photosensitizing drugs or if they become pregnant within 6 months after peeling, hyperpigmentation is more likely despite strict sun avoidance.[5] If this occurs, the areas may be repeeled 3 to 6 months later,[6] possibly but not necessarily with a less potent wounding agent. Nevi have been reported to hyperpigment after deep peeling,[7] but we have seen them survive the peel unchanged. Inadvertent minimal sun exposure may darken nevi and induce pigmentary disturbances.

Combinations of streaks or blotches of hyperpigmentation and hypopigmentation may result from inadequate skin preparation, uneven application of wounding agent, or inadequate mask adherence. In 1980, in a survey of 588 plastic surgeons using phenol, 2 out of 3 reported pigmentary problems, usually hypopigmentation.[8] A 50% TCA application will usually produce less hypopigmentation than phenol formulas in type IV to VI skin. Application of full-strength 88% phenol does not result in the same degree of hypopigmentation as the Baker's formula.

Hypopigmentation after Baker's phenol application is a function of patient selection and mode of application with subsequent wound care. The inherent color of the non–sun-damaged skin of the patient, the axillary skin, for example, may forecast the color after phenol peeling. Fitzpatrick type I photodamaged skin, redheaded patients, will be most likely to be the porcelain or alabaster white color after peeling, but this is close to their normal axillary skin color. Darker Hispanic skin, common in Florida, may have an after-peel appearance that is less hypopigmented in comparison to pretreatment skin tones than the very light English skin seen after peeling in Minnesota. Both skin types produce acceptable results when compared with nearby non–sun-damaged unpeeled skin. This skin must be appropriately treated. (See the box on page 166.)

Hypopigmentation after phenol is proportional to the amount of phenol applied, and a small pigment loss is an expected result and not a complication (Fig. 8-5). The role of the number of drops of croton oil in producing the degree of hypopigmentation in the Baker-Gordon formula is undetermined.[8a]

In preliminary observation, residual hypopigmentation occurring after laser resurfacing seems to be less noticeable or nonexistent in mild rhytides of photoaging III compared with usage of Baker's phenol, which is more likely to

Variable Factors in Pigment Loss in Baker-Gordon Peeling

Quantity of phenol applied relative to existing photodamage
Improper taping
Thymol iodine powder
Lighter Fitzpatrick skin type
Partial- or full-face peel comparison to adjacent unpeeled skin
Number of drops of croton oil

produce hypopigmentation in this setting of nonsevere rhytides. After severe rhytides of photoaging IV have been treated with the laser or Baker's phenol, residual hypopigmentation may be slight but not bothersome with both modalities. The rate of hypopigmentation with laser resurfacing seems to be lower than phenol but is unknown.

Stark porcelain white (alabaster) skin with clinical **depigmentation,** commonly seen around the mouth in the 1970s when only perioral peels were performed without blending neck or other areas with weaker peeling agents, may be more likely to result from larger amounts of Baker's phenol and greater occlusion. It is rarely seen today. The use of the original thymol iodine powder mask may have contributed to these appearances. Thymol is chemically related to phenol and may directly cause more melanocytic injury in addition to the nonwet reepithelialization of the mask itself. Depigmentation is more likely to occur with a heavy application of phenol to only mildly sun-damaged skin as opposed to heavily sun-damaged skin (Fig. 8-6). This improper patient selection was a major factor in producing depigmentation. Phenol produces hypopigmentation and not depigmentation by impairing melanin synthesis from melanocytes.[9] (See Chapter 2.) Therefore uneven freckling can occur with sun exposure after phenol peels. Uniform tanning does not occur, and burning has not been observed.[10]

Treatment of hyperpigmentation can be instituted by twice-daily application of tretinoin cream, 0.1%, and hydroquinone gel, 4% (Solaquin Forte or Viquin Forte gel). Optionally, corticosteroid cream no stronger than triamci-

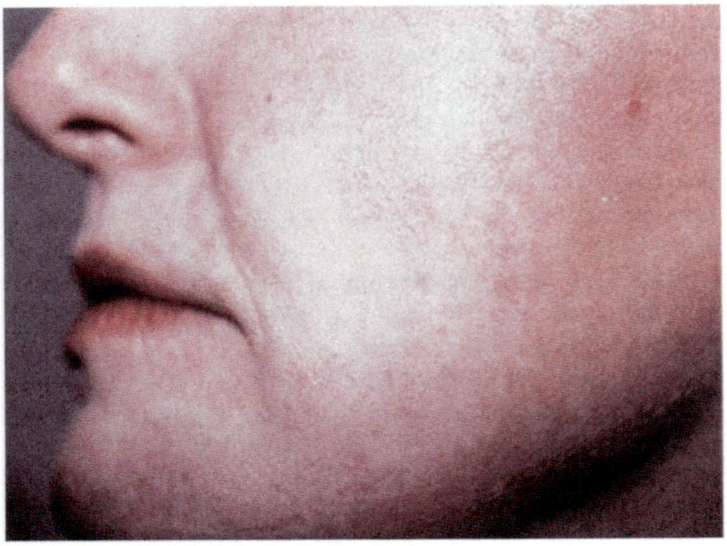

FIG. 8-5. Irregular hypopigmentation occurring after a Baker's peel.

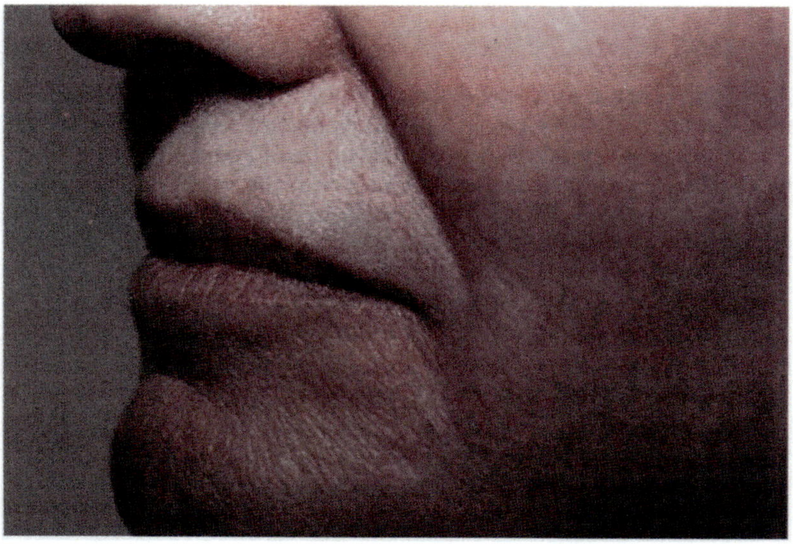

FIG. 8-6. Upper lip depigmentation from an occluded Baker's peel 12 years previously.

nolone, 0.1%, may be added. A modification of the traditional depigmentation formula is especially helpful after peeling for Fitzpatrick types IV through VI skin. (See the top box on page 168.) A small subset of patients may produce a better response when bleaching or prophylaxing against hyperpigmentation with the addition of glycolic acid lotion (e.g., Aquaglycolic astringent 11%—Herald Pharmacal) to their regimen.[11] (See the discussion on the rejuvenation regimen in Chapter 4.)

The compound should be used as soon after reepithelialization as tolerated and until the erythema is faint. If irritation occurs the frequency of application may be reduced to daily or every other day. Usually 3 to 6 months of therapy is required in patients at high risk.[12-14] It may be helpful to pretreat patients with hydroquinone and tretinoin for an unspecified period of time, usually 6 to 8 weeks, but we stress this subjectively only for skin types III to VI, the higher-risk groups. This has not been critically studied. Hyperpigmentation may resolve in time with sunscreens alone. Patients should be prepared to wear sunscreens with a sun protection factor of 15 or greater after peeling to ensure that the screen will adhere to the epidermis at all times.

If the peel is a success and all undesired pigmentation disappears but the patient begins to repigment in the immediate postpeel period within 2 to 4 weeks and postpeel bleaching creams fail, it may be prudent to repeel the skin before the melanophages integrate into the dermis. Jessner's solution is an excellent wounding agent with little risk and can be used to treat pigmentation after any TCA peel, especially in Fitzpatrick skin types III and IV. Repeeling with a weaker agent than the original TCA in the first month after reepithelialization has a small risk of scarring, but it can be very effective. The patient should be warned of the inherent risk because penetration will be enhanced from the recent peel, but the benefits may warrant local or complete repeeling with reassumption of strict bleaching and sun avoidance approximately after another 5 days.

We use hydroquinone, tretinoin, and the regimen outlined in Chapter 4 after peeling, especially in dark skin types. Realistically there is less need for them in Fitzpatrick skin type I and II because many of these patients retain the effects of their peels without tanning or refreckling in the absence of sun-

Bleaching Formula for Darker Skin Types: Bleach-eze

The initial concentration of hydroquinone is 6%. This may be increased if pigmentation returns after peeling. Ascorbic acid prevents the hydroquinone from oxidizing. Hytone (hydrocortisone) cream (Dermik) is paraben free. Creams with high concentrations of hydroquinone should be discontinued as soon as the appropriate amount of pigment loss is achieved to avoid paradoxic hyperpigmentation.

Hydroquinone, 6%-10%*
Ascorbic acid, 0.05%*
Retinoic acid, 0.1%*
Propylene glycol, 4%
Dissolve crystals* in propylene glycol and mix in Hytone cream, 2.5% (Dermik), 30 g
Sig: apply b.i.d.

This cream may be locally compounded or ordered for individual patients by prescription in concentrations up to 15% from Medical Center Pharmacy, 4600 N. Habana Ave, Tampa, FL 33614 at 1-800-226-7094; fax: 813-876-9095. Its potency decreases if not used in 2 months.

light. Physiologic freckles may return in the absence of the regimen, however, and the regimen will usually minimize these. It is impossible for everyone to completely abstain from the sun and adhere to the regimen. If lighter skin types are less diligent in their application, it is of less concern to the physician than darker skin types.

Scarring

Medium-depth and deep peels have the risk of scarring, but as of yet, the contributing factors are unresolved. (See the box below.) Heredity, darker skin types, smoking, inadequate topical hydration, constrictive taping, previous cosmetic undermining surgery, excessive facial chewing, and infection during healing may be contributory. Most scars in chemical peeling are hypertrophic scars and not true keloids. In contrast to keloids, scars from peeling occur soon after surgery and usually subside within several years. They may be improved with excisional surgery and are less common on the face than in keloid-predisposed areas such as the presternal or earlobe areas.[17] "Thin skin" has also been cited as an etiologic factor, but even thick-skinned individuals have "thin skin" at the temples or at the nasal bridges that may not scar. Perhaps the attempt to wound deeper to correct deep creases is the cause of scarring in "thin skin."[18,19] Any previous peels, dermabrasions, and isotretinoin use may be risk factors of uncertain degree for scarring. Medium-depth and deep dermal repeeling before the erythema has clinically resolved is also a hazard. Scarring is least likely to occur after **superficial peeling** because the dermis

Variations of Scarring

Formation of atrophic, hypertrophic, or keloidal scarring
Scarring or sloughing after cosmetic surgery from undermining
Ectropion after a peel with blepharoplasty
Cicatricial ectropion without blepharoplasty
Delayed healing

Perspective on Tretinoin Usage and Peel Complications

From a historical standpoint, before Kligman presented the use of tretinoin for photoaged skin and Mandy suggested its use before dermabrasion, and subsequently peeling to decrease healing time in the mid-1980s, we had peeled hundreds of patients with TCA preceded by dry ice with no preparatory creams except sunscreens. Theoretically, if the total number of days to reepithelialization is reduced due to preoperative tretinoin, there are less days present in the postoperative period for complications to occur. However, we can discern no difference in the scarring complication rate now or clinical improvement compared with the 7 years before 1986.[15] This does not include the scarring that is directly attributable to oral isotretinoin usage in concert with chemical peeling. There is no evidence that a more rapid reepithelialization after a peel is valuable. It is the dermis, not the epidermis, that determines the final cosmetic appearance of the skin.[16] Some of the most unsightly scars have a normal epidermis. More rapid reepithelialization may even decrease the amount of regenerated papillary dermis and may retard our goals in scar reduction. There is no dispute, however, that the postpeel use of tretinoin and its potentiation of hydroquinone have decreased postoperative hyperpigmentation.

is rarely penetrated, even when peeling these patients while erythematous, as in repetitive superficial peeling.

Some individuals who scar may have a mild variant of the mitis form of the Ehlers-Danlos syndrome.[20] This variant is purported to be present in as much as 9% of the population and is easily overlooked. However, Ehlers-Danlos scars are usually more atrophic than the more common hypertrophic and contractile variety seen after chemical peeling.

In **medium-depth peeling,** the risk of scarring is small. In a series of more than 3000 patients treated with solid carbon dioxide followed by 35% trichloroacetic acid (TCA) with rare local 50% TCA application to scars or individual rhytides, less than a 0.25% incidence of hypertrophic scarring was noted[5,14] (Fig. 8-7). Care should be exercised in using 50% TCA in combination medium-depth peeling because high-strength TCA is more caustic than full-strength phenol and may be more likely to produce scarring.[21-23] Fifty percent TCA alone is capable of unpredictable hypertrophic scarring; 35% TCA is relatively safe (Fig. 8-8). The combination of Jessner's solution followed by 35% TCA produced no scarring in 500 patients[24] (Fig. 8-9). No contractile scarring has been reported with any of the three published medium-depth combination peels.

For scarring occurring after the application of pyruvic acid, see the section on pyruvic acid in Chapter 6.

In **deep peeling** with a phenol formula, 21% of 588 plastic surgeons reported scarring, most frequently in the perioral area, and usually occurring in the first 3 months after peeling.[8] Racially dark individuals may have a higher incidence of hypertrophic scarring,[25] and a family history or a test area may be helpful to screen patients. Hair dyes or permanent wave solutions applied the week before a phenol peel may be factors that induce skin sloughing and hairline scarring.[6]

The incidence of scarring with the traditional Baker's phenol formula in the series of over 1000 patients peeled by Baker and Gordon is less than 1%. (Personal communication, Dr. Thomas Baker, April 1996.) We have noted no scarring in 100 patients peeled with the formula. These are patients who were

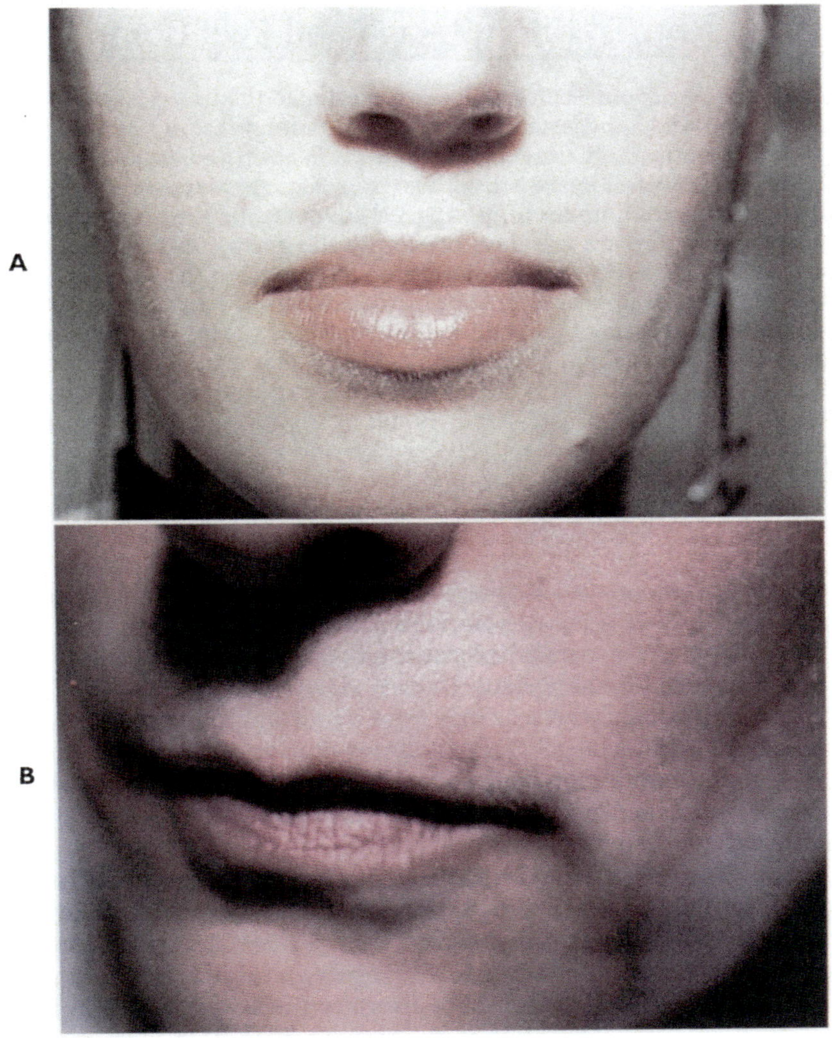

FIG. 8-7. Mild scarring in the perioral area after medium-depth peeling with CO_2 plus TCA, 35%, is minimized with intralesional steroids.

peeled without preliminary overtreatment with tretinoin or other topicals. The rate of scarring may increase with deviations from the original description of the peel, the use of preliminary treatments to increase absorption, improper patient selection, or other factors listed in this section. Preliminary comparison with CO_2 laser reveals equal safety.

Nonfacial skin is notoriously more difficult to peel. Areas such as the neck, back of the hands, forearms, and arms may be more prone to scarring, but these areas have been peeled less than facial areas. We probably do not have enough cases or adequate evidence to detail the exact risk. Certainly, superficial peeling can be performed in these areas with a very low risk. Poikilodermatous changes of the neck and sun-damaged skin of the hands resist therapy, and hypertrophic scarring with high-strength TCA may result.[21,26] Multiple superficial peels to reduce pigmentation, meticulous monthly electrosurgery, and the copper vapor or pulsed dye laser combined with chronic tretinoin therapy are the most reliable treatments. The pulsed dye laser may leave lines of demarcation. The dorsa of the hands can be spot peeled selectively with

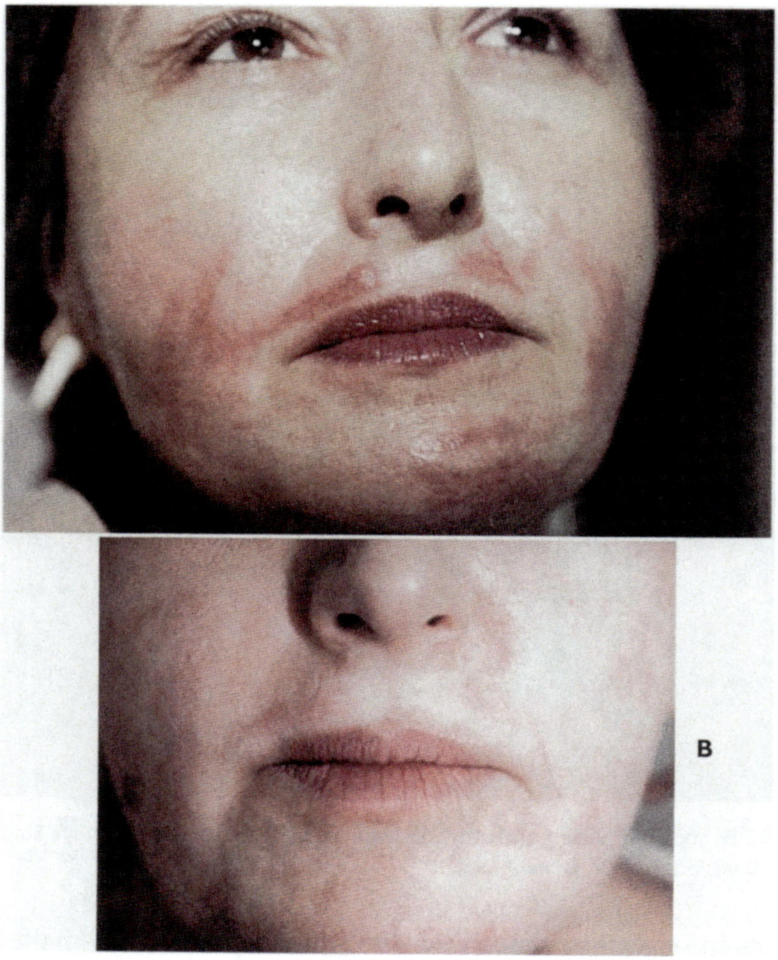

FIG. 8-8. A, Perioral scarring after 50% TCA peel. **B,** One year after intensive intralesional steroids.

phenol, but the skin does not respond as well as facial skin,[27] and scarring can occur. (See the section on exodermology in Chapter 10.)

Full-thickness skin sloughs are associated with simultaneous peeling and rhytidectomy, probably as a result of undermining and compromised skin vascular and lymphatic circulation. If this occurs, some recommend healing by secondary intention.[7] Others recommend excision of the affected areas and the use of a flap or graft to cover the defect.[28] A time interval of 1 to 3 months should separate deep or medium-depth peeling and rhytidectomy or brow lift. Peeling has been performed 2 to 3 months before rhytidectomy without scarring.[29] Localized perioral or periorbital peels can be performed at the completion of a face-lift if perioral surgery or a blepharoplasty is not done. A case of mild scarring in the area of undermining of a rhytidectomy performed 3 months before a medium-depth peeling with Jessner's solution plus 35% TCA has been observed resulting in only a permanent hypopigmented texture change (see Fig. 8-9). (Lack EB: Personal communication, 1991.)

Although simultaneous deep-plane face-lift and 35% TCA peeling has been reported by some physicians,[30] the combination is never risk free because the TCA application technique varies considerably among cosmetic surgeons. The

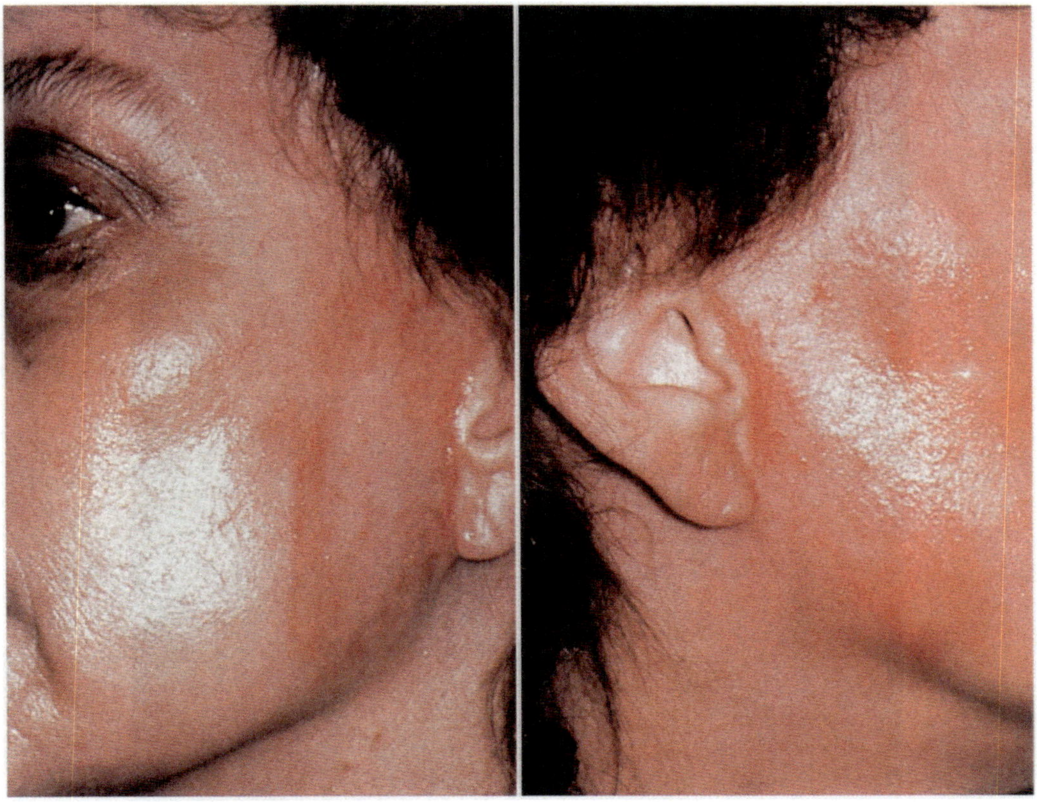

FIG. 8-9. A and **B,** Impaired healing after rhytidectomy in conjunction with Jessner's solution plus TCA, 35%. See the text. *(Courtesy of Dr. Edward Lack.)*

slight inconvenience associated with separating the peel from the surgical procedure is outweighed by the potential for scarring that might occur rarely if a complication arises or if these combined procedures are performed by a surgeon with limited TCA peeling experience.[31,32]

Both lidocaine injection with or without epinephrine and flap elevation are risk factors for increased penetration of Baker's solution in an animal model.[33] (See the discussion on dermal healing after skin flaps in Chapter 2.) The application to regional blocks before peeling in humans is uncertain.

Lower eyelid ectropion after chemical face peeling can develop if deep peeling is performed in conjunction with a blepharoplasty. It may resolve spontaneously in 3 to 4 months, but an interval of as long as 6 months has been suggested.[34] Cases of cicatricial ectropion have been reported in phenol-peeled patients who have not had a blepharoplasty.[35] The lower eyelids should be peeled with caution in individuals with subclinical or partial ectropion and minimal loss of apposition of the lid to the sclera. Less risk is apparent with transconjunctival blepharoplasty and peeling. (See the section on concurrent deep peeling and cosmetic surgery in Chapter 7.)

The role of isotretinoin (Accutane, Roche) in scarring after chemical peeling is uncertain. Cases of scarring have been reported after dermabrasion, but studies in the animal model have not demonstrated any increased risk.[36-39] The technique and depth of dermabrasion is highly operator sensitive, and therefore exact guidelines are difficult to establish. Scarring has been noted in patients who had discontinued isotretinoin use for as long as 6, 14, 24, and 36

A 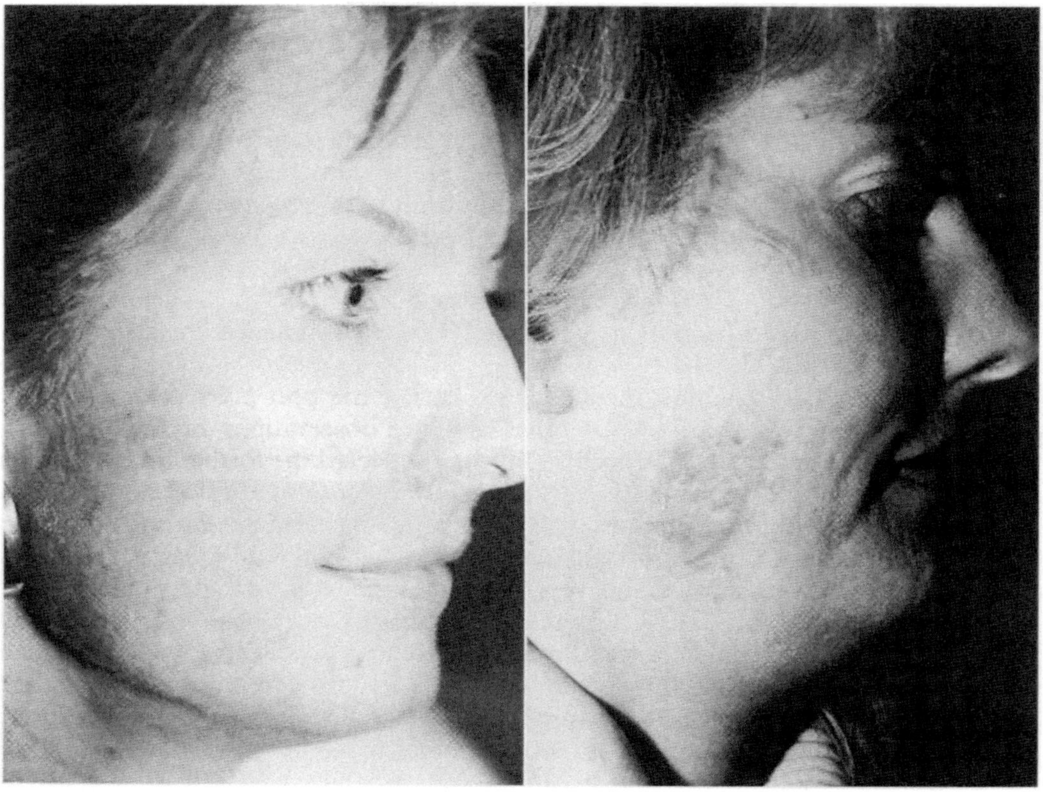 B

FIG. 8-10. A, Normal healing after a medium-depth peel. **B,** Scarring during the fourth month of isotretinoin therapy. (See the text.)

months before dermabrasion.[40] The generalization of a 6-month interval, for example, may or may not be appropriate, depending on physician technique and total drug dosage. (See the section on retinoids in Chapter 3.)

The incidence of scarring with chemical peeling in relationship to isotretinoin is rare at this time. Because wounds extending to the papillary dermis through the middermis can be reached with chemical peeling as well as with dermabrasion, performing a chemical peel on patients who have previously used isotretinoin should be approached with caution based on our knowledge of peel depth. In the time interval between 1982 when the drug was released and 1984 when scarring with dermabrasion was reported, we peeled a minimum of 100 patients who were taking the drug or had immediately completed a 4-month course. These patients underwent a CO_2 plus TCA upper dermal peel, and none of these patients experienced scarring.

Since that time, only one patient who received a medium-depth chemical peel with CO_2 plus 35% TCA experienced scarring directly related to the drug.[41] The quality of the scarring was different from the usual acne scarring but may have commenced with acne pustules (Fig. 8-10). The patient had received a 4-month course of isotretinoin 2 years before the peel. She healed uneventfully after the peel but spontaneously scarred when begun on a 4-month course of isotretinoin 3 months after reepithelialization.

There are at least two other cases of abnormal healing associated with isotretinoin use. Scarring resulted after two 50% TCA peels performed 4 months and 7 months, respectively, after completion of a course of isotretinoin.

(Boughton RS: Personal communication, July 1990.) Another patient was spot dermabraded 6 months after isotretinoin use without complication but scarred when peeled 4 to 6 months later with 25% TCA while taking 10 mg of isotretinoin daily. (Pinski KS, Roenigk HH: Personal communication, September 1990.) The use of the drug during the 6 months before or after a peel may be a factor in scar formation, perhaps because tissues have not returned to normal metabolism from insult with either the drug or the peel. The dose and duration of the drug and the depth of the peel are factors to consider when judging time intervals.

The phenomenon of **delayed healing** has been noted after both medium-depth TCA and deep phenol peeling.[42,43] The constellation of symptoms are listed in the accompanying box.

These patients give no indication during the peel process that they will have aberrant reepithelialization. Personal observations of the immediate frost in a case with TCA peeling have not reflected the forthcoming complication. Multiple or single friable stellate-bordered nonindurated slightly tender erosions with serous granulation tissue are present by the expected final days of the healing process. They are noticed by day 8 in medium-depth peeling and day 10 to 14 in deep peeling (Fig. 8-11, *A* and *B*).

To confirm the diagnosis and because these areas resemble bacterial infection, the lesions should be cultured and treated systemically for bacteria and yeast with oral antibiotics and antifungals. Moist nonhealing wounds after dermabrasion[44] or excision may provide a background for yeast infection,[45] but oral antifungals and antibiotics are ineffective in this entity.

Treatment of delayed healing with artificial wound dressing (Vigilon—Hermal Labs, Delmar, New York) is effective in reducing wound healing time. After 2 to 3 days Duoderm (ConvaTec, Bristol Meyers Squibb, Princeton, New Jersey) or Opsite (Smith and Nephew Research, England) may be substituted as less wet occlusive dressings are needed. These are changed daily until healing.[43] (See discussion in Chapter 3 on different biosynthetic occlusive dressings.) Because keloids have increased water content[25] and pathologic states such as eczema have increased transepidermal water loss,[46,47] this implies that the use of an artificial dressing will restore normal epidermal barrier function and facilitate epithelial cell migration and healing. Duffy has shown decreased wounding and more rapid healing with 30% TCA in photoaged forearm skin occluded with Vigilon for 24 hours before peeling (Duffy D, unpublished observation). Injection of the edge of the wound with very dilute intralesional triamcinolone (2 mg/ml in 1% xylocaine) will also reduce inflammation and speed epithelial migration with wound healing.

Without treatment these skin edges exhibit 6 to 8 weeks of delay in healing. They characteristically may heal with scars that resemble the smooth hypopigmented scars resembling cryosurgery. Phenol peeling may follow a similar sequence of wound repair to cryosurgery. Freezing destroys the cellular ele-

Delayed Healing

Friable, stellate, nonindurated painful unhealed erosions with serous granulation tissue
Persists 10 days after peeling
Unpredictable
May heal with hypopigmented flat scarring
Effective treatment with artificial wound dressings

A B C

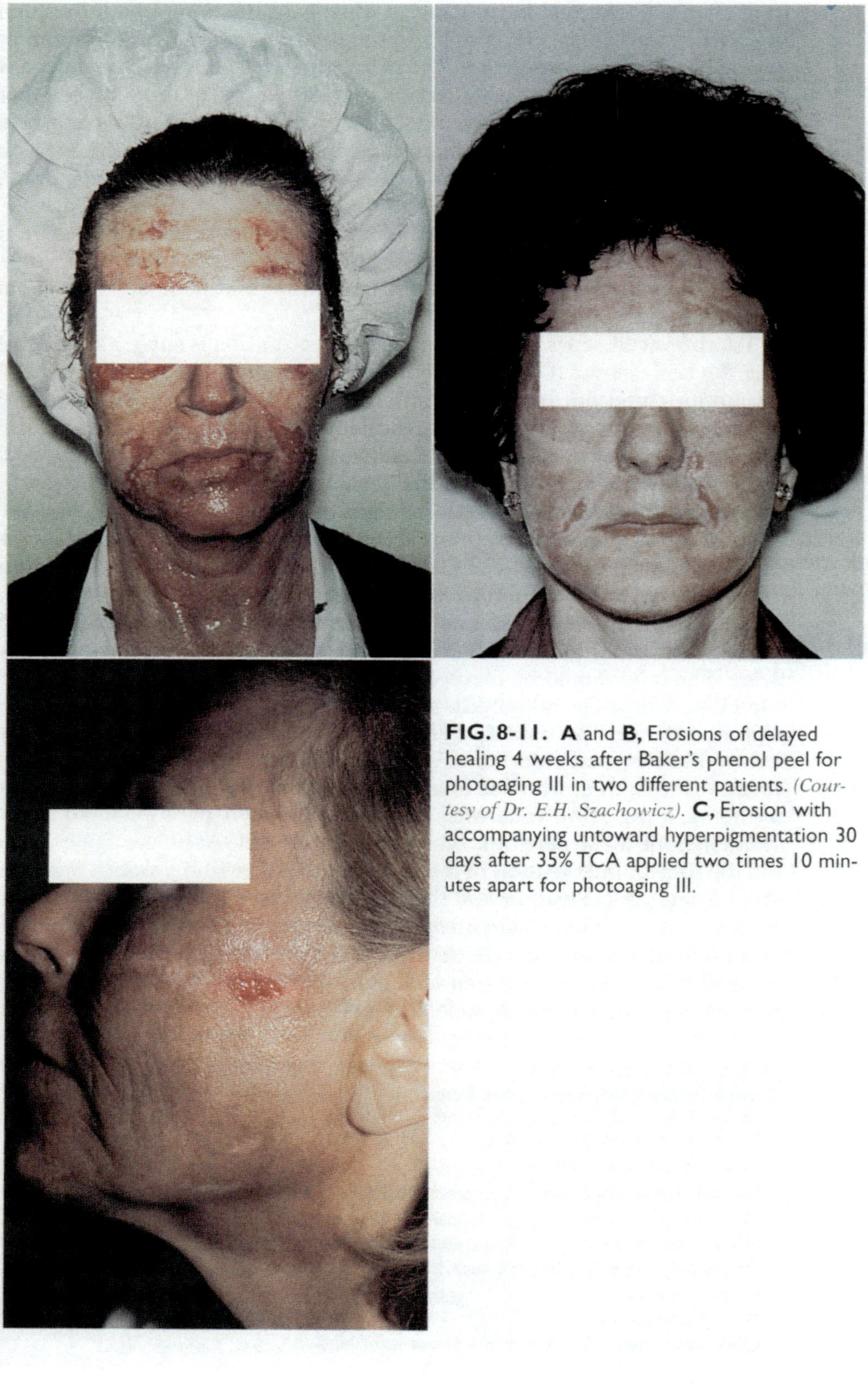

FIG. 8-11. A and **B,** Erosions of delayed healing 4 weeks after Baker's phenol peel for photoaging III in two different patients. *(Courtesy of Dr. E.H. Szachowicz).* **C,** Erosion with accompanying untoward hyperpigmentation 30 days after 35% TCA applied two times 10 minutes apart for photoaging III.

ments of the upper dermis while preserving the collagen matrix, which acts to prevent wound contraction, allowing gradual healing with nonhypertrophic textural change.[42] Thermal burns cause complete destruction of both the connective tissue matrix and cells, similar to the destruction occurring from an open wound, resulting in contraction. The delayed healing entity may be mixed with areas of deep dermal chemical invasion manifested first as indurated erythema. If deep dermal collagen matrix is disrupted and contractile scarring begins, intralesional injection with a minimum of 5 to 10 mg/ml of triamcinolone should be instituted at 2- to 4-week intervals. Deep erythema without induration should be treated with silicone gel sheeting as detailed in the following.

Other etiologies to consider include premature removal of occlusive tape before maximal edematous facial swelling, atopic skin (Alston LL, unpublished observation), factitial patient excoriation, and poor nutritional states in vegetarians.[48]

Treatment of scars during or after their formation is subject to judgment. (See the box below.) If only erythema without induration is present we favor a nonfluorinated but potent steroid cream such as (hydrocortisone valerate (Westcort—Westwood-Squibb Co., Buffalo, New York), alclometasone dipropionate (Aclovate—Schering Co., Kenilworth New Jersey), or desonide (Desowen—Galderma Labs, Ft. Worth, Texas) to avoid skin atrophy, and the patient and physican may watch for signs of induration. More aggessive topical and intralesional intervention is then indicated. The use of a class I topical steroid such as clobetasol (Temovate—Glaxo), or halobetasol propionate (Ultravate—Westwood-Squibb), diflorasone diacetate (Psorcon—Dermik), or a fluocinonide-impregnated tape (Cordran—Oclassen Pharmaceuticals, San Rafael, California) too quickly may reduce erythema but produce atrophy or striae. The tape should be used only at night, and signs of overusage necessitate close follow-up. Some physicians advocate aggressive treatment of any slightly indurated persistent erythematous linear or curved lesions with topical or intralesional fluorinated corticosteroids.[49] We feel that diluting the injection strength down to as low as 2 mg/cc for early questionable indurated erythema, 4 mg/cc for indurated erythema, and as high as 20 to 40 mg/cc of triamcinolone for hypertropic scarring is justified based on the aggressiveness and the time of intervention of the erythematous scarring process. Injection of an adequate concentration into the scar every 2 to 4 weeks to try to minimize the scar but not induce skin atrophy is based on the degree of erythema, the amount of induration, and the severity of the process. Injection pain is greatly reduced by local cryoanesthesia with light application of ethyl chloride, liquid nitrogen, or solid carbon dioxide. The antecedent use of EMLA may increase

Treatment of Hypertrophic Scars

Topical nonfluorinated steroids
Topical fluorinated steroids
Steroid-impregnated tape
Intralesional steroids
Silicone gel sheeting
Flashlamp-pumped pulsed dye laser, 585 nm
Surgical excision
Micropigmentation
Observation with or without the above intervention

Perspective on Scarring Complications

Scarring after peeling or dermabrasion occurs as a result of a combination of risk factors based on hereditary predisposition; the time interval between multiple peels or courses of isotretinoin; the concentration and application of specific wounding agent and peel depth; the location with varying appendages for healing, dermal actinic quality, and possible mobility of the skin being peeled (the perioral area, for example); the quality of wound care after peeling with the presence of infection[5,41]; and too short an interval between peeling and undermining from cosmetic surgery. Poor nutritional status in vegetarians may affect epithelialization and collagen reorganization after TCA or phenol peels.[48] Excessive dissolution of epidermal integrity from atopic dermatitis or overuse of abrasive scrubs or facials may cause undue absorption of wounding agents. Scarring occurs after CO_2 laser peeling and is compared and discussed in this chapter and Chapter 10.

With these factors, the inflammatory response is probably increased during the healing process. This may affect the wound healing stages of reepithelialization and collagen remodeling producing complications. (See the box below.) Chapters 2 and 3 contain more detailed discussions of the healing process.

tolerance for the injections. Time alone or compression and massage may resolve mild, small scars. Combined scar revision with intralesional steroids may be necessary in severe cases.[2]

A new approach to improve hypertrophic scars is with silicone gel sheeting, a semiocclusive scar cover made of cross-linked polydimethylsiloxane polymer.[17] The mechanism of action is unknown and is not related to pressure. Improvements in the texture, color, and height of some scars have been reported beginning about 3 months after use.[50-52] The silicone gel sheeting is cut to appropriate size and either self-adhered or taped to the potential area for a minimum of 12 hours of treatment daily. It can be washed and reused until deterioration necessitates replacement. (See the Appendix for availability.) The gel can be used in addition to intralesional steroids and may be initiated at night or even 24 hours a day at the first sign of deep erythema without induration.

Erythematous and hypertrophic scars can also be improved with the flashlamp-pumped pulsed dye laser (FLPDL), 585 nm, with or without intralesional triamcinolone.[53-55] Patients who receive combination treatment achieve greater resolution. Facial scars and scars less than 1 year old respond more readily to

Risk Factors for Scarring

Hereditary predisposition
Time interval between peels or isotretinion use
Concentration and application of the wounding agent
Location and actinic dermal quality of the skin
Quality of aftercare
Previous recent surgical skin undermining
Inadequate nutritional status
Disintegration of epidermal integrity

2 to 4 sequential monthly treatments. In patients with multiple rapidly evolving hypertrophic scars this may be an excellent treatment adjuvant.

Local depigmented macules remaining after scars have been treated and repigmented with color matching by microtattooing techniques (e.g., Permark, Micropigmentation Devices, Inc., Edison, New Jersey, 800-287-5228 or Lasting Impressions, Englewood, New Jersey 800-377-4088). This can blend with surrounding skin and soften the appearance of the residual scar.

Infection

Infectious complications of chemical peels are unusual. (See the box below.) Peeling ingredients are unlikely to be the source of infection because TCA and phenol are bactericidal[6,8] and surgical adhesive out of the package is sterile.[56] The best deterrent to infection after peeling is to minimize crusting by treating the skin with wet to dry soaks. Occlusive ointments may rarely promote folliculitis; this may become secondarily infected with *Streptococcus* or *Staphylococcus,* which are readily treated with penicillinase-resistant antibiotics. All suspected infections should be cultured for identification and sensitivity and the patient given appropriate antibiotics. In our experience, acne flare-ups after peeling respond best to an infectious approach with a culture and appropriate antibiotics first. (See the section on acne that follows.)

Pseudomonas infections (Fig. 8-12) are treated with the oral antibiotic ciprofloxacin and may occur from improper care during healing[19] or if the patient acquires a nosocomial hospital infection when the skin's barrier layer has been removed. Five percent acetic acid or white vinegar diluted 1:1 with tap water is a safe, effective, and inexpensive topical soaking agent for twice-daily use.[57] The presence of bacterial infection does not always cause scarring, as is the case with secondary impetiginization in patients with eczema.

Toxic shock syndrome, induced by an exotoxin elaborated by *Staphylococcus aureus,* has been reported after one unoccluded and two occluded Baker's phenol face peels.[58,59] Patients develop fever, syncopal hypotension, vomiting, or diarrhea 2 to 3 days after the peel; 2 to 6 days postpeel this is accompanied by a scarlatiniform rash with subsequent desquamation. Appropriate antibiotics with large volumes of parenteral fluids to prevent vascular collapse are necessary. The syndrome may include myalgias, mucosal hyperemia, and hepatorenal, hematologic, or central nervous system involvement.

Herpes simplex infection may be reactivated by peeling of any depth.[60] Unusual and unexpected postpeel pain may reflect the onset of viral infection. Patients with a positive history of herpes can be treated prophylactically during healing with 400 mg of acyclovir (Zovirax, Glaxo Wellcome, West Caldwell, New Jersey) three times daily if undergoing a deep peel beginning on the day of the peel. Valacyclovir HCl (Valtrex, Glaxo Wellcome, West Caldwell,

Infection with Chemical Peels

- Bacterial pyoderma
- Toxic shock syndrome
- Herpes simplex virus
- Epstein-Barr virus keratitis
- Candidiasis (rare)

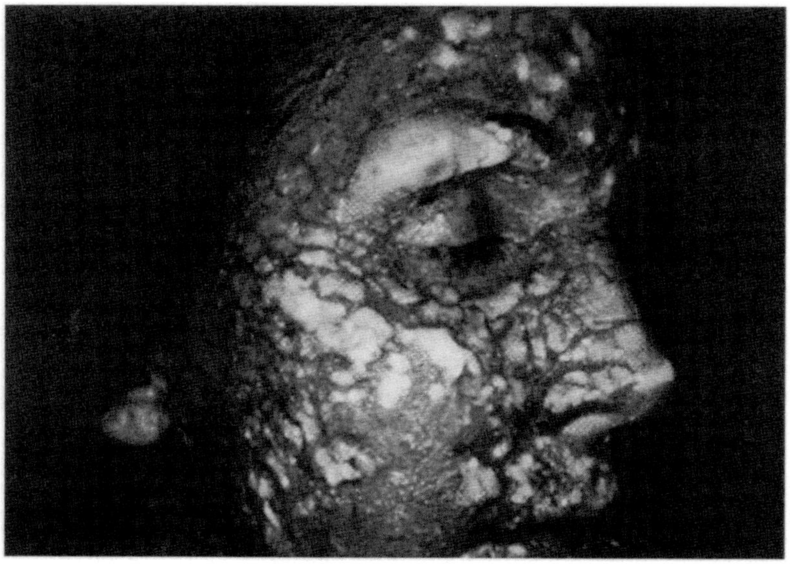

FIG. 8-12. *Pseudomonas* infection that has resulted from poor wound care after a Baker's chemical peel. *(Courtesy of Dr. Samuel Stegman.)*

New Jersey) 500 mg two times daily or famciclovir (Famvir, SmithKline Beecham, Philadelphia, Pennsylvania) 500 mg three times daily are effective alternative antivirals. We have never observed scarring from recurrent herpes with medium-depth or superficial peeling and do not routinely give prophylaxis to every patient with a rare history of "fever blisters" who is undergoing these peels. Active herpes during the postpeel period should be treated with appropriate increased therapeutic doses of antivirals (Fig. 8-13).

Before acyclovir, herpes activation was a feared complication and was treated with oral corticosteroids in attempts to decrease inflammation and antibiotics to prevent secondary infection. Trigger areas for herpes were not

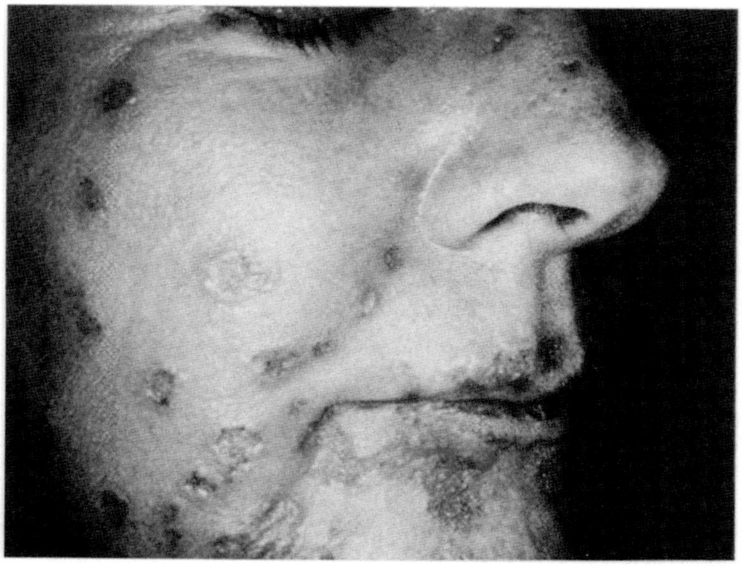

FIG. 8-13. Herpes simplex infection after a Baker's chemical peel. *(Courtesy of Dr. Samuel Stegman.)*

peeled or dermabraded until after the remainder of the face had healed. With these precautions, scarring from herpes infections was still rare, although the fear of dissemination of the herpes with oral steroids affected many a decision as to whether to use them.[5]

A patient that is exposed to herpes simplex for the first time during the healing period may become infected with primary inoculation herpes and experience severe pain with lymphadenopathy and fever. These patients are candidates for treatment with intravenous antivirals.

Epstein-Barr virus keratitis after a Baker's peel manifested as blurred vision with fever and joint pain 4 days after peeling.[61] The patient responded to prednisolone eyedrops, but recurrences that were manifested months later induced corneal stromal scarring and necessitated chronic acyclovir therapy. Croton oil may induce Epstein-Barr virus replication and reactivate the 10% of normal eyes of seropositive individuals for the virus.

Candidiasis (yeast) has been reported more frequently after dermabrasion and CO_2 laser resurfacing.[44,62] It is unusual and undocumented after peeling, although it is possible. The partially protective presence of a nonviable epidermis remaining intact after peeling and lack of occlusive dressings in peels make yeast less likely unless overuse of oral antibiotics or topical antibacterial or occlusive ointments predispose to its occurrence. All delayed healing wounds should be treated with a short course of systemic antiyeast drugs (e.g., ketoconazole 200 mg daily for 7 days) to establish a treatment course. (See delayed healing in previous section on scarring.)

A

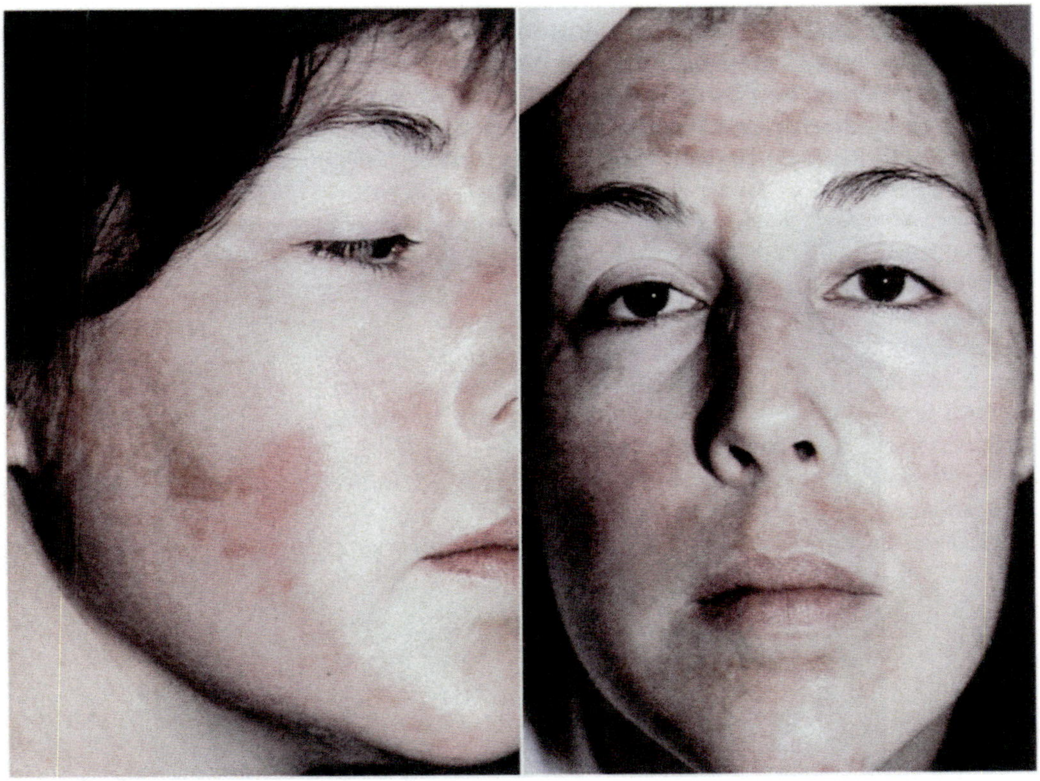

B

FIG. 8-14. Prolonged erythema 60 days after medium-depth peeling that has resolved without scarring or pigmentation. Note the linearity and configuration.

Prolonged Erythema or Pruritus

Erythema after peeling usually disappears in 30 to 90 days, depending on the wounding agent (Fig. 8-14.) Reasonable resolution times are 14 to 30 days after superficial peeling, 30 to 60 days after medium-depth peeling, and 90 days after deep peeling, but different patients may manifest longer intervals, especially if they are using tretinoin before and after peels.[5] Isotretinoin administration before peeling, genetic or atopic factors of the patient, rosacea, or minimal amounts of alcoholic beverages[7] may also affect redness. It is never permanent, but intermittent flushing may occur for as long as 4 years afterward. Persistent erythema with pruritis after multiple resorcinol peels should alert the physician to suspect contact dermatitis. Generally, the erythema after laser resurfacing is more prolonged than after chemical resurfacing. The same factors apply, but the number of passes with the laser, the laser system, and the energy used are additional variables.

The addition of 2.5% topical hydrocortisone lotion or other nonfluorinated steroid cream to the regimen as listed in the section on scarring (see the regimen discussion in Chapter 4) may be helpful. Oral antihistamines, short-term systemic steroids, silicone gel sheeting, and the application of a green foundation under base makeup can also be useful. Topical fluorinated steroids, which might produce atrophy or telangiectasia, and chronic systemic steroid use producing hypercortisolism are unwarranted. If induration is present treatment should be instigated for early scarring instead of persistent erythema.

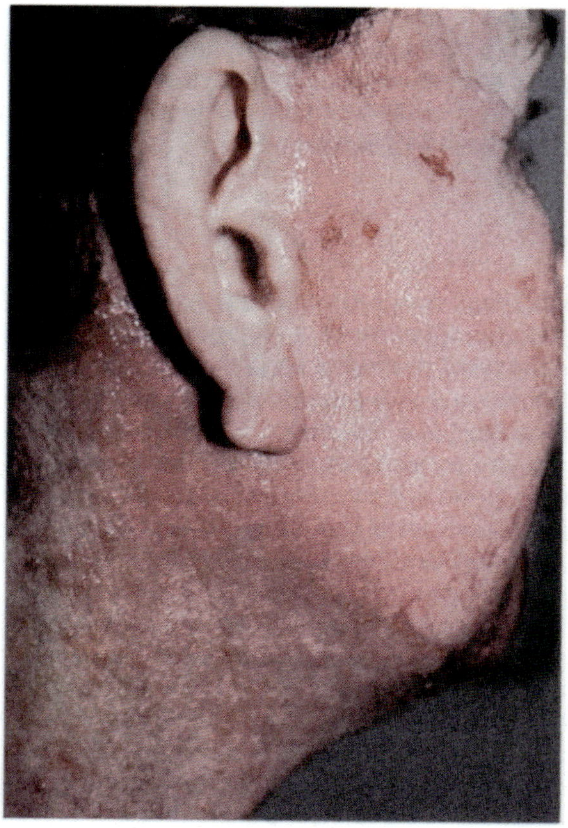

FIG. 8-15. Contact dermatitis resulting from Neosporin ointment, substituted by the patient.

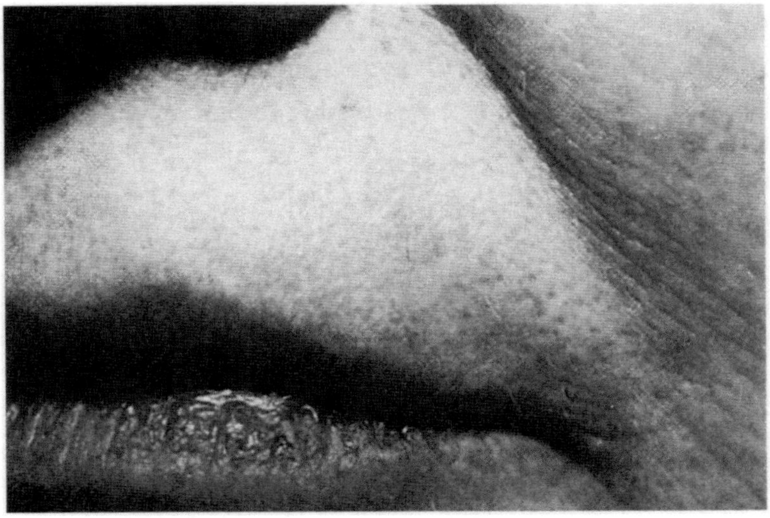

FIG. 8-16. Grainy, porous texture change after deep peeling.

Pruritus is a common occurrence after reepithelialization and typically persists for about 1 month. In addition to the aforementioned drugs, aspirin and propranolol in low doses will relieve some symptoms.[19] Pruritus occurring during the healing period can signal a **contact dermatitis** to the ointment used in wound care, especially when accompanied by slow healing, increased erythema, or follicular pustules on the neck or outside of the peel region (Fig. 8-15). In these cases, switching to Crisco vegetable shortening or petrolatum and administering 2 or 3 days of 40 mg oral prednisone can reset the healing course. Sensitivity to the fabric softener after washing a pillowcase can cause erythema and pruritus.

Textural Changes

Enlarged pores may result after peeling as a result of removal of the stratum corneum, but the appearance is temporary.[5] Pore size is not consistently changed by chemical peeling of any depth. Some patients may request chemical peeling of any depth for the treatment of enlarged follicles, and the result may be improved,[63] but the patient should understand that results may be unpredictable and enlargement may persist if repeeling is not performed. A diffuse, grainy, porous, peau d'orange texture can follow a chemical peel[19] (Fig. 8-16). We have seen this after 50% TCA, as well as phenol, but this change is not unique to these agents. It may be more noticeable in sebaceous patients. Temperature and wind sensitivity may occur.

If an agent is too weak to peel evenly below the defect, lacks the surfactant to provide an even depth of wounding, or has too high a surface tension, a texture change may be produced. Ideally, a wounding agent should penetrate just below the photodamage and produce no compromise in pigmentation. For example, solid CO_2 hard application, plus 35% TCA as a medium-depth agent, was unable to uniformly penetrate below severe actinically damaged perioral rhytides and produced an uneven texture that was corrected by repeeling with a deeper wounding agent (Fig. 8-17).

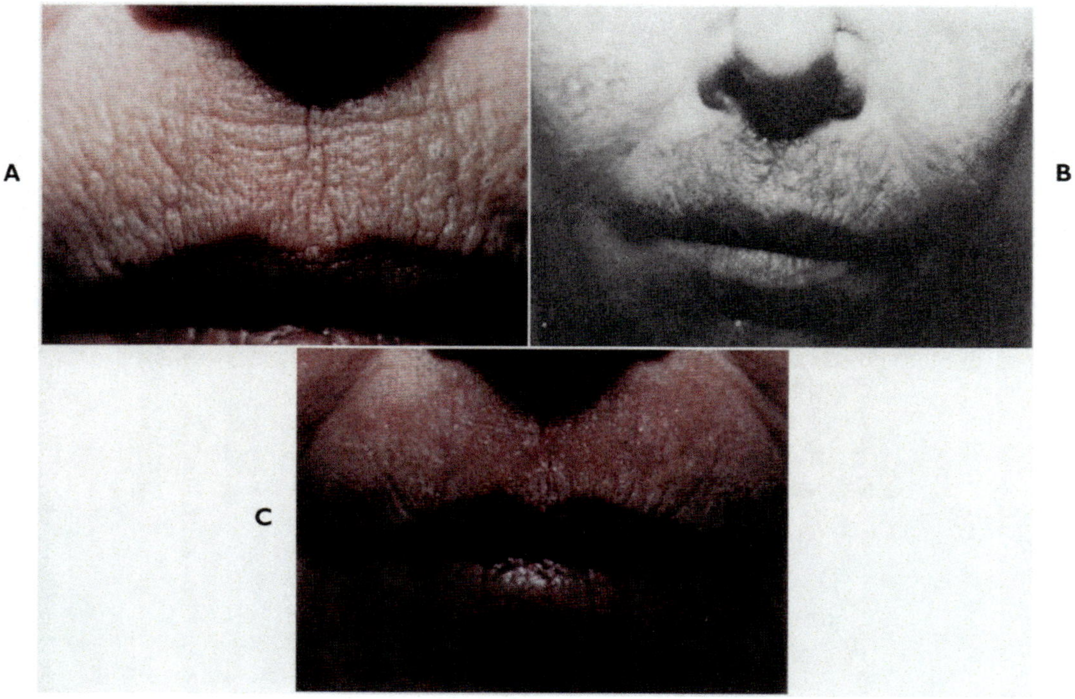

FIG. 8-17. A, Severe actinic and dynamic rhytides in Glogau photoaging group IV. **B,** Eight days after medium-depth CO_2 plus TCA, 35%, with an inability to penetrate defects. **C,** Irregular texture change 30 days after peeling.

Telangiectasia is not predictably altered by chemical peeling alone (Fig. 8-18). There may be an occasional patient who will complain of noticing them more after pigmentation has resolved from the peel. They may be more obvious after rhytidectomy in the undermined areas regardless of whether the patient has been peeled.

Milia

Milia, sometimes called inclusion cysts, appear as part of the healing process and are more common after dermabrasion than after chemical peeling (Fig. 8-19). They typically do not appear until 2 to 3 weeks after reepithelialization and may be aggravated by thick ointments that occlude the upper pilosebaceous units.[6] "Thicker-skinned" patients are said to be at greater risk,[19] but this has not been proved. In dermabrasion, saline scrubs immediately after surgery may minimize milia.[13]

After peeling, the use of gentle epidermabrasion (Buf-Puf, 3M, St. Paul, Minnesota) after reepithelialization or topical tretinoin both before and after peeling may decrease their occurrence.

Treatment with extraction by using a no. 11 scalpel blade or disposable lancet is effective, as is gentle electrodessication.[6] Spontaneous regression may occur.

Acne

The appearance of acne in the spectrum of pustular to cystic types during the healing process or immediately after reepithelialization is an alarming occurrence. It has been seen by the author in medium-depth peels using TCA alone

A

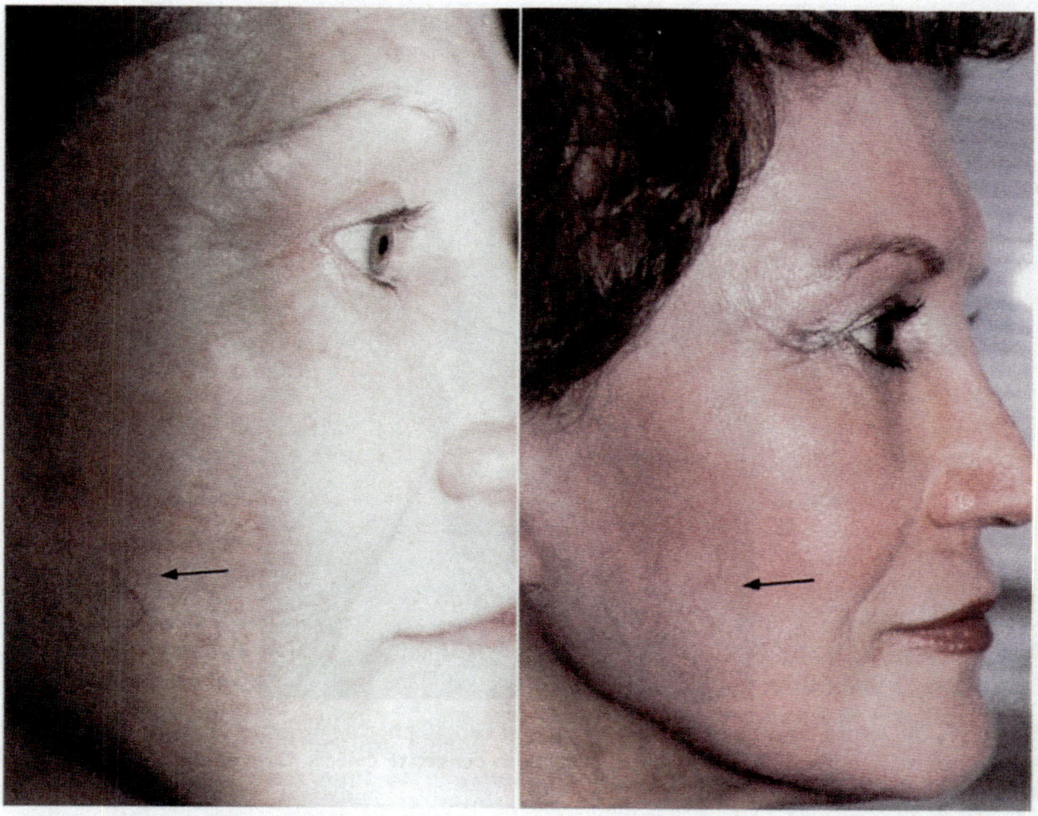

B

FIG. 8-18. Before **(A)** and after **(B)** pictures of a Baker's peel show no change in telangiectasia on the right cheek.

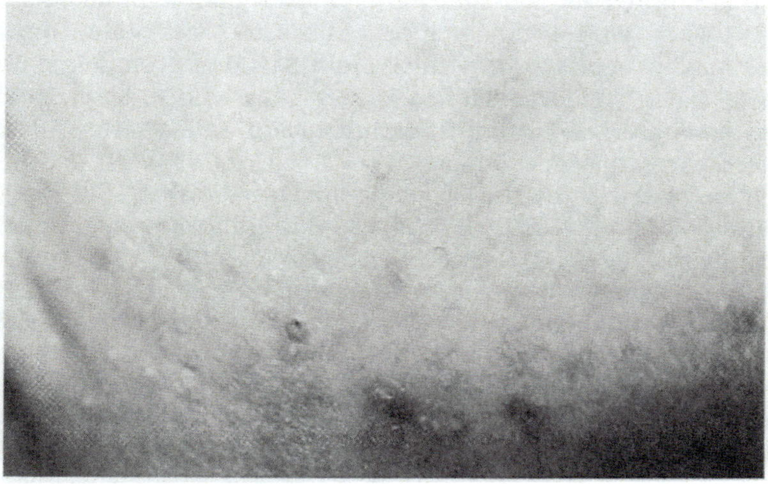

FIG. 8-19. Milia following deep chemical peeling.

or in combination with JS or CO_2. Its etiology may be multifactorial because a previous history of the disorder may not be present, and the lesions may produce scarring (Fig. 8-20). If the patient has only recently started to use tretinoin to pretreat the skin, the explosion of lesions anytime from day 3 through day 9 after peeling may be a temporary consequence of the drug, and the tretinoin should not be reinstituted immediately after healing. Overgreasing with irritant moisturizers or ointments during postoperative reepithelialization must be considered and discontinued.

The acneiform pustules must be distinguished from infection and aggressively treated. Culture and sensitivity should be obtained for bacteria and yeast, and the patient should be placed on treatment with topical and oral antibiotics for 5 days. For example, if oral cephalexin and ketoconazole have not been effective after this time and the cultures are negative, aggressive acne treatment in the form of tetracycline and topical antibiotics should be instituted. Intralesional triamcinolone acetonide 1 mg/ml and a rapidly tapering dose of prednisone for 1 week may be considered if cystic lesions are present to prevent scarring. The author has had two patients with no previous history of acne fail on this regimen and require treatment with low-dose isotretinoin (0.5 mg/kg per day) for 3 to 6 weeks to slow the progression of lesions and retard inevitable scarring. It is unlikely that any inhibition of the sebaceous apparatus would affect the wound-healing mechanisms when using a low dose for a short period of time in this setting, but the patient should be apprised of the potential risk.

Superficial peeling agents, glycolic acid or 15% TCA for example, are used for adjunctive acne vulgaris or acne rosacea therapy. When flaring of the disease occurs during the treatment, this is especially disconcerting. This different situation should not require the aggressive treatment detailed in this section.

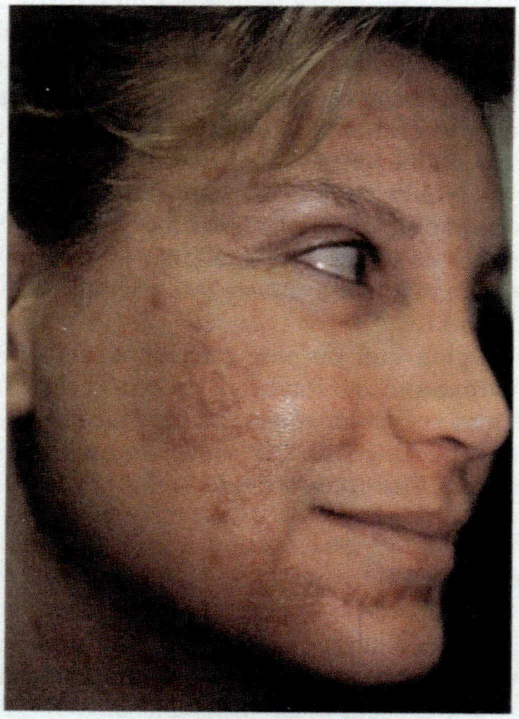

Fig. 8-20. Acne papules and pustules appearing 5 days after peeling with 35% TCA.

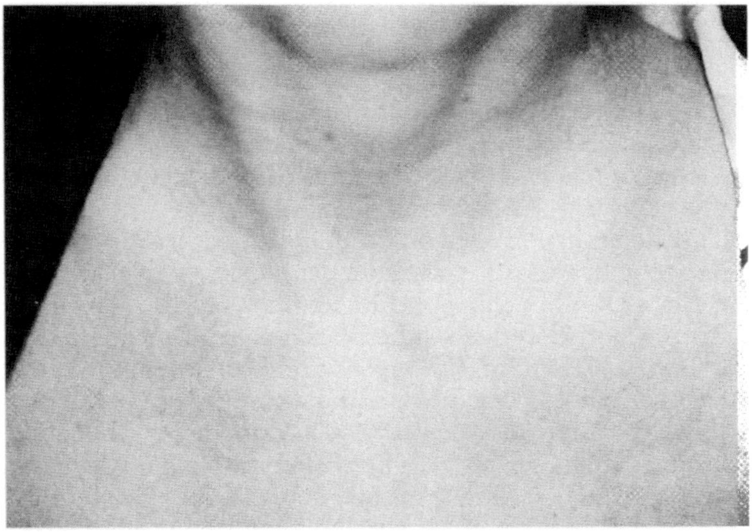

FIG. 8-21. Wheals distant from the peel site that were induced by solid CO_2 application.

Cold Sensitivity or Cold Urticaria

When using solid carbon dioxide (dry ice) to freeze the skin either alone or in combination with TCA in medium-depth peeling, transient swelling or urticaria can be produced in distant areas.[5] We have seen this in only 1 patient in whom the effect could be duplicated in a series of over 3000 patients (Fig. 8-21.) Because CO_2 has minimum temperature of only −78.5° C and because it is rarely concentrated in any one area for more than 20 seconds, it is limited in its ability to produce cold reactions. The freons, liquid nitrogen (−186° C), and prolonged cold immersion with water are more common precipitating factors.[64] The application of a 10-second liquid nitrogen spray to the entire face for acne scar treatment has resulted in full-thickness necrosis and scarring as a result of the presence of occult cryofibrinogenemia.[65] Increased serum levels of cryofibrinogens are found in about 4% of apparently normal individuals and may signal collagen-vascular disease, malignancy, pregnancy, oral contraceptive use, excessive smoking, or thromboembolic phenomena. Cryofibrinogenemia may be a transitory condition. This necrosis has not been reported with solid CO_2.

Transient stinging and burning sensations may occur during any freeze phase, and treatment to the forehead, especially if prolonged, may produce a headache that may persist for several hours. This responds to acetaminophen or ibuprofen. Facial freezing with CO_2, however, makes immediate application of TCA more tolerable. Reactions are rare, and cryopatch tests are unwarranted.

Poor Physician-Patient Relationship

Loss of confidence in the physician in the face of minor, manageable complications can result in a loss of follow-up and litigation. The physician-patient relationship is critical and must withstand any complication of the greatest gravity. Good preoperative counseling with thorough comprehension of the patient's desires by the physician and of the procedural risks by the patient is imperative. Patients must realize that they have priority during their recovery and can impose on office protocol at any time. Informed consent should be obtained. See the section on informed consent in Chapter 4

The average patient is not immune to the dismay of friends and neighbors as well as uninformed physicians during the postpeel period. Patients may be told that "something is wrong," "you aren't supposed to look like that," and "you're infected," with the insistence to see another physician. This physician in turn may not be aware of the entire spectrum of chemical peeling wounding agents or of the expected appearances in the ensuing weeks after peeling.

Patients with some psychiatric illnesses or untreated endogenous depression and patients who have unrealistic expectations should not be peeled or should have their primary disorders treated before peeling. Patients with major depressive disorders can exacerbate their diseases. The heighted excitement and trauma of the chemosurgery alone barring any unforeseen complications can aggravate or precipitate a mild tendency for depression. Being housebound for a week or more can be traumatic for some patients. Unrealistic expectations must be resolved before any cosmetic procedure. (See Fig. 4-14.)

COMPLICATIONS ARISING EXCLUSIVELY FROM DEEP PHENOL PEELS

Atrophy

Atrophy, or clinical loss of the normal skin markings in the absence of scarring, may occur after multiple deep peels with phenol but has not been observed after superficial or medium-depth peeling involving multiple applications of TCA. Atrophy may result also from applying a deep wounding agent on very thin, relatively non–sun-damaged skin. For example, using periorbital Baker's solution on a relatively non–sun-damaged 27-year-old produces almost transparent skin so that the muscle is seen when light is transmitted through the epidermis,[5] especially as chronologic aging proceeds (Fig. 8-22).

The examination of chemically peeled skin is not atrophic histologically. Brown and co-workers[66] in eyelid skin and Kligman and co-workers[9] in facial skin have shown that the epidermis usually returns to normal thickness, although it may be initially hyperplastic for more than 6 months after healing. The papillary dermis expands, and the dermis remains thickened even years after wounding. (See the section on middermal injury and deep wounding in Chapter 2.)

Cardiac Arrhythmias

Unlike phenol, TCA applied to the skin is neutralized by serum in the superficial dermal plexus and is nontoxic to internal body organs.[67] However, phenol and phenol formulas are cardiotoxic, and they can be hepatotoxic and nephrotoxic in high doses not encountered with proper chemical peeling. Seventy percent of phenol applied to the skin is absorbed within 30 minutes.[68] After absorption, 75% of phenol is either conjugated with glycuronic acid or sulfuric acid and excreted by the kidney, excreted unchanged by the kidney, or detoxified by oxidation in the liver to hydroquinone and pyrocatechin. The other 25% is metabolized to carbon dioxide and water.

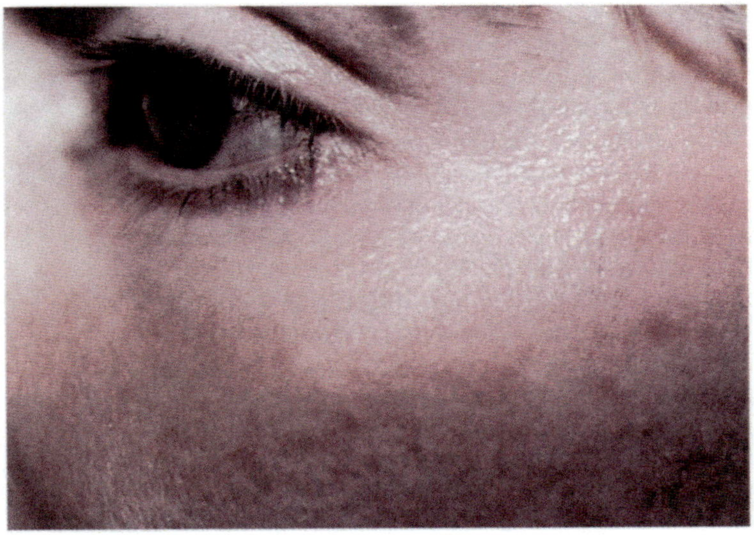

FIG. 8-22. Periorbital atrophy resulting from the application of Baker's solution to a relatively non–sun-damaged area for inappropriate dynamic changes.

Oral phenol poisoning by accidental ingestion has caused fulminant central nervous system depression, hepatorenal failure, and cardiorespiratory failure.[69] Industrial cutaneous exposure of phenol to large skin surface areas has caused hepatorenal toxicity. No hepatorenal or central nervous system problems have been reported in the literature with properly performed chemical peels. No reliable estimate of the mean lethal dose can be offered because of the wide variation in blood levels. There is a relative margin of safety between 0.68 mg/dl, the spectrophotometric blood level obtained on the entire facial application of 3 cc of a 50% solution of phenol, vs. 23 mg/dl measured in a man 15 minutes after ingestion who survived. It is not necessary to use more than 2 to 3 cc of phenol for each procedure.[70] Eight to 15 g is estimated to be the approximate toxic range. The extent of cutaneous absorption depends more on the total area of skin exposed than on the concentration of phenol. In humans, some evidence suggests that phenol may be less toxic by oral ingestion than by absorption from wounds, body cavities, or intact unbroken skin.[27,29,69]

Deaths attributed to phenol toxicity may have other causes. Stagnone and Stagnone[71] theorize that predisposed individuals may have idiosyncratic cardiac death from an adrenalin release resulting from facial pain transmitted from the trigeminal nerve to the cardiac vagal nerve or from the cerebral cortex directly to the cardiac sinoatrial node. This adrenal release could trigger a hypodynamic cardiac status or ventricular ectopic impulses.

Phenol is directly toxic to the myocardium. Studies in rats revealed slow electrical activity with an absence of myocardial contraction.[72] Phenol hypersensitivity may exist because fatal blood phenol levels varied widely in these studies, thus suggesting a wide variability in susceptibility to the cardiac effects of this agent.

In humans, cardiac arrhythmias have been associated with phenol application in full-face peeling. A survey revealed that 23% of phenol peel patients developed arrhythmias when 50% or more of the face was peeled in less than 30 minutes. However, no arrhythmias occurred when 50% or more of the face was peeled in 60 minutes. In patients deliberately peeled rapidly in 30 minutes' time, tachycardia was noted first, followed by premature ventricular contractions, bigeminy, paroxysmal atrial tachycardia, and ventricular tachycardia.[73] Atrial fibrillation has also been reported but was self-reversing after phenol serum clearance.[74] Of 588 plastic surgeons surveyed, 87% did not encounter any cardiac complications.[8] Neither sex, age, nor previous cardiac history were accurate predictors of cardiac arrhythmia susceptibility, and there was no relationship between serum phenol levels, the use of saponated or nonsaponated phenol, and arrhythmias.

Diuresis promotes metabolism and excretion of phenol and reduces arrhythmias. If minor supraventricular arrhythmias occur in spite of proper technique and pausing between cosmetic units to increase the time interval over which phenol is applied (see the section on application of phenol in Chapter 7), the application should be discontinued until normal sinus rhythm has returned for 15 minutes. The procedure may be resumed and the peel intervals extended for an additional 15 minutes.[75,76] If major ventricular arrhythmias occur, switching to 50% TCA may be prudent.

Holter monitor electrocardiographic (ECG) studies on 10 patients performed 24 hours before, during, and after Baker's phenol peels showed that there were many spontaneously occurring ventricular ectopic beats unrelated to the actual application of the chemical peel formula.[77] There was no correlation between a screening ECG and the Holter monitor tracings. In most patients there were more abnormalities in the preoperative data than in the intraoperative and postoperative data. Anxiety or exercise may have induced these changes. Sedation and relaxation during the procedure may have produced fewer ECG abnormalities during and after the procedure. Most ectopic beats occurred in the period after the completion of formula application, which suggests that the beats were random or spontaneous in nature or due to stress, anxiety, or unrecognized causes.

Spontaneously occurring arrhythmias in normal individuals are not uncommon. Infrequent ventricular ectopic beats occur in 25% of the normal population, with 10% showing supraventricular dysrhythmias and 5% showing varying arrhythmias.[78] Monitoring during the procedure and immediately thereafter allows the detection of possible cardiac complications, irrespective of cause.

As outlined in Chapter 7, the application of phenol to one cosmetic unit or less is equivalent to or less than the application of phenol into a nail matrix for chemical nail matrixectomy. Cardiac precautions and monitoring are not necessary for this, and oral hydration with 8 to 16 ounces of water can be given to the patient if the patient has not ingested an adequate amount of fluids on the day of the peel.

Resorcinol is chemically related to phenol. For specific complications of resorcinol peeling, see the discussion of resorcinol in Chapter 5.

Laryngeal Edema

Laryngeal edema associated with stridor, hoarseness, and tachypnea developed within 24 hours of phenol peeling in 3 of 245 women, approximately 1.2%.[79] All three women were heavy smokers, and their symptoms resolved within 48 hours with warm mist inhalation therapy. Antihistamines before peeling may have prevented this, but a previous history of urticaria was not known. Perhaps the cause was a hypersensitivity reaction to phenol or ether fumes in a larynx already chronically irritated by cigarette smoke.

Exacerbation of Concurrent Disease

A local pemphigus-like blister developed on the cheek of a 66-year-old woman 4 weeks after the second of two local phenol peels on the face within a 3-month interval.[80] Immunofluorescent-positive acantholytic lesions developed slowly months later on the body in the absence of oral lesions. These lesions responded to topical and intralesional steroids.

The physical trauma of the peel may have Koebnerized the disease, although she had no preexisting history. The isomorphic response of Koebner refers to the development of lesions in previously normal skin that has been traumatized. Patients with psoriasis, a much more common disease with an isomorphic response, have not been a problem during chemical peeling. This physically induced pemphigus-like response must be differentiated from delayed healing.

INHERENT ERRORS WITHIN THE PEEL PROCEDURE

In addition to the resultant complications in this chapter, inherent errors during the peel procedure may occur and can lead to complications. (See the box below.) With resorcinol combinations, TCA, or phenol formulas, errors in compounding or evaporation of the alcohol or water vehicle base can occur and inadvertently produce a stronger solution. Lactic acid and ethanol can both absorb water from moist air over time if unsealed (personal communication, Dermatologic Lab and Supply Inc., Council Bluffs, Iowa). Resorcinol and salicylic acid may sit on the pharmacy shelf for 10 to 15 years. Phenol solutions should be prepared fresh for each peel. Trichloroacetic acid solutions that are uncontaminated by cotton-tipped applicators are stable under natural office conditions for at least 6 months. (See the discussion of TCA and its preparation in Chapter 5 for details.) Jessner's solution might be prepared every 6 to 8 weeks, but this depends on the frequency of usage. It is best to pour all wounding agents into a 1-ounce glass cup to avoid touching applicators to the neck of a bottle that may contain evaporated crystals from solution (see Fig. 4-8).

The physician should take every precaution to avoid spilling a wounding agent on the patient, assistants, or himself or herself. Never hold an open container of the peeling agent, and never move the applicator or brush directly over the eye area. A syringe of saline or an eyewash bottle for dilution should be available for the eye if wounding agent is accidentally introduced (Fig. 8-23). Thirty-five percent TCA is not caustic enough to cause major corneal abrasions.[81] If phenol is spilled on the skin the most easily practiced decontamination procedure is to flood the area with propylene glycol or glycerol, the former being readily available. Polyethylene glycol, which is not readily available, is

Inherent Errors Leading to Complications

Incorrect wounding agent compounding or pharmacology
Accidental spillage of solution

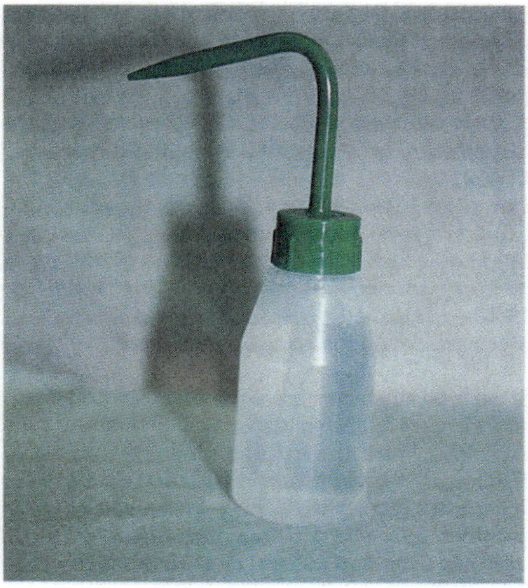

FIG. 8-23. Eyewash bottle for water irrigation if TCA or glycolic acid is accidentally introduced into the eye.

perhaps the best agent to decrease localized phenol entry and systemic intoxication through the skin. Olive oil, castor oil, and cottonseed oil may also reduce penetration.[18,19,69] Mineral oil in a dropper bottle should be available if phenol is placed into the eye inadvertently.

We live in a litigious society. This should not deter the dermatologic surgeon from performing chemical peels, but the risk-to-benefit ratio should be evaluated by both physician and patient. As long as this ratio can be weighed and balanced in the proper perspective, complications can be reduced to a minimum.

REFERENCES

1. Hendricks WM: The classificaton of burns, *J Am Acad Dermatol* 22(5, part 1):838-839, 1990.
2. Matarasso SL, Glogau RG: Chemical face peels, *Dermatol Clin* 9:131-150, 1991.
3. Swinehart JM: Test spots in dermabrasion and chemical peeling, *J Dermatol Surg Oncol* 16:557-563, 1990.
4. Pierce HE, Brown LA: Laminar dermal reticulotomy and chemical face peeling in the Black patient, *J Dermatol Surg Oncol* 12:69-73, 1986.
5. Brody HJ: Complications of chemical peeling, *J Dermatol Surg Oncol* 15:1010-1019, 1989.
6. Collins PS: The chemical peel, *Clin Dermatol* 5:57-74, 1987.
7. Spira M, Gerow FJ, Hardy SB: Complications of chemical face peeling, *Plast Reconstr Surg* 54:397-403, 1974.
8. Litton C, Trinidad G: Complications of chemical face peeling as evaluated by a questionnaire, *Plast Reconstr Surg* 67:738-744, 1981.

8a. Hetter GP: Facial peeling with different strengths of phenol and croton oil, *Am Soc Aesthetic Plast Surg*, p. 14, 1996 (abstract).

9. Kligman AM, Baker TJ, Gordon HL: Long-term histologic follow-up of phenol face peels, *Plast Reconstr Surg* 75:652-659, 1985.
10. Baker TJ, Gordon HL: Chemical peel with phenol. In Epstein E, Epstein E Jr, editors: *Skin surgery*, ed 6, Philadelphia, 1987, Saunders, pp. 423-438.
11. Rubin M: Symposium on AHAs, Orlando, Florida, December, 1994.
12. Kligman AM, Willis I: A new formula for depigmenting human skin, *Arch Dermatol* 111:40, 1975.
13. Stagnone JJ: Chemical peeling and chemabrasion. In Epstein E, Epstein E Jr, editors: *Skin surgery*, ed 6, Philadelphia, 1987, Saunders.
14. Brody HJ, Hailey CW: Medium-depth chemical peeling of the skin: a variation of superficial chemosurgery, *J Dermatol Surg Oncol* 12:1268-1275, 1986.

15. Humphreys TR, Werth V, Dzubow L, et al: Treatment of photodamaged skin with trichloroacetic acid and topical tretinoin, *J Am Acad Dermatol* 34:638-644, 1996.
16. Stegman SJ: Letter to the editor on chemical face peeling, *J Dermatol Surg Oncol* 12:432, 438, 1986 (letter).
17. Nemeth AJ: Keloids and hypertrophic scars, *J Dermatol Surg Oncol* 19:738-746, 1993.
18. Stegman SJ, Tromovitch TA: Chemical peeling. In *Cosmetic dermatologic surgery*, St Louis, 1984, Mosby, pp. 27-46.
19. Stegman SJ, Tromovitch TA, Glogau RG: Chemical peeling. In *Cosmetic dermatologic surgery*, ed 2, St Louis, 1990, Mosby, pp. 35-58.
20. Holzberg M, Hewan-Lowe K, Olansky A: The Ehlers-Danlos syndrome: recognition, characterization, and importance of a milder variant of the classic form, *J Am Acad Dermatol* 19:656-666, 1988.
21. Sperber PA: Chemexfoliation for aging skin and acne scarring, *Arch Otolaryngol* 81:278-283, 1965.
22. Ayres S III: Superficial chemosurgery, *Arch Dermatol* 89:395-403, 1964.
23. Ayres S: Dermal changes following application of chemical cauterants to aging skin, *Arch Dermatol* 82:578, 1960.
24. Monheit G: The Jessner's–trichloroacetic acid peel, *Dermatol Clin* 13(2):277-283, 1995.
25. Murray JC, Pollack SV, Pinnell SR: Keloids: a review, *J Am Acad Dermatol* 4:461-470, 1981.
26. Collins PS: Trichloroacetic acid peels revisited, *J Dermatol Surg Oncol* 15:933-940, 1989.
27. Litton C, Fournier P, Capinpin A: A survey of chemical peeling of the face, *Plast Reconstr Surg* 51:645-649, 1973.
28. Lober CW: Chemexfoliation—indications and cautions. *J Am Acad Dermatol* 17:109-112, 1987.
29. Litton C: Observations after chemosurgery of the face, *Plast Reconstr Surg* 32:554-556, 1963.
30. Dingman DL, Hartog J, Siemionow M: Simultaneous deep-plane face lift and trichloroacetic acid peel, *Plast Reconstr Surg* 93:86-93, 1994.
31. Baker TJ: Discussion on simultaneous deep-plane face lift and trichloroacetic acid peel, *Plast Reconstr Surg* 93:94-95, 1994.
32. Baker TJ, Gordon HL, Stuzin JM: Reply to letter to the editor on simultaneous deep-plane face lift and trichloroacetic acid peel, *Plast Reconstr Surg* 95:602, 1995.
33. Davies B, Guyuron B, Husami T: The role of lidocaine, epinephrine, and flap elevation in wound healing after chemical peel, *Ann Plast Surg* 26:273-278, 1991.
34. Litton C, Trinidad G: Chemosurgery of the eyelids. In Aston ST, et al, editors: *Third International Symposium of Plastic and Reconstructive Surgery*, Baltimore, 1982, Williams & Wilkins, pp. 341-345.
35. Wojno T, Tenzel R: Lower eyelid ectropion following chemical face peeling, *Ophthalmic Surg* 15:596-597, 1984.
36. Rubenstein R, Roenigk HH, Stegman SJ, et al: Atypical keloids after dermabrasion of patients taking isotretinoin. *J Am Acad Dermatol* 15:280-285, 1986.
37. Roenigk HH, Pinski JB, Robinson JK, et al: Acne, retinoids, and dermabrasion, *J Dermatol Surg Oncol* 11:396-398, 1985.
38. Dzubow LM, Miller WH: The effect of 13-*cis*-retinoic acid on wound healing in dogs, *J Dermatol Surg Oncol* 13:265-268, 1987.
39. Moy RL, Moy LS, Bennett RG, et al: Systemic isotretinoin: effects on dermal wound healing in a rabbit ear model in vivo, *J Dermatol Surg Oncol* 16:1142-1146, 1990.
40. Alt TH: Avoiding complications in dermabrasion and chemical peel, *Skin Allergy News* 21:2, 1990.
41. Brody HJ: Update on chemical peeling, *Adv Dermatol* 7:275-289, 1992.
42. Szachowicz EH, Wright WK: Delayed healing after full-face chemical peels, *Facial Plast Surg* 6:1:8-13, 1989.
43. Glogau RG: Delayed healing. Chemical Peel Symposium, American Academy of Dermatology, 1992.
44. Siegle RJ, Chiaramonti A, Knox DW, et al: Cutaneous candidosis as a complication of facial dermabrasion, *J Dermatol Surg Oncol* 10:891-894, 1984.
45. Giandoni MB, Grabski WJ: Cutaneous candidiasis as a cause of delayed surgical wound healing, *J Am Acad Dermatol* 30:981-984, 1994.
46. Aalto-Korte K: Improvement to skin barrier function during treatment of atopic dermatitis, *J Am Acad Dermatol* 33:969-972, 1995.
47. Ghadially R, Halkier-Sorensen L, Elias PM: Effects of petrolatum on stratum corneum structure and function, *J Am Acad Dermatol* 26:387-396, 1992.
48. Perez IR: Vegetarians may heal more slowly after chemical face peels. American Academy of Cosmetic Surgery, Los Angeles, Calif, Feb 1995.

49. Asken S: Unoccluded Baker/Gordon phenol peels: review and update, *J Dermatol Surg Oncol* 15:998-1008, 1989.
50. Mercer NSG: Silicone gel in the treatment of keloid scars, *Br J Plast Surg* 42:83-87, 1989.
51. Gold MH: A controlled clinical trial of topical silicone gel sheeting in the treatment of hypertrophic scars and keloids, *J Am Acad Dermatol* 30:506-507, 1994.
52. Katz BE: Silicone gel sheeting in scar therapy, *Cutis* 56:65-67, 1995.
53. Goldman MP, Fitzpatrick RE: Laser treatment of scars, *Dermatol Surg* 21:685-687, 1995.
54. Alster TS: Improvement of erythematous and hypertrophic scars by the 585-nm flashlamp-pumped pulsed dye laser, *Ann Plast Surg* 31:1-5, 1993.
55. Alster TS, Kurban AK, Grove GL, et al: Alteration of argon laser-induced scars by the pulsed dye laser, *Lasers Surg Med* 13:368-373, 1993.
56. Bundy AT: Sterility in unsterilized surgical adhesive tape, *Plast Reconstr Surg* 83:880, 1989.
57. Milner SM: Acetic acid to treat *Pseudomonas aeruginosa* in superficial wounds and burns, *Lancet* 340:61, 1992 (letter).
58. Dmytryshyn JR: Chemical face peel complicated by toxic shock syndrome, *Arch Otolaryngol* 109:170, 1983.
59. LoVerme WE, Drapkin MS, Courtiss EH, et al: Toxic shock syndrome after chemical face peel, *Plast Reconstr Surg* 80:115-118, 1987.
60. Rapaport MJ, Kamer F: Exacerbation of facial herpes simplex after phenolic face peels, *J Dermatol Surg Oncol* 10:57-58, 1984.
61. Pflugfelder SC, Huang A, Crouse C: Epstein-Barr virus keratitis after a chemical face peel, *Am J Ophthalmol* 110:571-573, 1990.
62. Fitzpatrick RE, Goldman MP, Satur NM, et al: Pulsed carbon dioxide laser resurfacing of photoaged facial skin, *Arch Dermatol* 132:395-402, 1996.
63. Alt TH: Occluded Baker/Gordon chemical peel: review and update, *J Dermatol Surg Oncol* 15:980-993, 1989.
64. Dowd PM: Cold related disorders, *Prog Dermatol* 21:1-7, 1987.
65. Stewart RH, Graham GF: A complication of cryosurgery in a patient with cryofibrinogenemia, *J Dermatol Surg Oncol* 4:743-744, 1978.
66. Brown AM, Kaplan LM, Brown ME: Phenol induced histological skin changes: hazards, techniques, and uses, *Br J Plast Surg* 13:158-169, 1960.
67. Ayres S: Superficial chemosurgery in treating aging skin, *Arch Dermatol* 85:125-133, 1962.
68. Wexler MR, Halon DA, Teitelbaum A, et al: The prevention of cardiac arrhythmias produced in an animal model by the topical application of a phenol preparation in common use for face peeling, *Plast Reconstr Surg* 73:595-598, 1984.
69. Gleason MD, Gosselin RF, Hodge HC, et al: Clinical toxicology of commercial products, Baltimore, 1969, Williams & Wilkins, pp. 189-192.
70. Litton C: Chemical face lifting, *Plast Reconstr Surg* 29:371-380, 1962.
71. Stagnone JJ, Stagnone GJ: A second look at chemabrasion, *J Dermatol Surg Oncol* 8:701-705, 1982.
72. Stagnone GJ, Orgel MB, Stagnone JJ: Cardiovascular effects of topical 50% trichloroacetic acid and Baker's phenol solution, *J Dermatol Surg Oncol* 13:999-1002, 1987.
73. Truppman F, Ellenbery J: The major electrocardiographic changes during chemical face peeling, *Plast Reconstr Surg* 63:44, 1979.
74. Gross D: Cardiac arrhythmia during phenol face peeling, *Plast Reconstr Surg* 73:590-594, 1984.
75. Beeson WH: The importance of cardiac monitoring in superficial and deep chemical peeling, *J Dermatol Surg Oncol* 13:949-950, 1987.
76. McCollough EG, Langston PR: *Dermabrasion and chemical peel: a guide for facial plastic surgery*, New York, 1988, Thieme Medical, pp. 53-112.
77. Price NM: EKG changes in relationship to the chemical peel, *J Dermatol Oncol* 16:37-42, 1990.
78. DeMaria AN, Amsterdam EA, Vismara LA, et al: Arrhythmias in the mitral valve prolapse syndrome: prevalence, nature, and frequency, *Ann Intern Med* 84:656, 1976.
79. Klein DR, Little JH: Laryngeal edema as a complication of chemical peel, *Plast Reconstr Surg* 71:419-420, 1983.
80. Detwiler SP, Saperstein HW: Physically induced pemphigus after cosmetic procedures, *Int J Dermatol* 32:100-103, 1993.
81. Morrow DM: Chemical peeling of eyelids and periorbital area, *J Dermatol Surg Oncol* 18:102-110, 1992.

9 Ethics in Chemical Peeling

A renaissance in chemical peeling occurred in dermatologic surgery in the late 1980s. This rebirth, initiated by the scientific investigations of the early 1980s, provided the hope that the less scientific and less reproducible results of the previous decades would be overshadowed by the honing of new techniques and wounding agents. The skills and basic knowledge of chemical peeling are part of the core curriculum for dermatologic surgery in residency programs and are taught in courses for dermatologic surgeons endorsed by the American Society for Dermatologic Surgery and the American Academy of Dermatology.[1] By the sharing of knowledge in medicine through the medical literature, the essence of the science in medicine is disseminated and subject to the criticism so essential to legitimizing the health of the public. Without the process of critical peer evaluation before publishing, we cannot accept the forceful impetus of the media bursting the newly published results of medical journals onto press and television barely before the mail in our offices is opened.

In the 1990s we have seen glamorization, sanctification, and unyielding praise of superficial peels by the television and print media. They have been portrayed as treatments that could be painlessly applied as a lunchtime process allowing immediate return to work with no "downtime" and with the production of younger and clearer skin. Glycolic acid at low to moderate concentrations is generally not dangerous and should be downgraded in its status as a miracle treatment modality until adequate comparative studies with the other long-proven superficial and medium-depth wounding agents are performed and until more relative predictability is secured.[2] Media attention has been instrumental in obscuring the fact that multiple superficial epidermal peels do not yield the same result as a single dermal peel. No one has demonstrated that the "induction of new collagen" in the upper papillary dermis will produce the histologic or clinical improvement from significant dermal cross-linked collagen rearrangement routinely achieved with TCA combinations or phenol. The sensationalism by the media before comparison studies have been performed is an injustice to the public. Many of the pseudoscientific touters of the benefits of the minipeels have no clinical experience with other parts of the chemical peel spectrum.

The employment of an aesthetician to apply superficial peeling agents in concert with dermatologists or other cosmetic physicians and surgeons has aroused some ethical controversy. The definition of peeling itself has been adulterated by those aestheticians and facial technicians performing dead skin "washes." The value of these exfoliants has been swollen to proportions that not only fail human understanding, but in addition the treatments and technicians have been accessed by the cosmetic physician directly or indirectly into his or her office to promote topical sales regimens and cosmetics. How ethical is a physician-supervised aesthetician when she or he is applying pumice and astringents, massaging, and repeatedly rubbing and "stimulating" the skin? In improving skin "quality, texture, feel, or look," subjectivity reigns supreme. What looks better in the qualitative eye of the beholder may be invisible to the scientific eye that quantitates coarse wrinkle lines, measures pigmentation with a melasma area and severity index (MASI) or colorimetry, or enumerates comedones. An aesthetician promoting treatment for acne and pigmentation without dermatologic sponsorship can prolong the time interval before established medical and acne-surgical treatment is initiated. This delay can be reflected by patient scarring and monetary waste. As long as the techniques are supervised by the physician and are grounded in scientific knowledge the liaison can be helpful for the patient. If not, the liaison can be more fruitful for the technicians and retailers.[2]

The marketing of the α-hydroxy acids in peeling has also led to the ethical issues of promoting cosmetics and "cosmeceuticals" through physicians' offices in concert with chemical peels. Assuming the doctor is honest, the sales of drugs in the physician's office could constitute a service to patients. Putting a physician's name on a bottle of cosmetic uncertainty, however, is perceived to be within the ethical bounds of some physicians and outside the boundaries of practice by the others' standards. This prostitutional promotion of non-drugs has ignited some cross fire between salon aestheticians and physicians or their paramedical aestheticians. How ethical is the office of a physician that resembles the cosmetics counter of a department store with the high-sell pressure to match?

Cosmeceutical is a term that has no standing in U.S. regulatory law. The term was coined by Dr. Albert Kligman to connote a cosmetic product that exerts a pharmaceutical therapeutic benefit but not necessarily a biologic therapeutic benefit, classifying it as a drug.[3,4] Such products fall outside the regulations of the existing classifications. The classification of a product depends on the claims that a manufacturer or distributor makes for a product to reflect its intended uses. A suntan preparation is classed as a cosmetic, but a sunscreen to prevent sunburn with a specific sun protection factor (SPF) that blocks ultraviolet radiation is subject to regulation as an over-the-counter drug. The α-hydroxy acids exemplify the dilemma based on concentration in a product. Lower strengths have been present in cosmetics for years. Higher concentrations are classified as drugs.

The resurfacing trends of the late 1990s are a reflection of the introduction of the new resurfacing CO_2 laser. The technical ease of this modality has led to premature advertising and promotion both by laser companies and by physicians. Biased and unscientific claims accompanied by puffery in the legal sense make inadequate or nonexistent comparisons with chemical peeling and dermabrasion. There is a lack of long-term follow-up and a lack of adequate comparative data with all techniques. The next decade will elucidate the advantages and disadvantages of all resurfacing techniques.

The field of chemexfoliation for the celebrated cause of rejuvenation is becoming the breeding ground for the sycophant physician as well as nonphysician. Some of these individuals feed the media with the assistance of public relations firms deceiving the public with claims of nonsurgical face-lifts, miraculous before-and-after pictures, claims of peeling all skin types with impunity, claims of being exclusive in their ability to peel nonfacial skin, and miracle self-invented restorative regimens before peeling, sometimes claimed to be the invention of the trademarked procedure itself. The utter disgrace of the debacle is when the individual is himself or herself a dermatologist. Under the guise of better health care or better appearance for the public, some of these individuals may attract the consumer by an attractive brochure, a free party with refreshments, or a reward for bringing in new prospective customers. They may attract physicians as franchised dealers by offering lucrative contracts and figures to nondermatologists who may not be financially successful in their own eyes, especially because cosmetic surgery is no longer tax deductible, or by promulgating uniqueness in the form of secret formulas, scientifically unproven peel additives, or miracle results. The physicians who pay to subscribe or succumb to these schemes may be equally as guilty as the originators.

When we examine the truth of the matter, **chemical peeling is a surgical procedure**. Invasion of the skin by a chemical is no less invasive than by cold steel, liquid nitrogen cryosurgery, or the laser. Implications that the procedure is a "face-lift" connote a misunderstanding of the surgical correction of the effects of gravity vs. the improvement of skin quality ravaged by actinic radiation and age. This is the public's misconception. The before-and-after pictures are invalid when edema is still present in the after pictures or when the dark-skinned pigmentation is seemingly improved because of inadequate photography or makeup. Dermatologic chemical peeling has always been able to peel the darker skin types and nonfacial areas such as the hands or chest, with greater risk of complications.[5-7] Most galling is the promotion and sale to the nondermatologist of skin bleaches such as hydroquinone and "miracle creams" such as tretinoin under the umbrella of the promoter as his own inventions. These agents have been used by the dermatologist since the seventies and incorporated in chemical peeling regimens since the early eighties.[8-10]

In the mid-1980s, the American Academy of Dermatology filed a complaint with the Federal Trade Commission against the peeling procedure exodermology-endodermology, a phenol peel franchise using a fictitious, meaningless name that misappropriated the name recognition of our specialty to deceive the public. (See the section on proprietary peels in Chapter 10.) Congressional hearings on cosmetic surgery chaired by Congressman Wyden in 1989 began the task of demonstrating the inability of the public and medicine to protect itself when confronted with an environment of duplicity and untruths. Two deaths and two cases of permanently impaired vision have emerged from this procedure, which was founded by a layman and was taught sometimes by unlicensed physicians. Physicians of any specialty were taught improper peeling techniques for the sum of $50,000. This sum included marketing techniques and insistence on secrecy of the mechanism of the procedure because any procedure that is shrouded in the mystique of secrecy is somehow more appealing—not only to the consumer but also to the uninformed physician-operator. Alarmingly, some of these ill-trained physicians still advertise and promote these techniques.

And what is the real cost of these marketing schemes in the hands of uninformed physicians who do not understand or take the trouble to research the spectrum of already existing peels that provide excellent cosmetic correction?[11-13] Complications and more complications in the form of scarring and irreversible pigmentary anomalies amplified by brochures that minimize risks and paint rosy portraits of peeling as "safe, nonsurgical face-lifts." The lawyers, who through depositions provide us with the actual knowledge of the logistics of some of these peel operations and who also enlist scientific knowledge to show the illegitimacy of the schemes, are the real beneficiaries.

Representatives of the American Academy of Dermatology, the American Society for Dermatologic Surgery, the American Society of Plastic and Reconstructive Surgeons, the American Academy of Facial Plastic and Reconstructive Surgery, the American Academy of Otolaryngology–Head and Neck Surgery, the American Medical Association, and the Federal Trade Commission met to solidify guidelines for truthful advertising of physician services. Physician advertising with respect to false, misleading, and deceptive statements in peeling are addressed. Substantiation of claims must be supported by, for example, publication in a peer-reviewed medical journal. Puffery or the tenor of an ad accompanied by the exaggeration of ordinary commercial advertising for household products may be deceptive in a medical context. Appeals to emotional vulnerabilities may reach the anxieties, fears, and hopes of patients. Pictures can be misleading and may not reflect the true degree of recovery after peeling. Patient testimonials and endorsements may not reflect the average patient experience, especially with respect to comfort, ease, or pain. Adverse effects must be addressed. Physician qualifications and training must be presented or available.[14]

These guidelines are almost completed but have been delayed because of controversy within the surgical specialties regarding the advertising of board certification. Will they enable us to prevent a return to the nonscientific methodology of the fifties? Will they be enforceable?

If statements made in advertising are misleading or deceptive, they may be used as evidence to prove a lack of informed consent. In addition to oral communications and signed consent forms, information in advertising or endorsements provides additional evidence for lack of patient information for consent.[15] Informed consent may be advised for prescribing medications for off-labeled use. However, if the medicine is used for treatment rather than research, "innovative therapy" appears to be within the physician's ethical and legal prerogative supported by the FDA.[16]

At the present time, grounds for disciplinary action by many state medical boards include false, deceptive, or misleading advertising; paying or receiving any commissions for patients referred to providers of certain health care goods; making untrue or fraudulent representations in the practice of medicine; and soliciting patients through the use of fraud, undue influence, or a form of overreaching.[17] Secret formulas or formulas of unspecified composition are not suitable for publishing in reputable medical journals. The American College of Physicians states in its ethical guidelines that "secret remedies" are not allowed by its members; this alludes to the historical development of medical education and appropriate patient care.[18] Because physicians have an ethical obligation to share medical advances, it is unlikely that a physician will have a truly exclusive technique. Claims that imply such a skill can therefore be deceptive. Advertisements that claim unique skills must be true and capable of substantiation, according to the Ethics Guidelines of the American Society for Dermatologic Surgery and the American Academy of Dermatology.[19] The intentional withholding of new medical knowledge, skills, and techniques from colleagues for reasons of personal gain is detrimental both to the medical profession and to society and is to be condemned.[20] Efforts to prohibit patents on medical procedures and therefore on medical chemical peeling techniques are in evolution within organized medicine and in Congress.[21,22]

The original techniques of superficial and medium-depth peeling in dermatologic surgery are now being recognized and used by other specialties for the safety and beauty that the procedures provide. This sharing of knowledge through the legitimate peer-reviewed literature has also been the backbone of the growth of dermatologic surgery as we know it today. We perform flaps, grafts, and other procedures pioneered by different specialties but refined and simplified to suit our own specialty. We pioneered treatments of venereal disease, infectious disease, and connective tissue disease, but we now share them with other medical specialties. This is well and good, as long as the information is obtained scientifically and legitimately. When information is propelled by the media and disseminated like the plague to other specialties and the public without the benefit of criticism in medical forums and when legitimate physicians in other specialties embrace this "knowledge" in ignorance, the loss is shared by everyone. In the face of deceptive advertising in media-sparked publicity campaigns performed in the interest of financial remuneration, the real challenge of our professionalism emerges now as we convince our patients that dermatologic surgeons are among the original experts in chemical peeling.[23]

When the lion fawns upon the lamb,
The lamb will never cease to follow him.

SHAKESPEARE: *HENRY VI*, PART III, ACT 4, SCENE 8

REFERENCES

1. Hanke CW: *Fundamentals of dermatologic surgery for the dermatology resident,* Evanston, Ill, 1992, Association of Academic Dermatologic Surgeons, Dermatology Services.
2. Brody HJ : Current advances and trends in chemical peeling, *J Dermatol Surg Oncol* 21:385-387, 1995.
3. McNamara SH: "Cosmeceutical," *Cosmet Dermatol* 7(3): 28-29, 1994.
4. Terezakis N: Cosmeceuticals: a new breed of cosmetic products, *Cosmet Dermatol* 6(4):40-41, 1993.
5. Pierce HE, Brown LA: Laminar dermal reticulotomy and chemical face peeling in the Black patient, *J Dermatol Surg Oncol* 12:69-73, 1986.
6. Collins PS, Farber GA, Wilhelmus SM, et al: Superficial repetitive chemosurgery of the hands, *Am J Cosmet Surg* 1:22-24, 1984.
7. Lotter AM: Human pigment factors relative to chemical face peeling, *Ann Plast Surg* 3:3, 1979.
8. Kligman AM, Willis I: A new formula for depigmenting human skin, *Arch Dermatol* 111:40-48, 1975.
9. Stagnone JJ: Chemical peeling and chemabrasion. In Epstein E, Epstein E Jr, editors: *Skin surgery,* Philadelphia, 1987, Saunders, pp. 412-422.
10. Brody HJ, Hailey CW: Medium-depth chemical peeling of the skin: a variation of superficial chemosurgery, *J Dermatol Surg Oncol* 12:1268-1275, 1986.
11. Stagnone JJ: Superficial peeling, *J Dermatol Surg Oncol* 15:924-930, 1989.
12. Brody HJ, editor: Special issue on chemical peeling, *J Dermatol Surg Oncol* 15:912-1024, 1989.
13. Brody HJ, Alt TH: Chemical peeling. In Coleman WP, Hanke CW, Alt TH, et al, editors: *Cosmetic surgery of the skin: principles and techniques,* Philadelphia, 1991, Decker, pp. 65-88.
14. *Guidelines for truthful advertising of physician services,* draft prepared by the Office of the General Counsel of the American Medical Association, Chicago, Ill, 1995.
15. Hirsh BD: The ethical and legal status involving informed consent, *Cosmet Dermatol* 7(8):25-30, 1994.
16. Torres A: The use of Food and Drug Administration–approved medications for unlabeled uses, *Arch Dermatol* 130:32-36, 1994.
17. Department of Health, State of Florida Statutes, Chapter 458, Medical Practice.
18. Greenway HT: Commentary, *Adv Dermatol* 7:275-289, 1992.
19. *Ethics in medical practice with special reference to dermatologic surgery,* Schaumburg, Ill, 1994, American Society for Dermatologic Surgery.
20. *Current Opinions. The Council on Ethical and Judicial Affairs of the American Medical Association, including principles of medical ethics,* articles 5.02 and 9.08, Chicago, 1992, AMA Publications.
21. Groups move to bar patents on medical procedures, *Skin Allergy News* 26:23, 1995.
22. Morain WD: Patently unethical, *Ann Plast Surg* 36:334, 1996.
23. Brody HJ: Ethics in chemical peeling, *J Dermatol Surg Oncol* 17:620-621, 1991.

10 Peel Combinations and Other Peels

Some physical processes such as dermabrasion, dermasanding, or the CO_2 laser can be legitimately combined with peeling and performed simultaneously. Some peeling procedures have not been demonstrated to be superior to existing procedures presented in the preceding chapters or have not been subjected to peer review. This is not to say that some of the procedures are not capable of producing an effective chemical peel.

Other peels have been marketed in an unprofessional and proprietary fashion and do not, therefore, have the credence that accompanies those shared within the medical community. Some of the details herein have been obtained by reviewing depositions of lawsuits that forced some physician-operators to reveal details. For the sake of completeness, this information is for the cosmetic surgeon who is confronted with the need for additional knowledge of other procedures within the broadest definition of chemical peeling.

COMBINING CHEMICAL PEEL AND DERMABRASION ON THE SAME AREA

The performance of a Baker's phenol chemical peel immediately followed by dermabrasion has been reported as an alternative to taping a chemical peel.[1,2] Originally, results were thought to be more sustaining for the removal of acne scarring and for fine rhytides. Phenol provided its own topical anesthesia, depth control was reportedly more precise, and tape removal was obviated. Histology was similar to comparable deep chemical peeling. Claims have been made that the procedure is superior to either procedure alone.

Spira[3] described the treatment of acne pitting and scarring by performing a phenol peel followed by dermoplaning the scarred areas with a dermatome as a split-skin graft. Occlusion of the peeled, surrounding, unscarred skin to overlap the dermoplaned and chemopeeled areas would avoid lines of demarcation and blend color changes. Scarring was reported where the two procedures overlapped.[4]

Lusthaus and co-workers[5] utilize the same concept by using sterile and disposable diathermy head cleaner sandpaper (Surgikos, Inc.) after performing a phenol peel. The device is composed of three different layers with two external faces and a third one interposed between them. One external face is sandpaper and the opposite face has an adhesive film to secure the device to the surgeon's finger. Rotary motions to desired depth may improve selected scarring or rhytides.

Stagnone[6,7] coined the term **chemabrasion** to combine rapid application of trichloroacetic acid (TCA), 50%, to the entire face of a heavily sedated patient followed by dermabrasion with light topical cryoanesthesia. The dermabrasion is more rapid because it is easier to abrade coagulated tissue, and better visualization is afforded by the whitening and lack of hemorrhage resulting from the cauterizing effect of the acid.

All of these procedures require extra time, usually additional sedation, and expertise for dermabrasion or skin sign recognition after sanding. They are legitimate procedures and efficacious. No one has shown long-term results in prophylaxis of actinic damage in these combination procedures as compared with either peel or dermabrasion alone. None of the combination procedures used for actinic damage or scarring have been demonstrated to be superior to the peel or the dermabrasion procedure performed alone when the proper indication has been selected.

COMBINING CHEMICAL PEEL AND DERMABRASION ON DIFFERENT AREAS

Combining chemical peel and dermabrasion on different areas is appealing because patients are afforded the advantage of experiencing deeper local resurfacing techniques such as dermabrasion only where it is required.[8] Many patients have minimal photodamage outside of the perioral area, and dermabrasion is an alternative here to deep peeling. In patients who are very sun damaged in one cosmetic unit or less and are fair skinned this may offer little advantage over using unoccluded Baker's phenol in this area. Hypopigmentation may occur with either procedure and may be cosmetically acceptable.

This should not be confused with the concept of simultaneous peel followed by dermabrasion on the same area. Dermabrasion may cause deeper injury than medium-depth chemical peels. It is more effective in treating upper lip rhytides or localized acne scarring. Use of tumescent anesthetic techniques decreases bleeding and allows good visualization of the depth of abrasion, especially for scarring.[9] Chemical peeling is an excellent method to blend the areas between dermabraded and nondermabraded skin. It may be easier to perform the peel first and the dermabrasion second, but the two techniques may be performed in either sequential order as long as care is taken not to apply peel solution to dermabraded areas. Chemical peeling is useful also to blend areas in partial dermabrasions after punch grafting or repeat localized dermabrasion (Fig. 10-1).

COMBINING CHEMICAL PEELING WITH MANUAL DERMASANDING

Combining chemical peeling with manual dermasanding has been described for elimination of 70% to 90% of fine to moderately deep rhytides in a series of over 300 patients.[10] Silicone carbide wet-or-dry sandpaper from fine to coarse grades is cut into 2 × 3–cm pieces and autoclaved. After acetone or alcohol scrub, the patient is sedated with oral diazepam and intramuscular meperidine. Lidocaine nerve blocks or EMLA (Astra, Inc., Westborough, Massachusetts) can be used for local anesthesia. After gentian violet marking, rhytides are manually sanded by wrapping the sandpaper around a cone of 2 × 2 gauze pads and wetting the sandpaper-gauze roll (Fig. 10-2). While the area is stretched, the skin is gently abraded back and forth or in a circular motion until glistening and fine bleeding points are reached within 30 to 45 seconds. More actinically damaged skin requires coarser grades of sandpaper. After abrading, iced compresses are

A 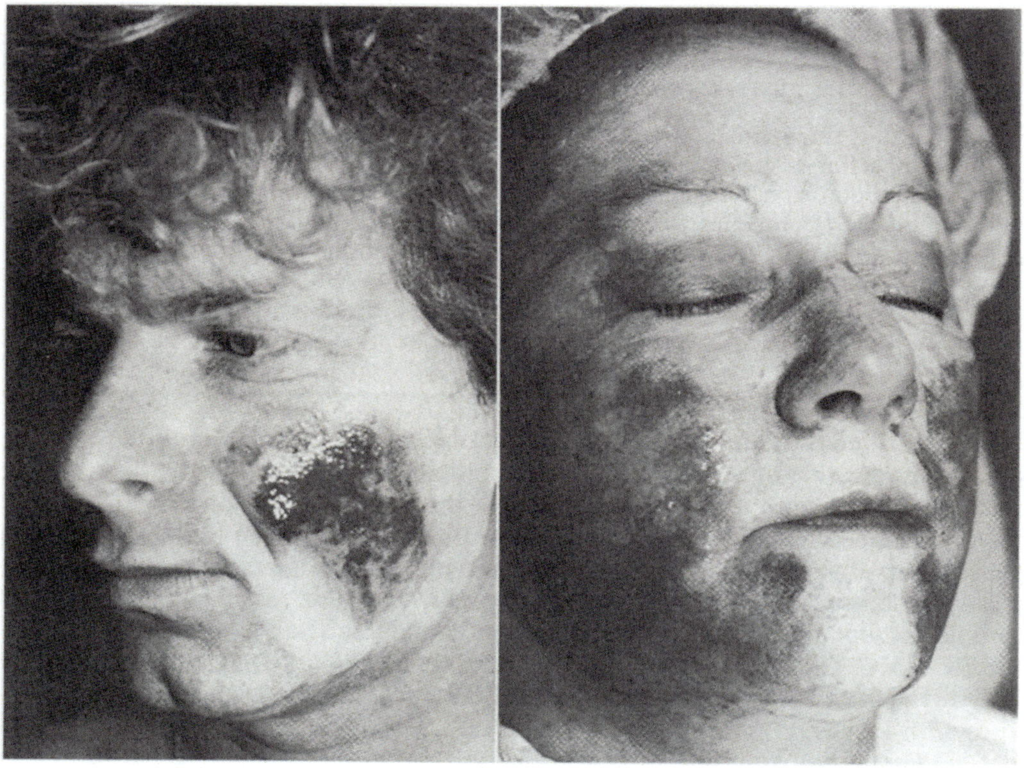 B

FIG. 10-1. Medium-depth peeling with CO_2 plus TCA or Jessner's solution plus TCA will blend areas of partial dermabrasion used to treat scarring or photodamage.

applied for about 5 minutes for hemostasis. Twenty-five percent TCA is then applied using 2 × 2–inch gauze pads. The denuded skin is rubbed vigorously until an even, white frost occurs. The burning is relieved by pretreatment with EMLA or 30% lidocaine jelly under occlusion for 1 hour before the procedure. Aquaphor after wet soaks promotes healing in the usual fashion.

This procedure avoids splatter associated with dermabrasion, and dermal injury sufficient to eliminate rhytides can be achieved. Scarring and hypopigmentation are rare but have been produced in an incidence of approximately 2%. In dark-skinned patients a test area can be performed, but good results have been obtained with antecedant and subsequent hydroquinone application.

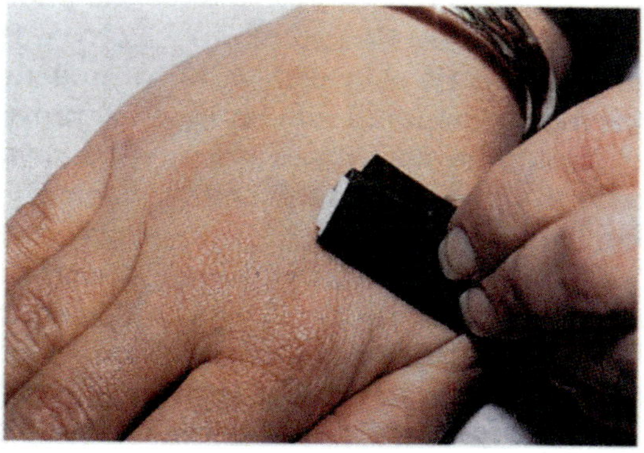

FIG. 10-2. Two 2 × 2–inch gauze pads are rolled up into a cylinder, over which silicone carbide sandpaper is wrapped or folded.

Perspective on Peeling Versus Dermabrasion

If scarring is the primary indication, dermabrasion is the more efficacious treatment. If fine wrinkles are the primary indication, either procedure is acceptable, but peeling may be superior. If actinic damage is the indication, either procedure is acceptable, but dermabrasion may have more sustaining results.[11-14] There are multiple approaches to attain the same result in patient care. One path may deviate slightly from the other, but the destination is the same. (For additional information on actinic damage persisting after peeling, see the middermal injury—deep peeling section in Chapter 2 and the discussion sections on JS + TCA and 50% TCA peeling in Chapter 6.)

This procedure describes the use of sandpaper on the skin followed by the application of TCA. If the TCA is applied first and the sandpaper is used afterward, the process is also effective. In the preceding section sandpaper is used immediately after the application of Baker's solution. In both cases the sandpaper avoids the splatter of blood and the setup of mechanical dermabrasion.

COMBINING CHEMICAL RESURFACING WITH LASER RESURFACING OR COMBINATION SKIN RESURFACING

Carbon dioxide laser ablation of the skin with the blending of affected and unaffected skin using TCA has been reported in the past,[15] but it is only with the introduction of the resurfacing pulsed or scanned CO_2 laser with minimal thermal tissue damage that the laser has ignited the hearts and minds of the American public in precisely removing thin layers of skin. Most experience with this new modality has been through two venues. The Coherent UltraPulse laser and the Sharplan SilkTouch system have similar courses of instruction, spot sizes, depth gradients, scanner devices, clinical effectiveness, and undetermined exact complication rates. Other, newer laser system models and scanners are forthcoming. The value of this type of CO_2 laser in reducing scars and eliminating rhytides is considerable, especially in the perioral and periorbital areas,[16,17] but at this time its efficacy cannot be adequately compared with deep peeling or dermabrasion until unbiased comparative clinical and histologic studies have been performed on all indications, including actinic keratoses. Preliminarily and perhaps oversimplified, the ultra short–pulsed laser seems to be able to reduce rhytides by one photoaging group for each treatment.[18-20] A very severe Glogau photoaging type IV patient's skin will be reversed to photoaging III skin with mild to moderate wrinkling. Multiple laser touch-ups may be required for continued improvement. Baker's solution will usually eliminate the vast majority of severe rhytides in one treatment. Neither procedure will have bothersome pigmentary abnormality. In photoaging III skin with mild wrinkling, the laser may reverse to a photoaging II without rhytides and no pigmentary change; Baker's solution may also give a good clinical result but may leave slight hypopigmentation.

The depth of injury is enhanced by the number of passes with the laser until the desired depth is reached. The number of passes to achieve a selected depth will vary with the specific laser being used and the energy being delivered. Depth variation will also depend on operator-dependent determination of the chamois color of the dermis that is observed immediately after laser resurfacing as a stopping point. Interpretation of this color gradient between light or heavy will make interpretation, comparison, and evaluation of complications slow to be analyzed. Anesthesia for the laser consists of local nerve blocks, ring blocks, tumescence of the facial skin, or even sedation similar to deep peeling if full-face resurfacing is performed.

Rates of complications when compared with peeling are undetermined at this time until long-term studies have been performed. Hyperpigmentation in darker skin types in both modalities is usually temporary. Delayed hypopigmentation and hypertrophic scarring can occur with both procedures and are dependent on operator technique, among other factors. Preliminary comparable scarring rates of less than 3% for both procedures prevail in comparing the Baker-Gordon peel formula with the CO_2 laser. (See the sections on hypopigmentation and scarring in Chapter 8.)

Candidiasis and contact dermatitis are more common with the laser because of the lack of nonviable epidermis that serves as partial protection in peeling. There are more factors to consider in performing a chemical peel as opposed to the laser. However, care with simple operator technique in applying peeling agents and in performing the number of laser passes with or without overlapping may be the single most important factor in preventing complications.

Resurfacing with medium-depth chemical peeling techniques to minimally photodamaged or unlasered skin seems to be as efficacious in blending cosmetic units as with dermabrasion, dermasanding, and different peeling techniques on separate cosmetic areas. The chemical peel takes less time to perform than laser resurfacing and is less painful and less expensive (Fig.10-3). The healing time and residual postoperative erythema after the laser generally are more prolonged than those after medium-depth chemical peeling combinations. Operator technique with the number of passes, the laser system, and the energy settings as additional variables make definitive evaluation difficult. Comparable duration of results is unknown.

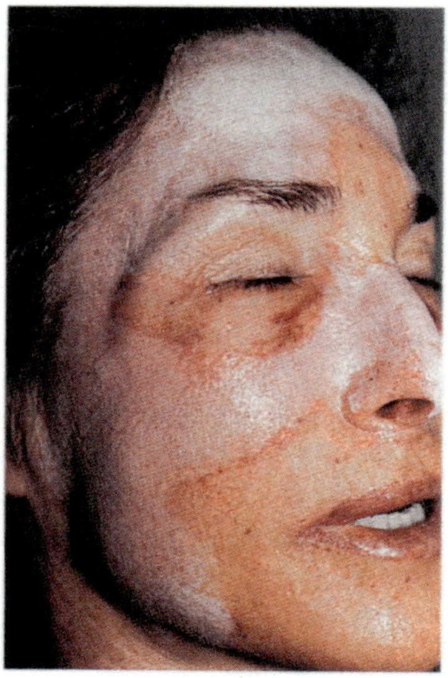

FIG. 10-3. After ultrapulse laser techniques to the periorbital, perioral, and glabellar areas, JS plus TCA is applied immediately afterward to unlasered mildly photodamaged skin for blending. Healing reveals no discernible difference in skin texture. The peel may be performed before the laser, but the patient may find this less tolerable when using only local or tumescent anesthesia and nerve blocks.

For additional related discussion see the perspective on deep peeling (p. 137) in Chapter 7. For histologic correlation, see the section on comparison of dermal peeling with the CO_2 laser in Chapter 2. For complications comparison, see Chapter 8.

TRICHLOROACETIC ACID PEEL WITH METHYL SALICYLATE

The "hot rod" TCA peel[21] is a 35% TCA peel with the addition of 5% to 10% methyl salicylate to "augment" the TCA and 1% polysorbate 20 as a surfactant. It is purported that the additives make TCA "potent enough to do a phenol-type peel."[21] However, the method is not effective in removing all perioral or periorbital rhytides, and dermabrasion of these residual areas within 4 to 6 weeks after the peel is advocated, which may not be enough time for collagen reorganization to occur. The peel is advocated for local scarring treatment. The solution, available from Delasco, is aggressive, will pull TCA through a latex glove, and will erode a plastic bottle after a year. Repeated consecutive application and nonfacial application are not recommended. Rabbit skin studies showed increased inflammation with methyl salicylate, but wound-depth studies at peak wounding and after 90 days have not been performed on the human face. Intravenous sedation is recommended for this peel, and healing is allegedly promoted by the drinking of 20 ounces of aloe vera juice daily and topical aloe vera gel followed by Polysporin ointment. Adequate preparation of the skin with tretinoin in the usual fashion is emphasized. (See the regimen discussion in Chapter 4 and the discussion on aloe vera in Chapter 3.) For discussion on additives to TCA, see the section on frosting and additives to TCA in Chapter 4.

The incidence of scarring, pigmentary complications, and infection with this peel is greater than those with TCA alone because of the increased penetration. The exact frequency is unknown, and its advantages are uncertain.

Severe contact dermatitis to aloe vera juice after a Baker's solution peel has been reported.[22]

PROPRIETARY PEELS

Exodermology or endodermology connotes a direct association with dermatology by the sound of its name, but it is not endorsed by the specialty. A complaint was filed by the American Academy of Dermatology to the Federal Trade Commission in the middle 1980s because the exodermology marketing organization was operated by a nonphysician in Florida and employed some physicians who had had their medical licenses revoked. Doctors who never received training in chemical peeling, such as rheumatologists, pathologists, psychiatrists, and allergists, each paid $50,000 to attend a seminar on how to perform phenol peels on patients, along with franchising, advertising, and marketing advice. The Congressional Subcommittee Hearings on Outpatient Cosmetic Surgery, which investigated questionable franchising of chemical peels and was chaired by Congressman Ron Wyden of Oregon, were directed toward this same group in 1989.[23]

Improper techniques employed by these groups included occlusion of Baker's solution down to the eyelash cilia, application and occlusion of Baker's solution to the entire neck, absence of cardiac monitoring and intravenous

A

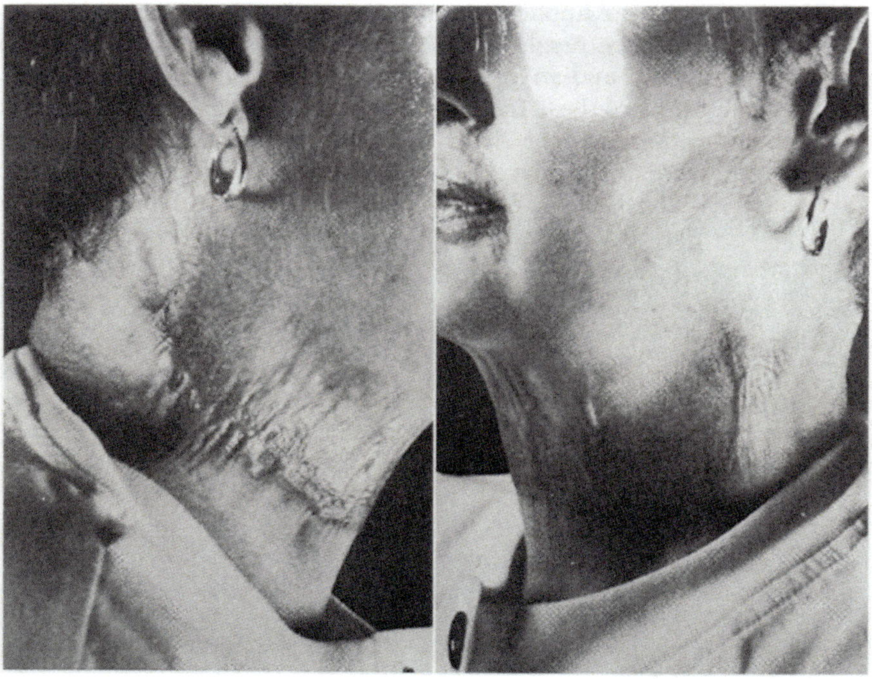

B

FIG. 10-4. Neck scarring resulting from exodermology peeling with Baker's solution. *(Courtesy of Dr. David Duffy.)*

A

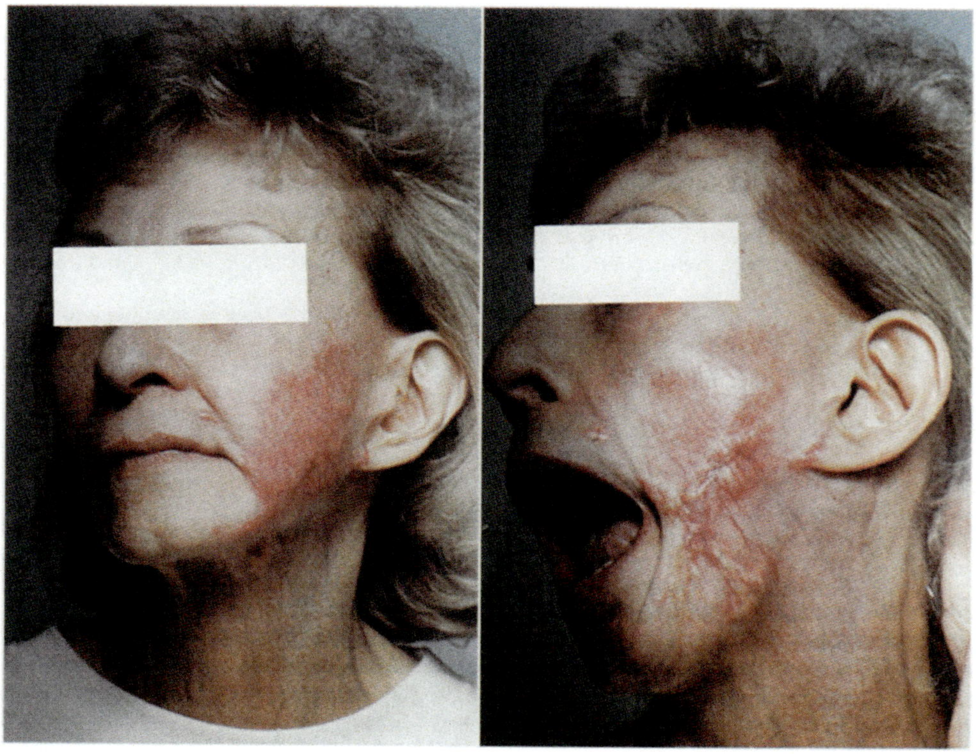

B

FIG. 10-5. Severe scarring resulting from a TCA peel performed by a graduate of a proprietary program.

hydration, and rapid application with large cotton swabs over too short a time interval. These have resulted in at least two cases of permanently impaired vision, two deaths, and an unknown number of cases of face and neck scarring (Fig. 10-4). Some of these franchises are still in operation. (See Chapter 9.)

Other proprietary peels with claims of unproven efficacy or superiority marketed by unnamed physicians in brochures under meaningless nomenclature such as "Live Cell Novadermy" or "La Peau Nouvelle" might be variations on techniques in this book or even the same techniques, but their main thrusts are attempts at unique marketing. Reluctance to be specific in advertisements and outrageous claims in their promotion may make them vulnerable to investigation by the Federal Trade Commission (Fig. 10-5).

REFERENCES

1. Dupont C, Ciaburro H, Prevost Y, et al: Phenol skin tightening for better dermabrasion, *Plast Reconstr Surg* 50:588-590, 1972.
2. Horton CE, Sadove RC: Refinements in combined chemical peel and simultaneous abrasion of the face, *Ann Plast Surg* 19:504-510, 1987.
3. Spira M: Treatment of acne scarring by combined dermabrasion and chemical peel, *Plast Reconstr Surg* 60:38, 1977.
4. Szalay LV: Treatment of acne scarring by combined dermabrasion and chemical peel, *Plast Reconstr Surg* 79:307, 1987, (letter).
5. Lusthaus S, Benmeir P, Neuman A, et al: The use of sandpaper in chemical peeling combined with dermabrasion of the face, *Ann Plast Surg* 31:281-282, 1993.
6. Stagnone JJ: Chemabrasion: a combined technique of chemical peeling and dermabrasion, *J Dermatol Surg Oncol* 3:217-219, 1977.
7. Stagnone JJ, Stagnone GJ: A second look at chemabrasion, *J Dermatol Surg Oncol* 8:701-705, 1982.
8. Coleman WP, Roenigk HH: Combining dermabrasion and chemical peel, *Face* 2:89-94, 1994.
9. Coleman WP, Klein J: Use of the tumescent technique for scalp surgery, dermabrasion and soft tissue reconstruction, *J Dermatol Surg Oncol* 18:130-135, 1992.
10. Harris DR, Noodleman FR: Combining manual dermasanding with low strength trichloroacetic acid to improve actinically injured skin, *J Dermatol Surg Oncol* 20:436-442, 1994.
11. Field LM: Dermabrasion and chemical exfoliation, *J Am Acad Dermatol* 10:521-522, 1984, (letter).
12. Spira M, Freeman R, Arfai P, et al: Clinical comparison of chemical peeling, dermabrasion, and 5-FU for senile keratoses, *Plast Reconstr Surg* 46:61-66, 1970.
13. Benedetto AV, Griffin TD, Benedetto EA, et al: Dermabrasion: therapy and prophylaxis of the photoaged face, *J Am Acad Dermatol* 27:439-447, 1992.
14. Coleman WP, Yarborough JM, Mandy SH: Dermabrasion for prophylaxis and treatment of actinic keratoses, *Dermatol Surg* 22:17-21, 1996.
15. David LM, Glassberg E, Lask G: Combined carbon dioxide laser resurfacing and TCA chemical peel, *Am J Cosmet Surg* 9(2):153-158, 1992.
16. Waldorf HA, Kauvar ANB, Geronemus RG: Skin resurfacing of fine to deep rhytides using a char-free carbon dioxide laser in 47 patients, *J Dermatol Surg Oncol* 21:940-946, 1995.
17. Ho C, Nguyen Q, Lowe NJ, et al: Laser resurfacing in pigmented skin, *Dermatol Surg* 21:1035-1037, 1995.
18. Hruza GJ, Dover JS: Laser skin resurfacing, *Arch Dermatol* 132:451-455, 1996.
19. Fitzpatrick RE, Tope WD, Goldman MP, et al: Pulsed carbon dioxide laser, trichloroacetic acid, Baker-Gordon phenol, and dermabrasion: a comparative clinical and histological study of cutaneous resurfacing in a porcine model, *Arch Dermatol* 132:469-471, 1996.
20. Fitzpatrick RE, Goldman MP, Satur NM, et al: Pulsed carbon dioxide laser resurfacing of photoaged facial skin, *Arch Dermatol* 132:395-402, 1996.
21. Fulton JE: Step-by-step skin rejuvenation, *Am J Cosmet Surg* 7:199-205, 1990.
22. Hunter D, Frumkin A: Adverse reactions to vitamin E and aloe vera preparations after dermabrasion and chemical peel, *Cutis* 47:193-196, 1991.
23. Wyden Congressional Hearings on Cosmetic Surgery; the Subcommittee on Regulation, Business Opportunities and Energy of the Committee on Small Business; House of Representatives, Washington, DC, November 2, 1989.

11 *Special Cases*

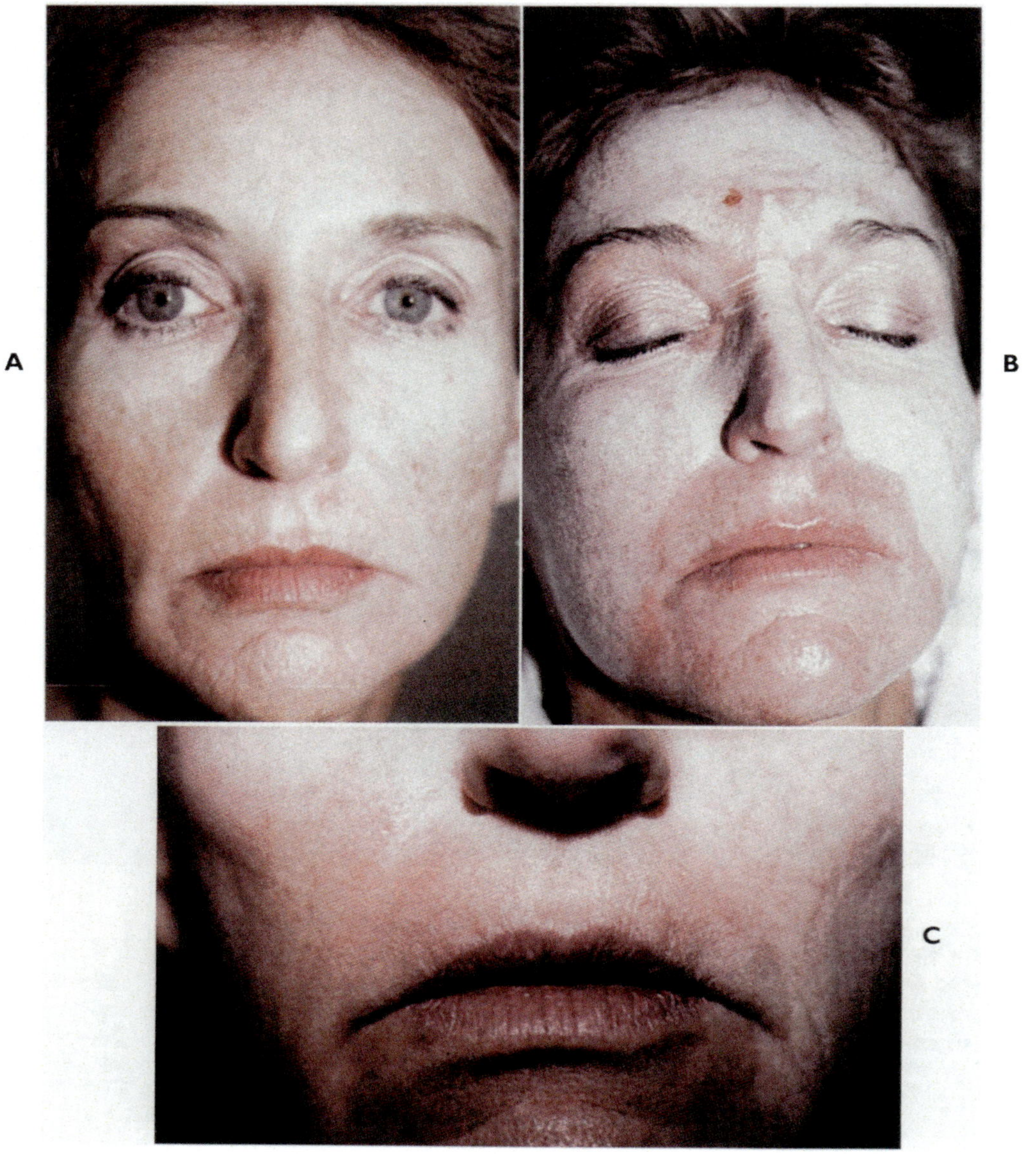

CASE 1

FIG. 11-1. (A) This is a Fitzpatrick type III, Glogau photoaging type III patient with minimal sebaceous activity and only moderate vertical rhytides in the perioral area. She was peeled with an unoccluded Baker's phenol peel in this area and medium-depth CO_2, hard, plus trichloroacetic acid (TCA), 35%, elsewhere **(B)**. Her response was satisfactory **(C),** with no color change between the cosmetic units, but there are still several very fine vertical rhytides in her lipstick lines. She will benefit from local repeeling, but a more aggressive coating of solution in this area or taping of the vermilion area only might have made this a more effective peel in one procedure. This is a common occurrence for the beginning or experienced physician.

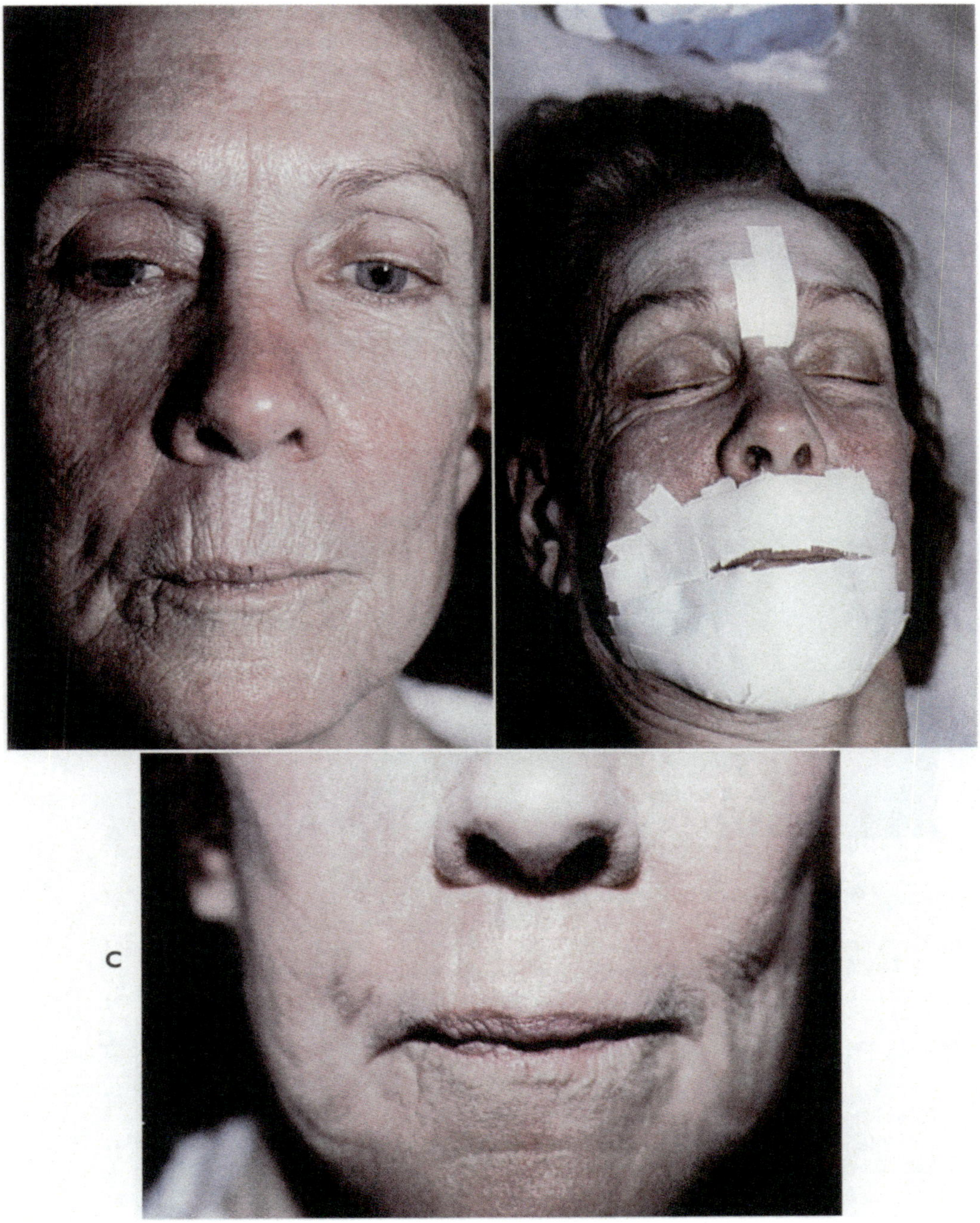

A B C

CASE 2

FIG. 11-2. (A) This is a Fitzpatrick type II, Glogau photoaging type III patient with severe perioral and glabellar actinic elastosis and a full-thickness vertical scar of 20 years' duration on the right upper and lower lip. The remainder of the cheeks were moderately sun damaged, but she did not have a history of skin cancer. She was peeled with occluded Baker's phenol in the perioral and glabellar areas, with 50% TCA on the cheeks, and CO_2 plus TCA, 35%, elsewhere **(B)**. Her response was excellent 6 months later **(C)**, with no discernible color change between areas and eradication of most rhytides.

The scar itself, while certainly no worse, perhaps even improved, is more obvious in the absence of the many vertical rhytides. Perioral dermabrasion might have provided a more uniform improvement, although the patient and physician are mutually pleased.

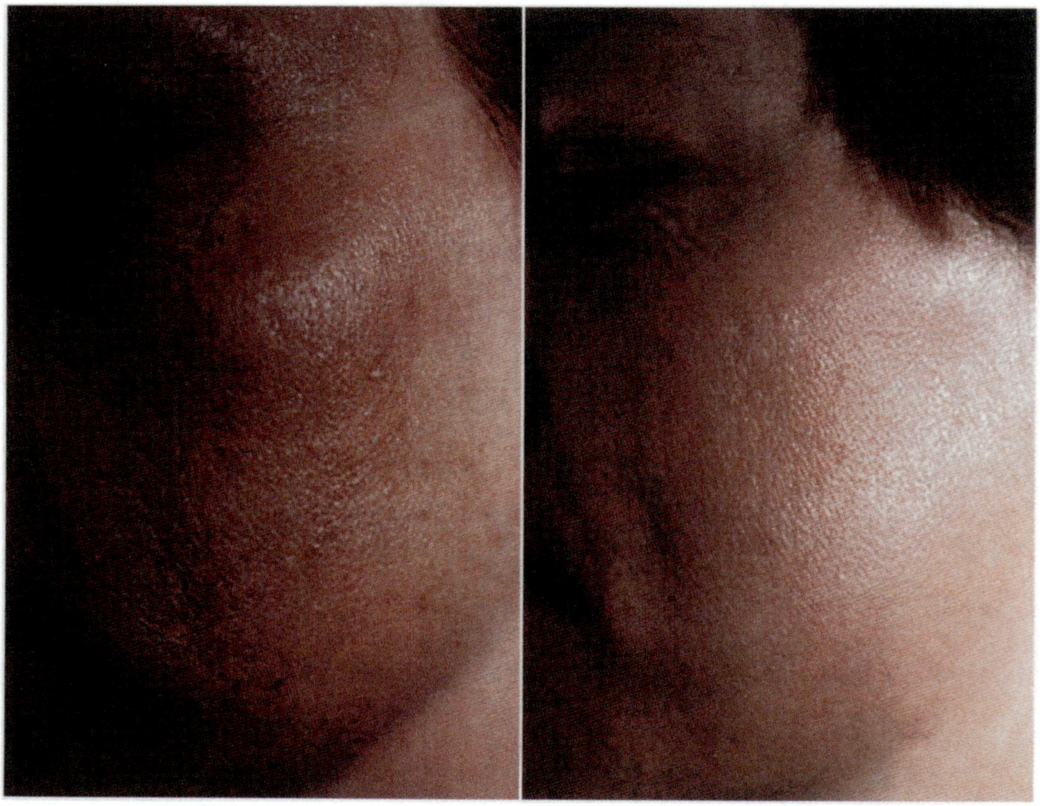

A B

CASE 3

FIG. 11-3. This is a Fitzpatrick type IV, Glogau photoaging type II, 26-year-old young female with increasing light freckling on the cheeks **(A)**. She very rarely burns, and her eye color is light brown. She achieved significant improvement **(B)** with Jessner's solution (JS) application to the freckled areas with one cotton-tipped applicator and 35% TCA to the entire face with one cotton-tipped applicator. She followed the traditional regimen.

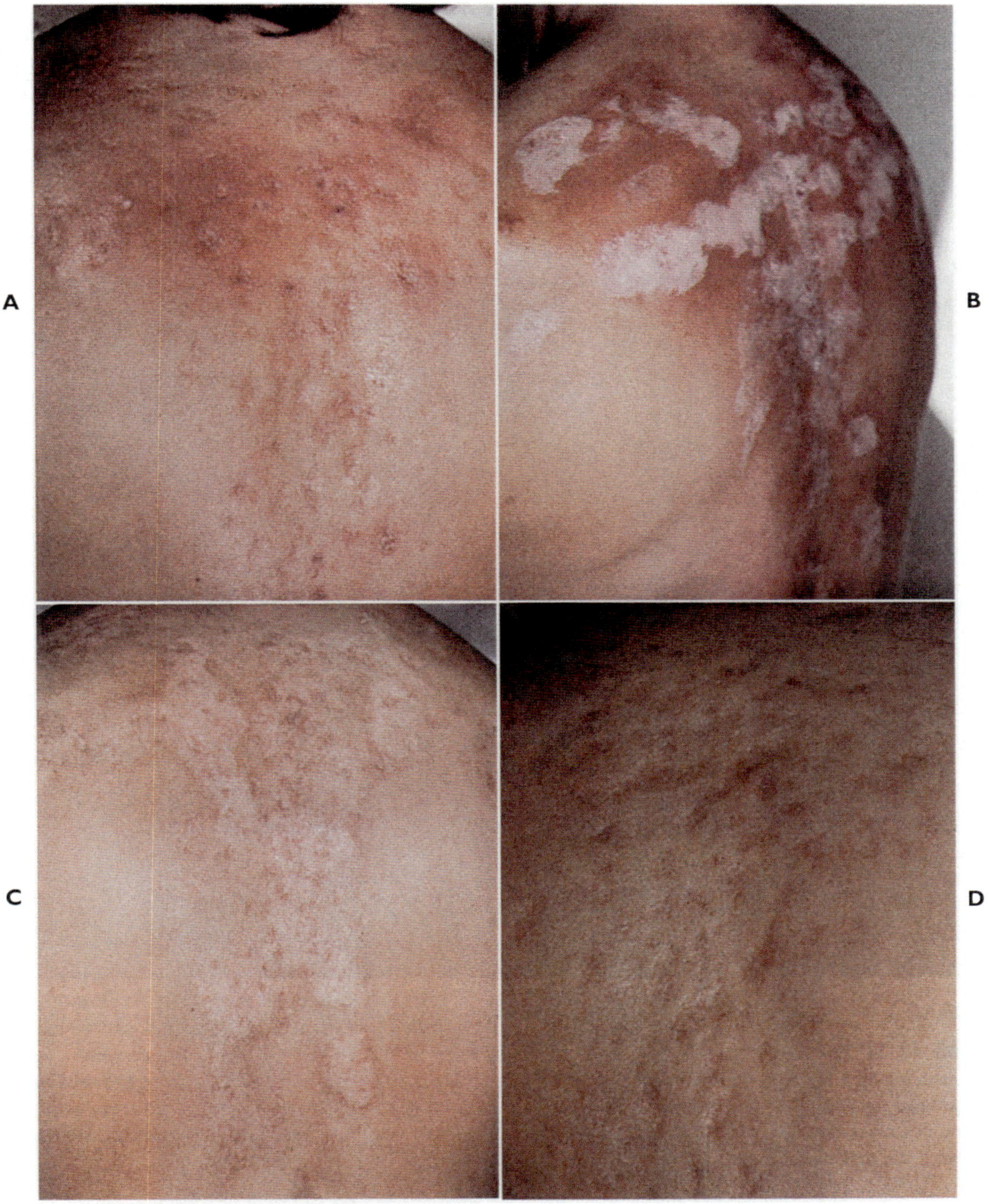

CASE 4

FIG. 11-4. This is a Fitzpatrick type IV, Glogau photoaging type I, 28-year-old male with severe acne scarring on the back of greater than 10 years' duration. His eye color is dark brown, and he has no history of sunburns. The scars were frozen with CO_2, hard, **(A),** followed by TCA, 35%, **(B),** and 3 months after shows flattening of the scar rims with appreciable hypopigmentation and hyperpigmentation of the peripheral peeled areas, **(C)**. Characteristically, the areas repigmented evenly in 18 to 24 months, **(D)**. Because there are cases that may not ever pigment entirely evenly, this should be discussed thoroughly with the patient to form an excellent physician-patient relationship. This patient was peeled twice over a 5-year period with success. A lighter Fitzpatrick skin type might tolerate 50% TCA to the scar rims without color compromise.

A

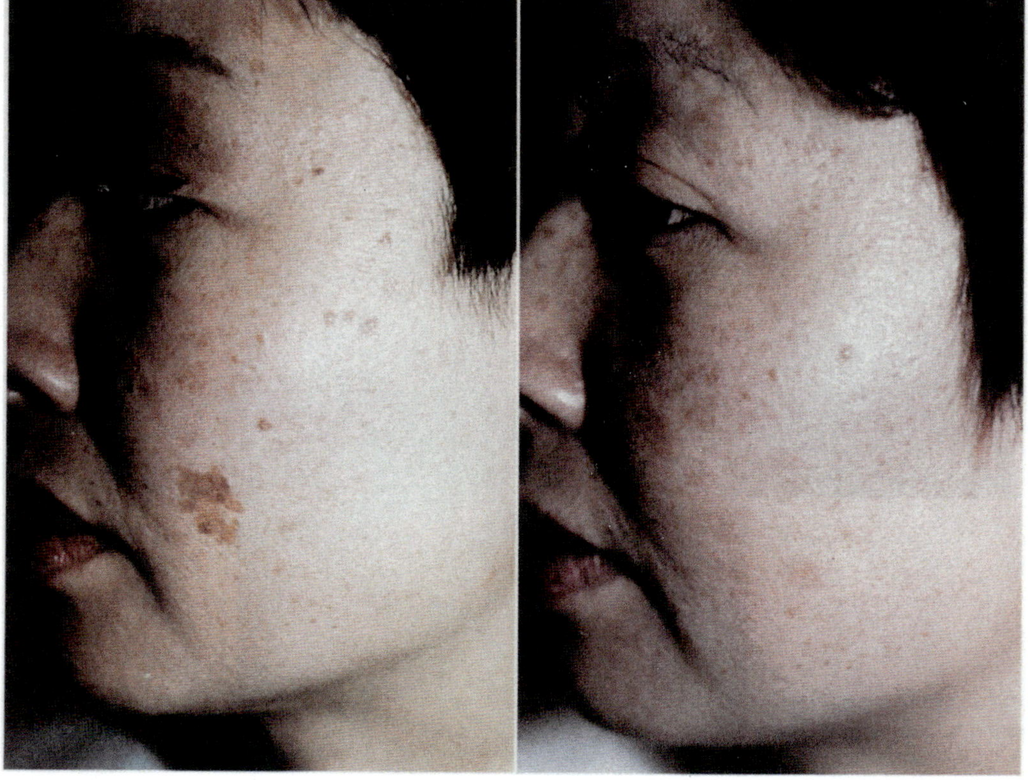

B

CASE 5

FIG. 11-5. This Fitzpatrick type V, Glogau photoaging type I female has epidermal keratoses over the face, **(A)**. Her test spots hyperpigmented initially, but all faded after 3 months with CO_2 mild, a 7-second application of liquid nitrogen on a cotton swab with light pressure, and JS. Her largest keratosis was treated with liquid nitrogen, and the remainder of the small keratoses were treated locally with CO_2 mild. The remainder of the entire face was then treated with JS with two cotton applicators; this was repeated in 6 weeks. **(B)** Nine months after healing. The patient followed the traditional regimen but was warned of the possibility of dyschromia as a complication. Some freckling persists.

Skin type V is the most difficult to peel for pigmentation. Every patient may respond differently. Choosing an agent on the basis of histology with gradual peeling of individual pigmented areas and later blending can be valuable. Obviously, types V and VI sustain little photoaging, and wounding agents are chosen on the basis of the local lesion depth rather than the degree of actinic damage per cosmetic unit. Following the regimen before and after peeling is mandatory.

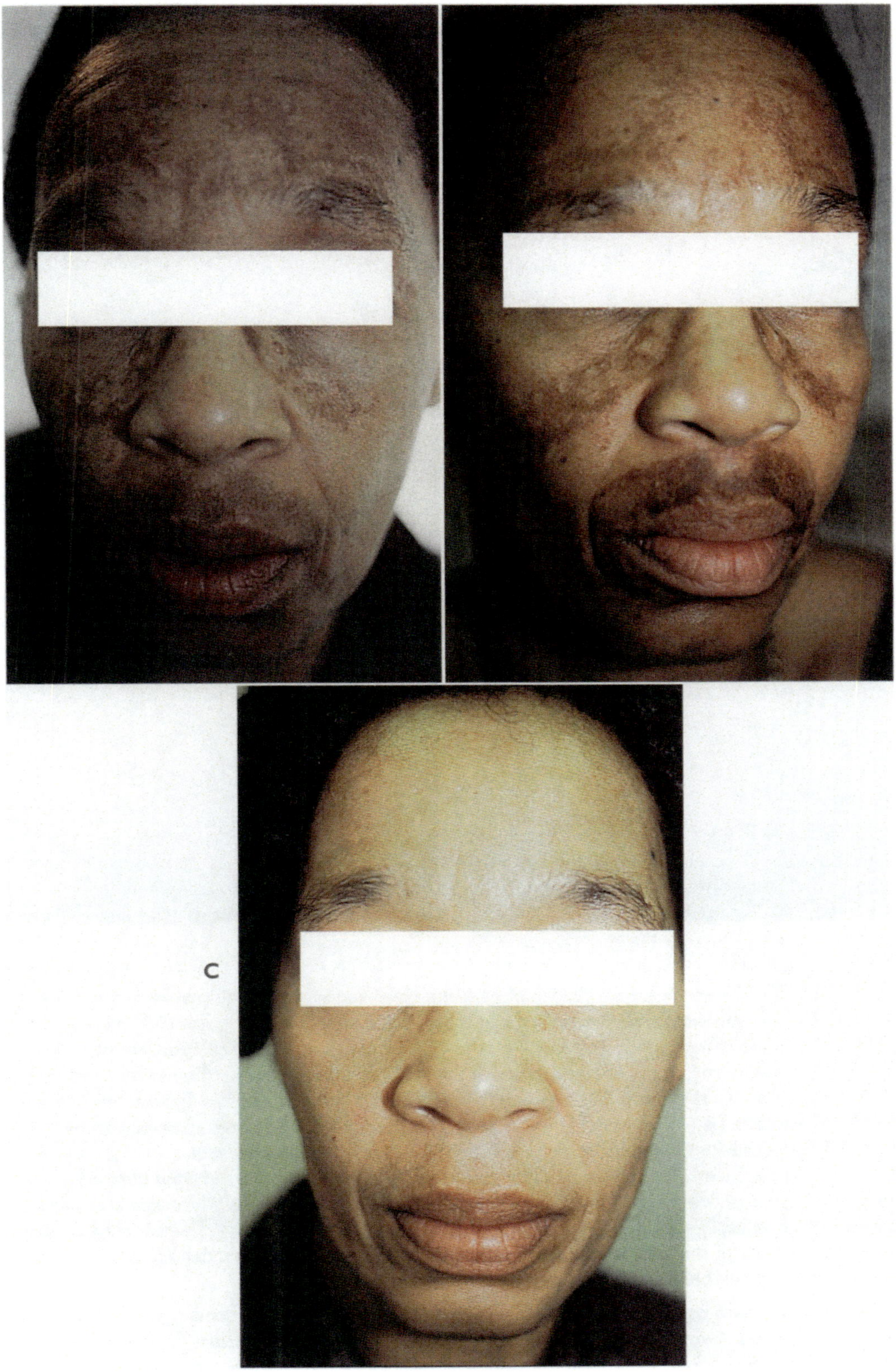

CASE 6

FIG. 11-6. This Fitzpatrick skin type V patient illustrates the routine and aggressive procedural attack for melasma in skin types from III to VI. **(A)** Before peeling. **(B)** One day after application of two coats of Jessner's solution with a sable brush. **(C)** After two monthly treatments with Jessner's solution showing good resolution of pigmentation.

Skin types I and II may be peeled with little risk with superficial or medium-depth peels and sometimes optional adherence to the regimen. The Fitzpatrick type V or VI patient must use the regimen for his or her skin type as discussed in Chapter 4. Dark-skinned patients should be told that their faces will be a lighter complexion after treatment.

The first peel of **serial repetitive increasing-strength peels** essentially retinizes the patient's epidermis if the patient has not been using or is not using enough tretinoin. The initial peel with a superficial agent, one or two coats of JS, for example, will serve this purpose. This may be performed on the first visit or about 4 to 6 weeks after the patient has begun the regimen. It is repeated up to three times on a monthly basis, and the degree of improvement is assessed. In addition, the patient should be asked if the pigment came off and returned or if it never changed. If it came off and returned, the concentration of hydroquinone must be increased to 6% or later 8% from 4%. The same strength peel is then repeated. Concentrations of up to 15% hydroquinone can be used for only 1 week and then immediately tapered if effective under close follow-up to avoid ochronotic pigmentation. The peels permit some deeper penetration of the bleaching agents.

If no pigment has been removed, a heavier peel is needed. Progressing to 35% TCA, the lightest peel for papillary dermal penetration, is indicated, and if no improvement is noted in 2 to 3 months, GA plus TCA or JS plus TCA medium-depth peels may be used.

If pigmentation is not substantially improved after these trials and almost 6 months have elapsed, peeling with Baker's solution can be performed with resulting hypopigmentation. Rebound hyperpigmentation can always occur with any peel.

After the patient is stable 2 months after peeling, reduction in frequency of application of the bleach may be attempted. Application from twice daily to once daily and then from every other day to weekly can be achieved over months with possible eventual elimination or irregular indefinite use, depending on inadvertent sun exposure. Patients must be willing to work with the physician for months in improving and maintaining their pigmentation problem, and an excellent physician-patient relationship is imperative.

The wounding agents sited previously are the author's preferences. Other superficial or medium-depth wounding agents or techniques as outlined in Chapters 4 and 5 may be used in sequence.

A B C D E

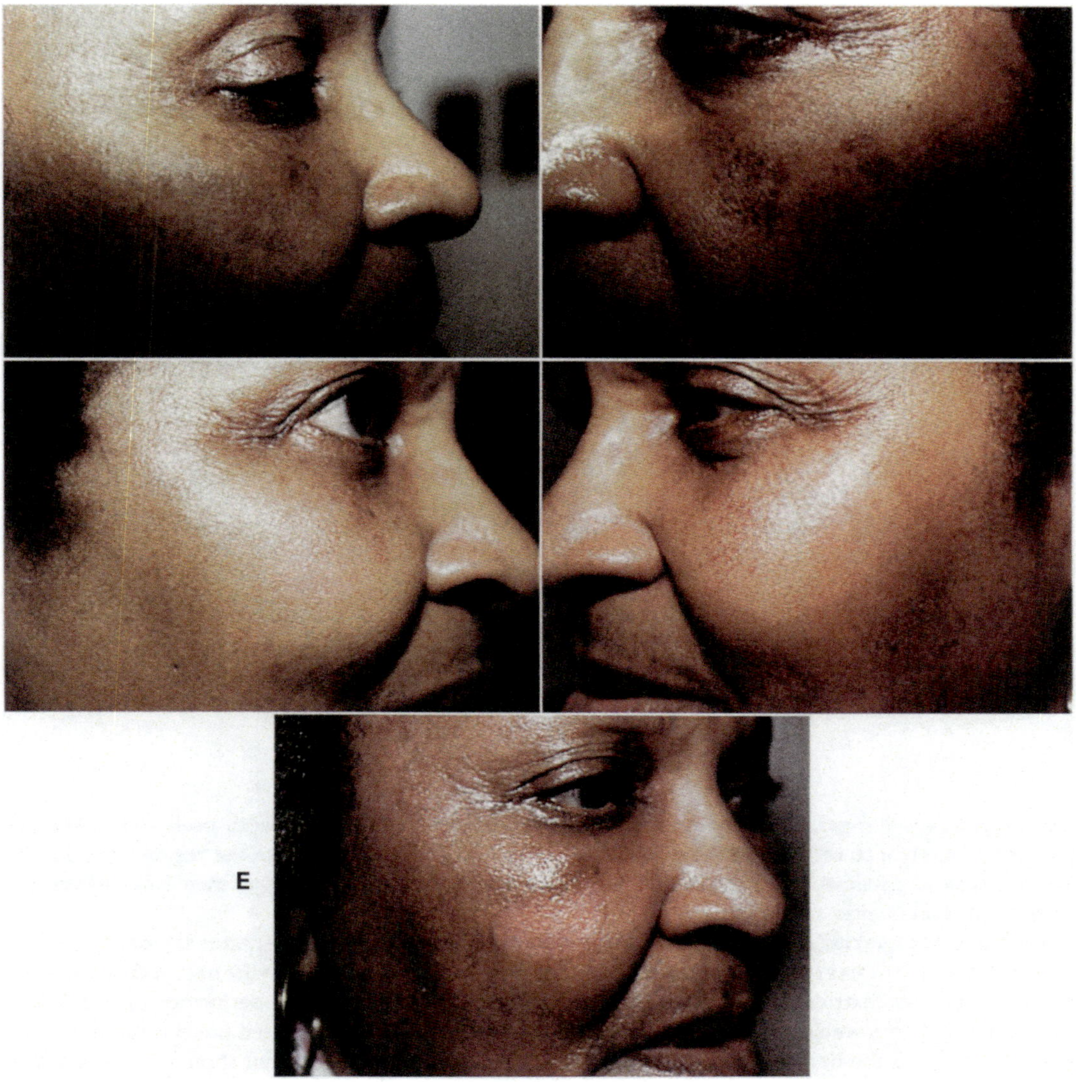

CASE 7

FIG. 11-7. This Fitzpatrick type VI female has both melasma and postinflammatory hyperpigmentation, (**A** and **B**). All test spots to JS, 35% TCA, and Baker's solution exhibited repigmentation in 4 months, the latter slightly hypopigmented and the most effective. The patient used the standard regimen before and after all peeling. She was peeled twice with JS to the individual lesions at 2-week intervals and showed only mild improvement. She was then peeled with 35% TCA to the individual lesions only. **(E)** Four days after peeling. She reachieved her pigment in 3 months and continues the regimen, and the lesions are slightly hypopigmented from the surrounding skin but are satisfactory, (**C** and **D**).

Darker skin types may improve with serial repetitive increasing-strength peels applied to only the darkest pigmented macules rather than a single medium-depth or deep procedure.

In Fitzpatrick skin types V and VI, if entire cosmetic units are normal and non–sun-damaged, these uninvolved units need not be peeled, but the regimen should be used on the entire face. If only a small area within the unit is darkened, that pigmented area may be peeled selectively because peeling is performed for the indication of photodamage. If over 50% of a cosmetic unit is irregularly pigmented, the entire unit may be peeled.

A

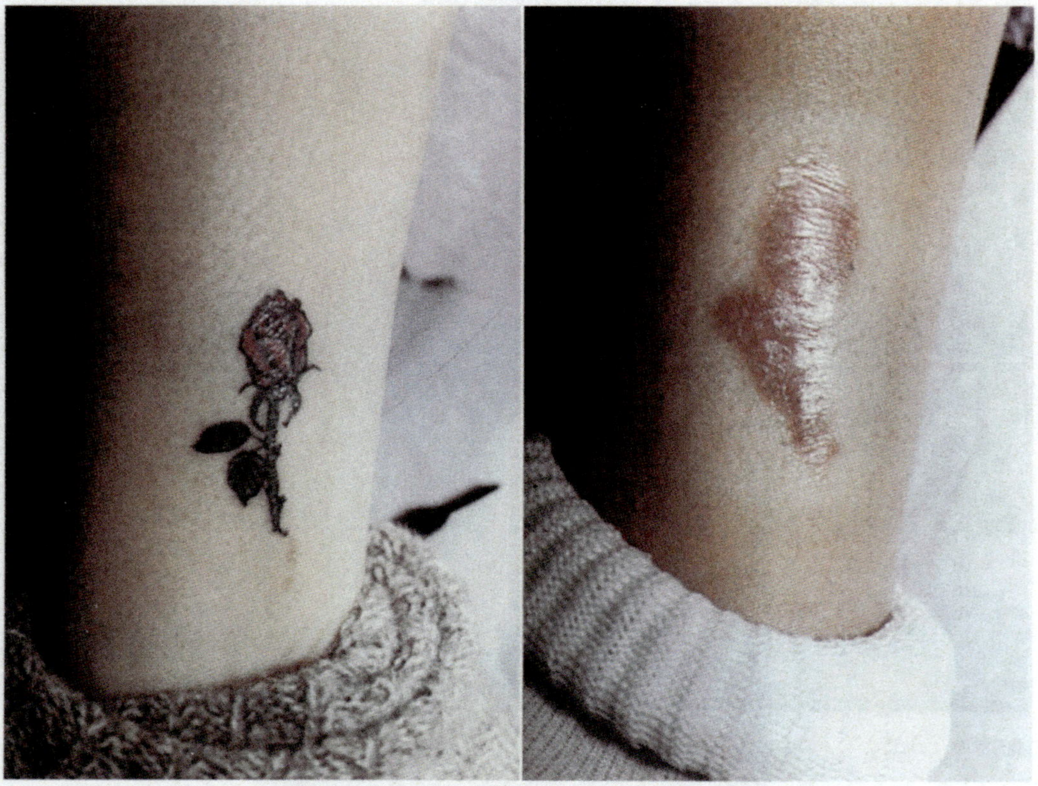

B

CASE 8

FIG. 11-8. Tattoo on the ankle of a 22-year-old white female, **(A)**. The area was peeled successfully with Dr. David Duffy's technique of light electrodesiccation and curettage of the epidermis after local anesthesia followed by three consecutive applications of 75% TCA at 5-minute intervals. **(B)** A nonpigmented scar 2 months later improves with time and intralesional steroids.

Although this is not a chemical peel in the strict sense, it illustrates the destructive potential of high-strength TCA. We have seen this procedure fail on amateur tattoos that have been impregnated too deeply into the dermis. (See the section on 50% TCA in Chapter 6.)

A B C D

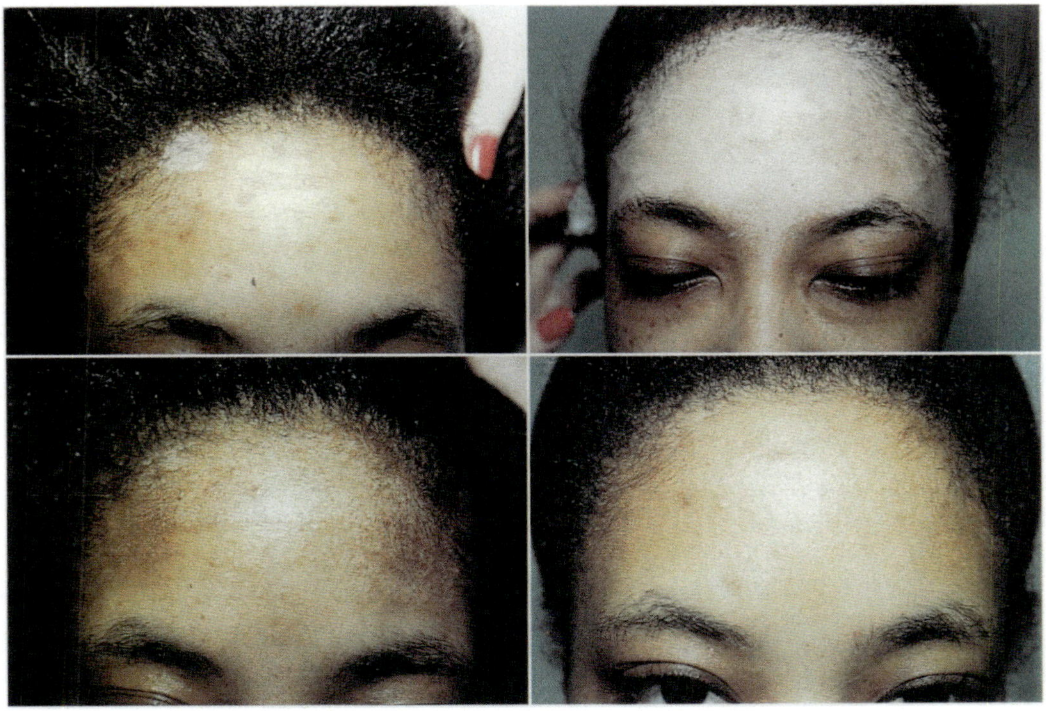

CASE 9

FIG. 11-9. **(A)** This Fitzpatrick skin type V patient has postinflammatory hyperpigmentation from acne and excoriations on the forehead. She was peeled twice on a monthly interval with Jessner's solution and skin tested with 35% TCA. **(B)** After 2 months she was peeled with 35% TCA applied with a single 4 × 4–inch gauze pad to a uniform frosting. **(C)** Four weeks later the skin was reepithelialized but dyschromic. **(D)** After using the regimen for her skin type the skin was uniform and clear of pigmentation in 6 months. Several indented scars remain.

This case illustrates the expected dyschromia after peeling Fitzpatrick skin types V and VI. The skin may not return to normal until 6 to 18 months after peeling. The patient should be warned in advance to expect this side effect.

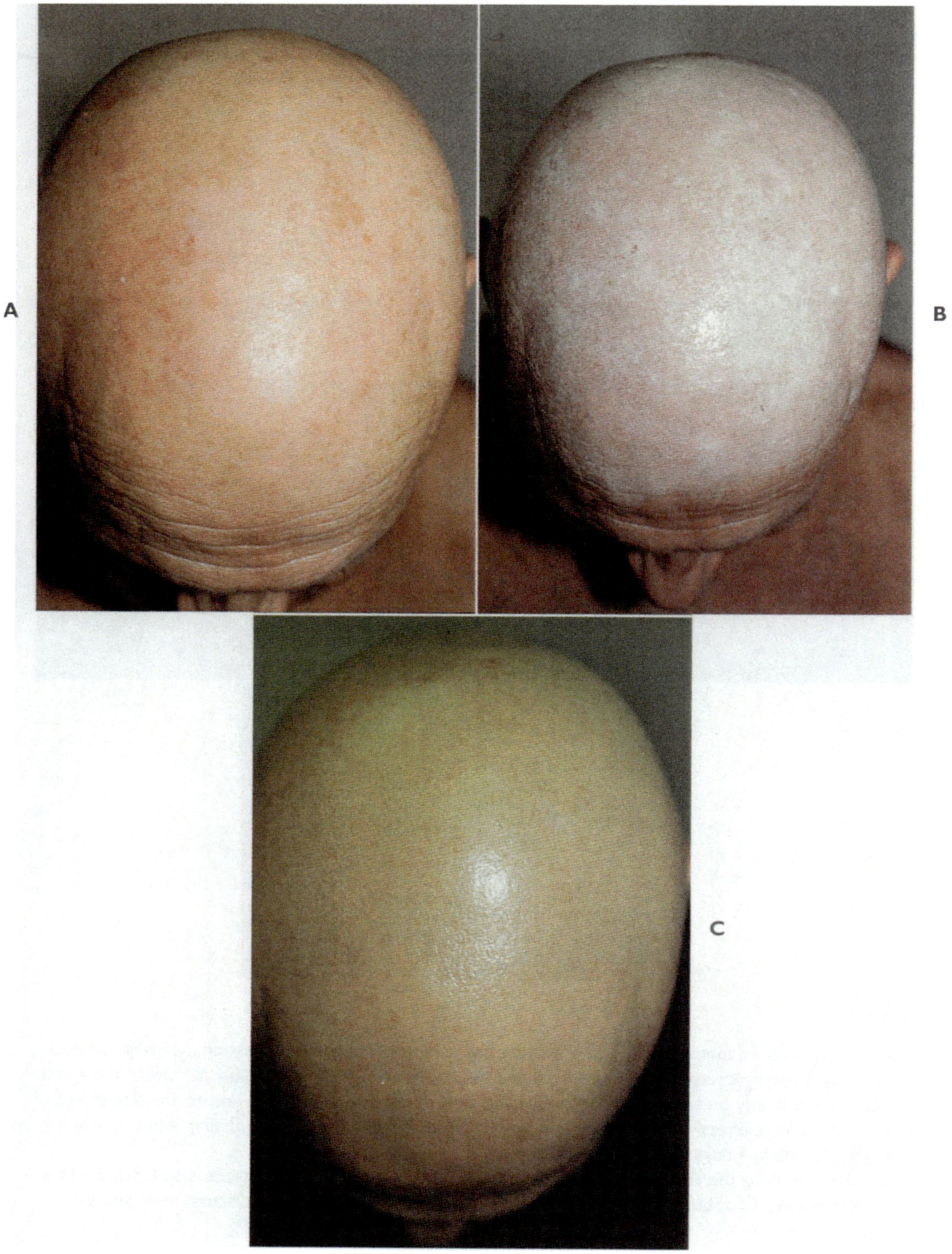

CASE 10

FIG. 11-10. This Fitzpatrick skin type II patient exhibits Glogau photoaging type III with actinic keratoses, lentigines, and freckling over an alopecic scalp before peeling, **(A)**. Hypertrophic actinic keratoses were gently debrided with a curette after local anesthesia and covered with a light application of Monsel's solution. The skin was peeled with a liberal coating of JS applied with a sable brush followed by 35% TCA applied with a wet 4 × 4–inch gauze pad and reapplied a second time 10 minutes later. **(B)**, Immediately after peeling. Excellent improvement of the scalp is seen 9 months after the peel, **(C)**. Resulting eradication of all pigmented lesions has persisted for 2 years with strict sun avoidance. No regimen was used before or after the peel in this skin type, although the patient was encouraged to use tretinoin after peeling as often as he could remember.

With less adnexal structures on the scalp for reepithelialization the risk of delayed healing or scarring is increased with strengths of greater than 40% TCA. Combination peeling outlined in Chapter 6 is effective.

A B C

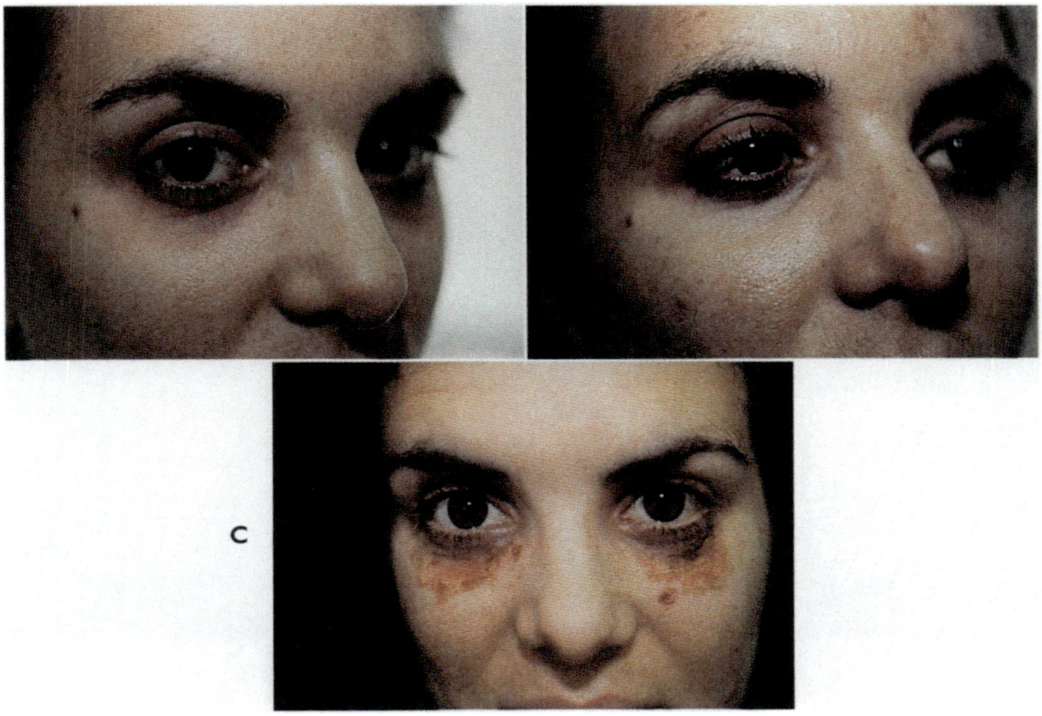

CASE 11

FIG. 11-11. This Fitzpatrick skin type V patient has periorbital hyperpigmentation, partially hereditary and partially photoaggravated, **(A)**. Superficial and medium peeling will predictably fail under the eye in this skin type but may be tried first. The safe application of Baker's phenol solution to the lower half of the cosmetic unit is effective in reducing the pigmentation. Nine months after peeling when erythema has faded, **(B)**. Crusting 4 days after peeling, **(C)**.

The patient is using the regimen for dark skin three times weekly as maintenance. See Chapter 4 for periorbital peeling, Chapter 7 for deep peeling techniques, and Chapter 8 for discussion of phenol hypopigmentation.

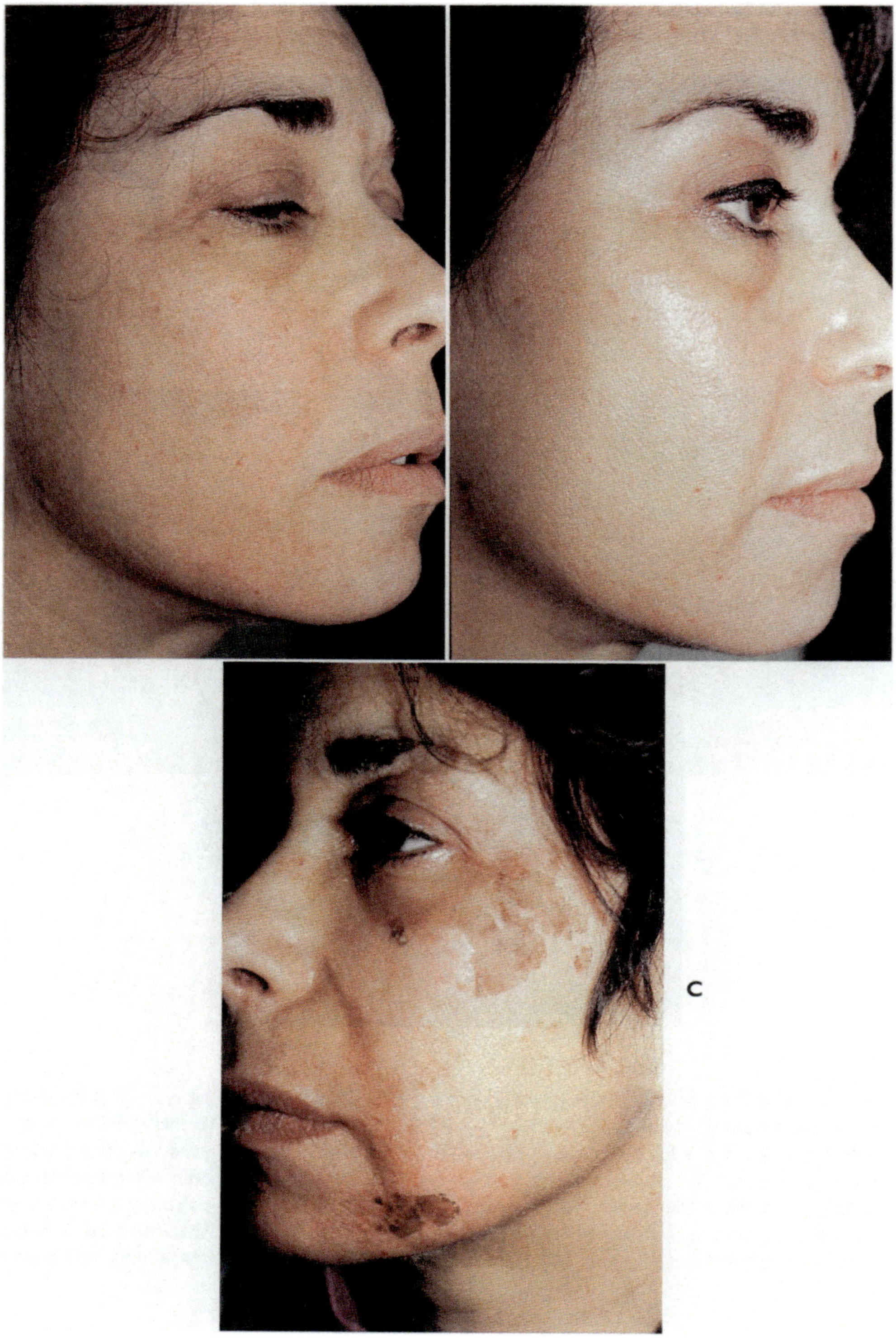
A
B
C

CASE 12

FIG. 11-12. This Fitzpatrick skin type III, Glogau photoaging type II patient has mottled actinic dyschromia responding to two monthly treatments with Jessner's solution, two coats applied with a sable brush. The patient is using the regimen for dark skin between peels. Swelling with considerable peeling occurred after the second application. The patient should be warned that it may be difficult to completely apply makeup over this type of superficial peel even though vesiculation does not occur. If the skin is erythematous from the regimen before peeling or the patient is rarely sensitive to the resorcinol, untoward swelling with prolonged peeling may be intensified. **(A)** Before peeling. **(B)** One month after the final peel. **(C)** Three days after the second peel with unexpected swelling and protracted peeling.

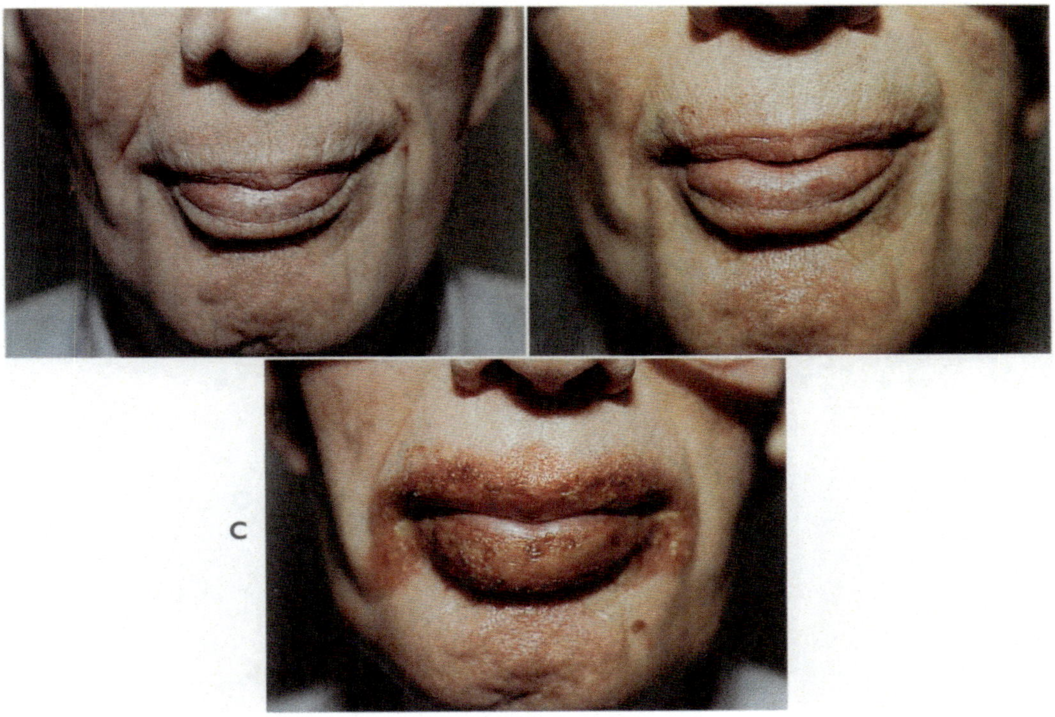

CASE 13

FIG. 11-13. This Fitzpatrick skin type II male with perioral Glogau photoaging type IV skin exhibits actinic rhytides responding well to application of the Baker's phenol solution to the vermilion area. Although the patient has a habit of pursing his lips, the actinic component overshadows the dynamic component of the unit. The perivermilion skin is always hypopigmented and never reflects perceptible color change or a line of demarcation after peeling. This technique is excellent also for a female whose lipstick is bleeding into vermilion rhytides. **(A)** Before peeling. **(B)** Three months after peel showing good resolution of vermilion rhytides. **(C)** Four days after peeling with erythema, edema, and crusting.

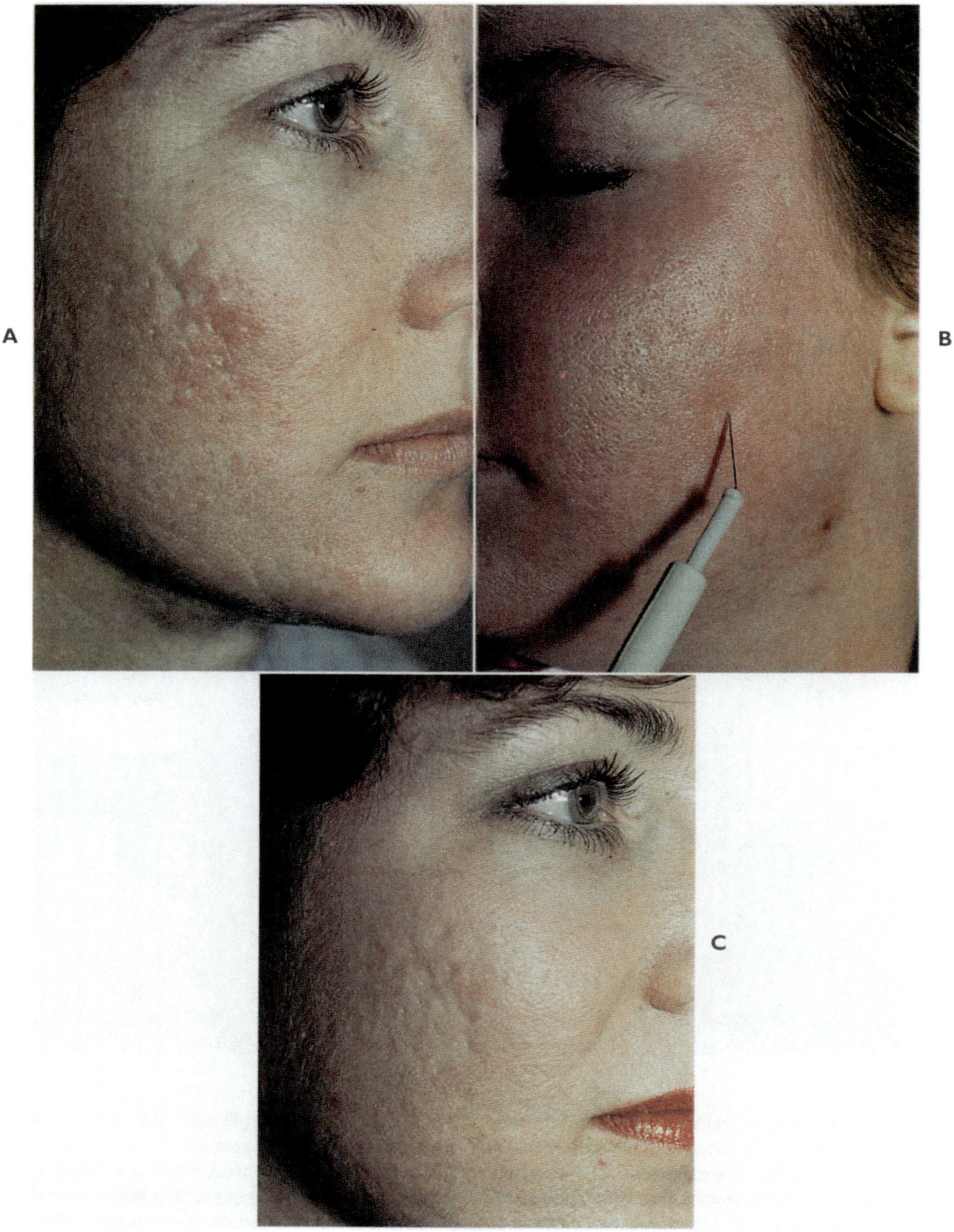

CASE 14

FIG. 11-14. This Fitzpatrick skin type II patient has depressed scarring on the cheeks without any pitted component, **(A)**. She is peeled with CO_2 hard, immediately electrodesiccating the edges of the scars, **(B)**, and then fifty percent TCA is applied to the edges with the broken end of a wooden cotton-tipped applicator. 35% TCA is then applied liberally to the entire face with a single 4 × 4–inch gauze pad. Improvement is substantial 3 months later, **(C)**. The combination CO_2 plus TCA peel is the only peel that is effective for scarring because it employs a physical modality. (See Chapter 6.)

A
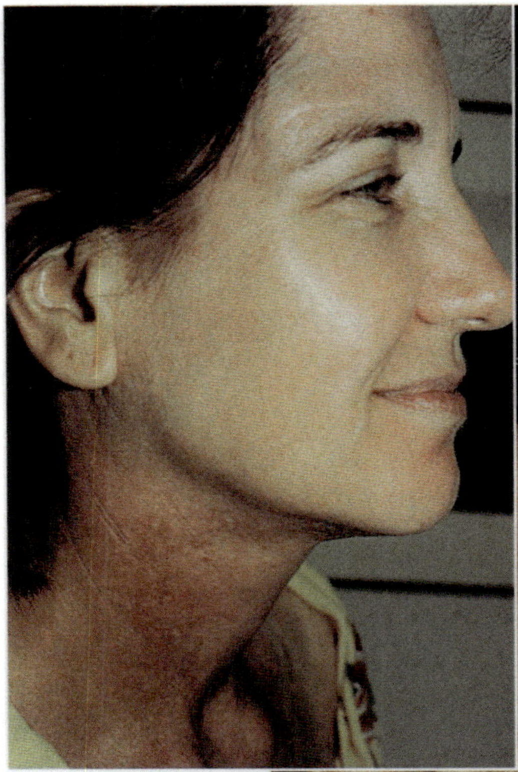
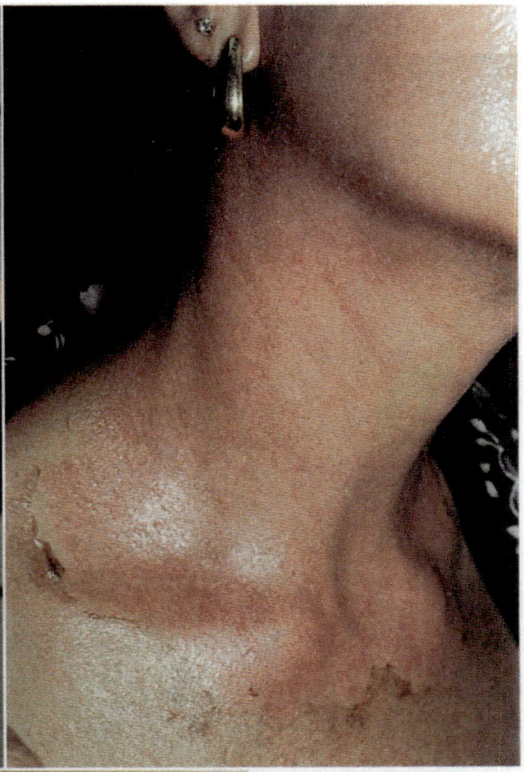
B

C
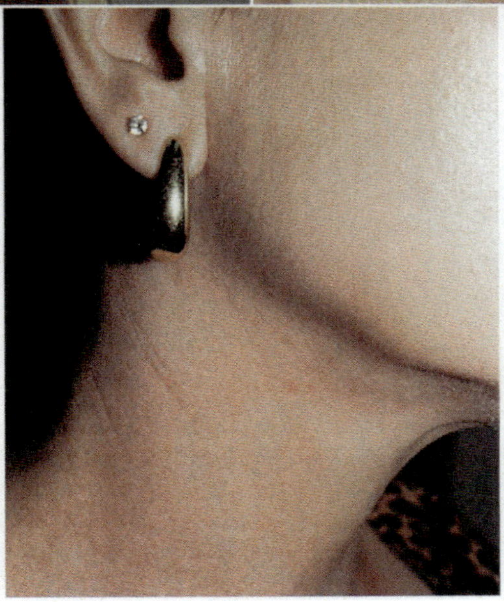

CASE 15

FIG. 11-15. This Fitzpatrick skin type II, Glogau photoaging type II patient has extensive poikilodermatous (atrophy, hyperpigmentation, telangiectasia) changes on the neck from chronic sun exposure with the pigmentary component in the majority, **(A)**. Two consecutive peels with Jessner's solution failed to fade the pigment. After a test spot with 20% TCA showed little reaction she was peeled with one coat of 35% TCA applied with two-cotton tipped applicators. The patient is using the regimen for dark skin. **(B)** Five days after application showing diffuse peeling. **(C)** Five months after healing shows excellent improvement of all components of photodamage.

Informed consent was obtained and the patient was advised of increased risk of scarring on nonfacial mobile areas such as the neck. Telangiectasias are unpredictably affected by peeling agents and are generally not substantially improved. See the section on neck peeling with TCA in Chapter 5.

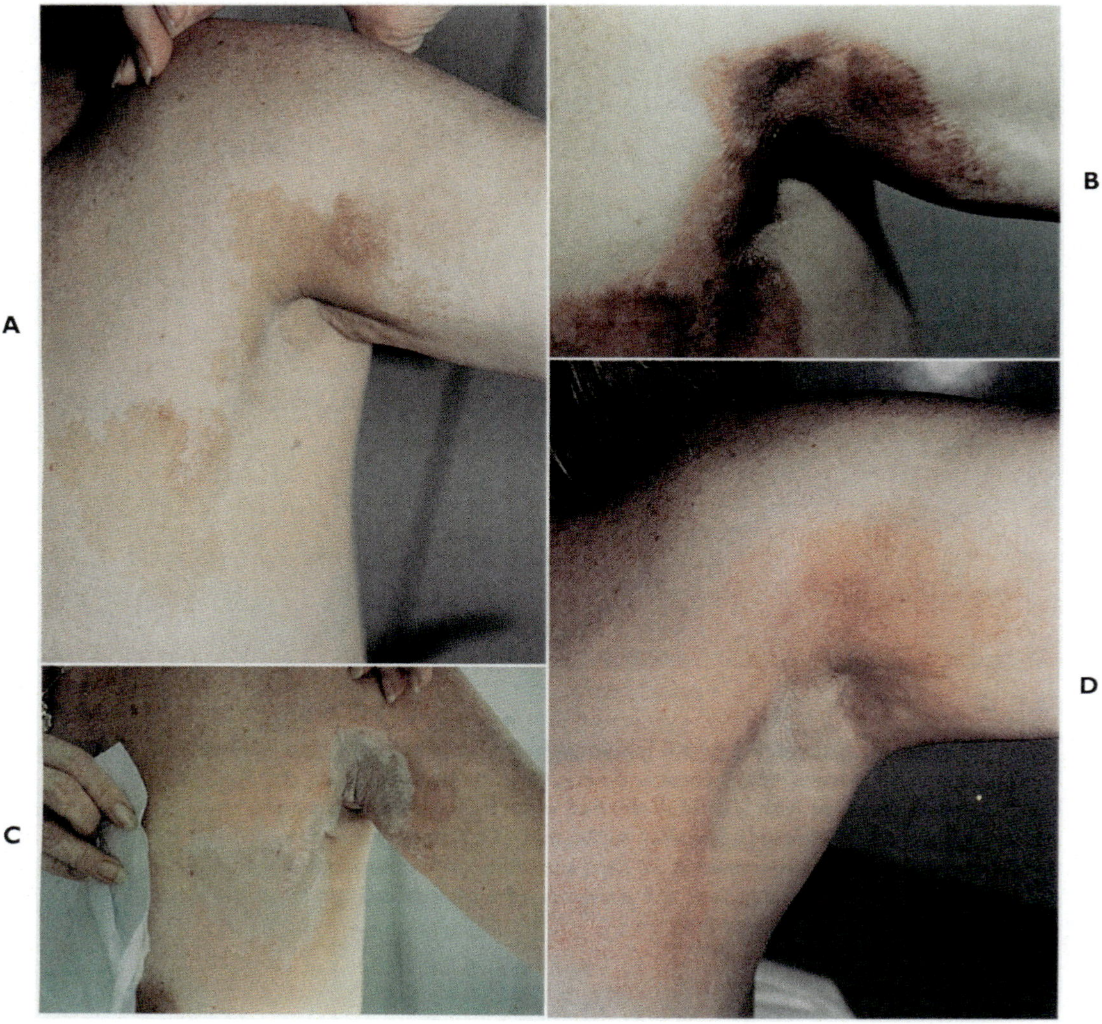

CASE 16

FIG. 11-16. (A) This Fitzpatrick skin type II female with no history of neurofibromatosis or neurologic disorder has a café au lait patch near the left axilla. Skin biopsy showed increased basal cell layer hyperpigmentation without giant melanin granules. She is peeled with CO_2 moderate with 35% TCA applied with two cotton-tipped applicators and reapplied 10 minutes later. **(B)** Immediately after peeling. **(C)** Four days later, crusting occurs. **(D)** After 9 months the area is clear and mildly erythematous from nightly tretinoin, 0.1%.

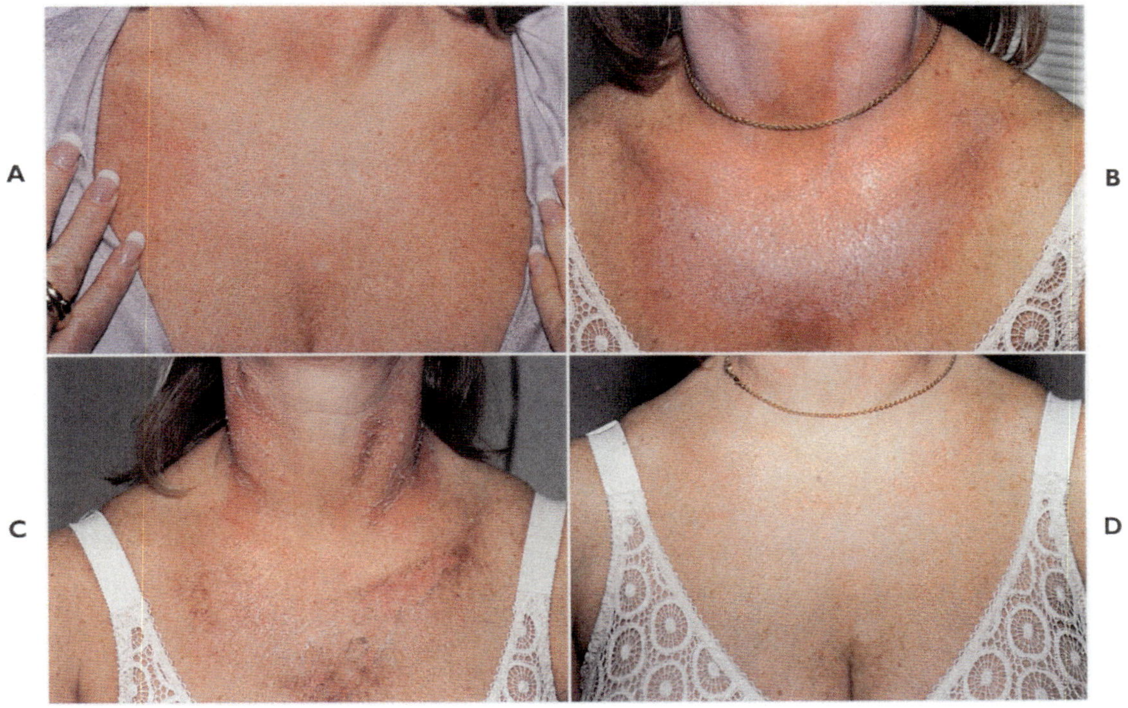

CASE 17

FIG. 11-17. This Fitzpatrick skin type II female with Glogau photoaging type II skin has dyschromia and scattered pigmented macules of the chest and neck, **(A)**. She had been using the regimen for bleaching light skin types. A test spot with 20% TCA showed white frosting. The agent was applied with a moist 4 × 4–inch gauze pad. **(B)** Immediately after application. **(C)** Considerable desquamation ensued at 7 days. **(D)** Minimal erythema remained at 30 days, and although another peel could be performed for further fading of pigmentation, the patient and physician were pleased and agreed to simply maintain the application regimen for the present time.

Appendix

Chemicals and Products Available for Purchase

The following is a partial list and does not claim to represent all products available. Proprietary companies are not listed.

Delasco/Dermatologic Lab & Supply, Inc. 608 13th Ave. Council Bluffs, IA 51501 800-831-6273 712-323-3269 Fax: 712-323-1156	All peeling solutions and accessories
Dermatopics or Pharmatopix Pharmagen Inc. 155 Knickerbocker Ave. Bohemia, NY 11716 800-445-2595 516-563-9349 Fax: 516-567-1025	Pharmatopix has Glycolic Acid with or without sodium fluorescein Highlighter Prepeel degreasers TCA Jessner's solution with sodium fluorescein Glycolic acid Neutralizer Postpeel balm
Dermatologic Cosmetic Laboratories 20 Commerce St. East Haven, CT 06512 800-552-5060 203-467-1570 Fax: 203-467-1573	Exclusively private labeling for physicians
Donell DerMedex Donell, Inc. 342 Madison Ave. New York, NY 10173 212-697-3800 Fax: 212-697-8908	CATRIX cream
Gly-Derm, Inc. 800-321-4576 Fax: 313-642-2798	Glyco citrate esters

Herald Pharmacal A division of Allergan Herbert 1701 Touchstone Rd. Colonial Heights, VA 23834 800-253-9499 Fax: 804-524-3194	Over-the-counter glycolic acid products
Humatech Laboratories 4800 N. Federal Highway #204D Boca Raton, FL 33431 800-593-SKIN Fax: 407-338-7513	Private Label skin care
Jan Marini, Inc. 6951 Via del Oro San Jose, CA 95118 800-347-2223 408-266-2478 Fax: 408-362-0140	Kojic acid and others
M.D. Formulations/Herald Pharmacal, Inc. 1701 Touchstone Rd. Colonial Heights, VA 23834 800-MD-FORMULA Fax: 804-524-3194	M.D. Forte line sells glycolic creams up to 15% for physicians only
Murad 8570 South Sepulveda, #1212 Los Angeles, CA 90045 800-242-1103 408-723-4480 Fax: 408-448-7206	
NeoStrata, Inc. 4 Research Way Princeton, NJ 08540 800-628-9904 Fax: 609-520-0849	Glycolic acid creams 8%-15% (15% to physicians only)
Physician's Choice of Arizona (PCA) 14807 North 73rd St. #103 Scottsdale, AZ 85260 800-758-8185 602-998-7733 Fax: 602-998-7808	Pigment lightening gel with kojic acid Lactic and citric acids with 2% hydroquinone Aloe vera–based products PCA peel (patented); places salicylic, lactic, citric, and kojic acids in a Jessner's ethanol base with or without hydroquinone or resorcinol
Alpha Hydrox Neoteric Co.	8% glycolic

ProPeel
Vivant Skin Care, Inc.
James E. Fulton, MD
714-722-1802

PRODUCTS

Cellex-C (vitamin C lotion)
2631 Commerce St., Suite C
Dallas, TX 75226
214-747-3310
800-423-5539
Fax: 214-747-3314

Ethocyn
Stanson Medical Corporation
8885 Venice Boulevard, #205
Los Angeles, CA 90034
800-579-7990

Kelocote silicone gel topical
Allied Biomedical Corporation
3850 Ramada Drive
Paso Robles, CA 93446
800-276-1322

Meshed Omiderm
Doak Dermatologics Wound Care
383 Route 46 West
Fairfield, NJ 07004-2402
800-405-DOAK

Silicone Gel Sheeting
Epi-Derm (Biodermis)
3753 Howard Hughes Pkwy.
Las Vegas, NV 89109
800-322-3729
Fax: 702-369-2607

Cica-Care silicone gel sheeting
Smith & Nephew, Inc.
11775 Starkey Rd.
Largo, FL 34643
800-876-1261

Solaquin Forte gel (4% hydroquinone) and Viquin Forte cream or gel (4% hydroquinone and 12% glycolic acid)
ICN Pharmaceuticals, Inc.
3300 Hyland Ave.
Cosa Mesa, CA 92626
800-7BLEACH (725-3224)
714-545-0100

TCA Masque, Inc.
ICN Pharmaceuticals, Inc.
3300 Hyland Ave.
Cosa Mesa CA 92626
714-545-0100

Vigilon Wound Dressing
Hermal Dermatology Group
163 Delaware Ave.
Delmar, NY 12054
1-800-HERMAL

Index

Note: Page numbers followed by "f" indicate figures; page numbers followed by "t" indicate tables.

T

Made in United States
Orlando, FL
05 November 2026

90199220R10159